Advance Praise for

"*Bouncebacks! Pediatrics* is an absolutely ar ... and clinicians. By delving into real cases and featuring the ac... ...entation, we learn from the pitfalls others have endured. Reading the commentary from Dr. Greg Henry will improve your charting, but more importantly, will help you think more critically to ensure the best possible care of children.

Anand K Swaminathan MD, MPH
Assistant Professor of Emergency Medicine
Assistant Residency Director
NYU/Bellevue Emergency Department

"Mike and his team have done it again! The ***Bouncebacks!*** series has truly been practice changing and now with this pediatric version, Peds and Adult Emergency Medicine physicians alike are in for a REAL treat! ***Bouncebacks! Pediatrics*** brings you to the bedside and makes you ask yourself 'What would I have done?' It gifts you with the opportunity to learn from others' mistakes, so that you don't have to relive the same ones! A must-have for any Emergency Physician who takes care of kids!"

Mizuho Spangler DO
Assistant Professor of Emergency Medicine LA County + USC
Editor in Chief Pediatric Reviews and Perspectives (PC RAP)

"***Bouncebacks! Pediatrics*** is the third offering of lessons in emergency care. The superstar panel of authors provides insight into the anatomy, physiology, and toxicology of the emergency care of children.They offer further insight into why 'bouncebacks' are the friend of emergency care, and probably even more so for young ones. Children are not just little adults!

After their stomach settles (That child could have been the one I saw in the last 5 shifts), readers will find this an enlightening look at thoughtful care, and effective communications, with children and their caregivers.

Another must read for emergency physicians, and those who aspire to be emergency physicians."

James J Augustine, MD
Director of Clinical Operations, EMP Ltd, Canton, Ohio
Assistant Clinical Professor
Wright State University, Department of Emergency Medicine
Fire EMS Medical Director

"***Bouncebacks! Pediatrics*** is a fascinating book that focuses on the process of medical decision making through the use of case-based stories of emergency department patient 'bouncebacks.' This unique format presents important teaching points of the subtleties of patient presentations. The cases, written by experienced physicians with expert commentary by the illustrious Dr. Greg Henry, provide for a memorable learning experience. I recommend all emergency physicians read this book.

David C. Seaberg, M.D.
Dean and Professor
Chairman, Department of Emergency Medicine
University of Tennessee College of Medicine Chattanooga

"***Bouncebacks! Pediatrics*** has an exceptional format that is easy to read and provides practical pearls that are guaranteed to change your current practice. This book resonates with the phrase "By the grace of God, go I" which springs to mind with every startling yet familiar case. In the current litigious medicolegal environment, ***Bouncebacks!Pediatrics*** is a must read for all practicing emergency medicine clinicians."

Ghazala Q. Sharieff, MD, FACEP, FAAP, FAAEM
Corporate Director, Physician Outreach and Medical Management, Scripps Health, San Diego, CA Clinical Professor, University of California, San Diego

"***Bounceback Pediatrics*** is an educational yet frightening read. These patients may present as a benign illness, only to become a disastrous, life-threatening event. Learn the pitfalls and missed clues so that you can prevent your own 'bounceback.' This is a must read for any provider who treats pediatric patients."

Fred Wu, MHS, PA-C
Lead Physician Assistant, Department of Emergency Medicine
Kaweah Delta Medical Center, CEP America
Visalia, California

"***Bouncebacks! Pediatrics*** is gut wrenching, reality-based, clinically relevant and motivating. The cases are disturbing and accomplish exactly what the authors intend – to demonstrate how a seemingly simple, straightforward pediatric case can go bad, and sometimes, disastrously bad. While reading each case, looking for the clues to the underlying etiology, I recognized just how easily a well meaning, mildly fatigued, and occasionally distracted practitioner can be lulled into a false sense of complacency and overlook a sometimes subtle, but critical, life threatening sign or symptom. Every case encourages the reader to look deeper and to avoid the 'decision-making shortcuts' that are so common in a busy high-acuity practice.

These are not invented cases, but 'actual' pediatric presentations, exactly as they appeared to the clinicians. Knowing that each case involves some form of bias, shortcut, or lack of full consideration of the available information, we are given the opportunity to do what we should always do—think beyond the obvious and take a second look. These are great lessons for any practitioner who cares for ill children.

And so, to the authors and many contributors of this stunning set of cases, who have provided perspective and wisdom, I can only say,

Thank you for helping me to be a better clinician."

Robert W. Strauss, MD, FACEP
Chief Editor, Strauss and Mayer's: ED Management
Vice President of Program Development, TeamHealth
Director: ACEP's Emergency Department Directors Academy

"The book series that changed the way we think about patients returning to the ED has done it again, this time with a series of real-life pediatric cases. The bounce backs series has become a standard in Emergency Medicine circles and this new offering will only extend and enhance the series as fundamental for the informed clinician. A must read text!"

Mel Herbert, MBBS (MD) BmedSci, FACEP
Professor of Emergency Medicine
Editor in Chief EMRAP

"As if I didn't have enough to worry about at this stage of my career! Just when I thought I had most of Pediatric Emergency Medicine mastered, these authors come along and have the audacity to debunk that myth.The cases in this text are real, pertinent, and instructive. The lessons presented are useful, concise, and in some cases, may save a life. Buy this book!"

Richard M. Cantor MD FAAP/FACEP
Professor of Pediatrics and Emergency Medicine
Director of Pediatric Emergency Medicine
Medical Director, Upstate Poison Center
Golisano Children's Hospital
Syracuse, NY

"***Bouncebacks! Pediatrics*** is the latest in this extraordinarily popular series, starting off with easy-reading sections on the care of children and general legal issues. Following are 28 detailed cases solicited by the authors from all walks of Emergency Medicine. In Michael Weinstock's customary fashion many of the cases drill down to the actual patient records and medical testimony. Then, Greg Henry gets to 'Monday Morning' critique the case drawing on his experience from reviewing over 2,000 cases. Bottom line—every emergency clinician can pick up a ton of great deal from ***Bouncebacks! Pediatrics*** whether a relative newbie or a seasoned pro.

W. Richard Bukata, MD
Medical Director
The Center for Medical Education, Inc.
Clinical Professor of Emergency Medicine
Department of Emergency Medicine
Los Angeles County / USC Medical Center
Los Angeles, California

Reviews from specialists in Family Medicine:

Like ***Bouncebacks! ED Returns*** and ***Bouncebacks! Medical and Legal, Bouncebacks! Pediatrics*** will prove an invaluable tool for pediatricians, family physicians and ED personnel who wish to avoid common, but often overlooked problem cases presenting to emergency departments, walk-ins and primary care offices. Informative and fascinating. Enjoy!

Ivan S. Wolfson, MD, FAAFP, FASAM
Clinical Assistant Professor of Family Medicine
Alpert Medical School, Brown University
Medical Director
Discovery House of RI
Providence, RI

"Imagine for a moment the crushing, dark sickness that would descend upon you, if a colleague, seeing you as you're coming in the ED door, said quietly, 'Remember that kid you saw last night?'... 'Came back in full arrest.'

For those of you who are familiar with the ***Bouncebacks!*** series, this is yet another gem, but amplified by the poignant wrench that these cases all involve children. For those who are unfamiliar, this is a gripping introduction.

Dr. Weinstock and colleagues have assembled 28 fast-paced mysteries, taken verbatim from actual case files. For each, all you know is that a bad outcome awaits. For each, you see what the ED physician wrote, and you instinctively put yourself in his or her shoes. Then, in the space of about 10 minutes reading, the mystery is revealed, the case analyzed by an expert, and the subtle clues uncovered. It is simultaneously entertaining, and for dedicated clinicians, often distinctly disturbing.

This particular series is prefaced by a set of expert tips on treating children in the ED that highlights common traps and pitfalls, and helps us orchestrate the delicate choreography that a pediatric emergency creates. It's must reading for not only for ED staff, but also for family physicians and pediatricians who see many similar cases in the office."

Rob Crane, MD
Associate Professor—Clinical
Department of Family Medicine
The Ohio State University

What the journals say about the *Bounceback!* series

Bouncebacks! Medical and Legal &
Bouncebacks! Emergency Department Cases: ED Returns

"***Bouncebacks! Medical and Legal*** takes the reader along an enlightening educational journey beginning with deceptively well patient visits, followed by the feared patient 'bouncebacks'with their unexpected bad outcomes, and ultimately revealing the courtroom proceedings that arose from the encounters ... ***Bouncebacks! Medical and Legal*** should be mandatory reading for all involved in emergency medicine."

Annals of Emergency Medicine, 2012

"I would recommend this book [***ED Returns***] for both residents and practicing physicians. For residency programs it can serve as an adjunct to case discussions and as a model for morbidity and mortality conference. For practicing emergency physicians it can provide excellent continuing education as an engaging and occasionally terrifying reminder of the high risk cases that masquerade as benign problems."

Annals of Emergency Medicine, 2007

"***Bouncebacks! Medical and Legal*** is an insightful and pragmatic analysis of emergency department malpractice litigation. ...The lessons presented are a good reminder for any practicing physician."

JAMA, 2012

"***Bouncebacks!*** is a collection of cases that all emergency physicians dread, or should."
Academic Emergency Medicine, 2007

Bouncebacks!

Pediatrics

Michael B. Weinstock, MD

Kevin M. Klauer, DO, EJD, FACEP

Madeline Matar Joseph, MD, FAAP, FACEP

Case by Case Commentary by:

Gregory L. Henry, MD, FACEP

Illustrations by:

Hannah Schumick

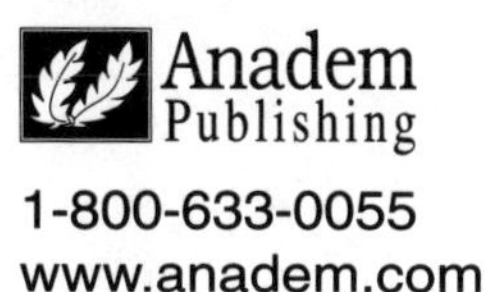

1-800-633-0055
www.anadem.com

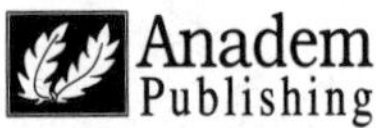

Anadem Publishing
3620 North High Street
Columbus, OH 43214
Tel: 1 (800) 633-0055
www.anadem.com

Bouncebacks! Pediatrics

Michael B. Weinstock
Kevin M. Klauer
Madeline Matar Joseph
Commentary by Gregory L. Henry

Illustrations by Hannah Schumick

Bouncebacks! is based upon information from sources believed to be reliable. In developing this book the publisher, authors, contributors, reviewers, and editors have made substantial efforts to make sure that the regimens, drugs, and treatments are correct and are in accordance with currently accepted standards. Readers are cautioned to use their own judgment in making clinical decisions and, when appropriate, consult and compare information from other resources since ongoing research and clinical experience yield new information and since there is the possibility of human error in developing such a comprehensive resource as this. Attention should be paid to checking the product information supplied by drug manufacturers when prescribing or administering drugs, particularly if the prescriber is not familiar with the drug or does not regularly use it.

Readers should be aware that there are legitimate differences of opinion among physicians on both clinical and ethical/moral issues in treating patients. With this in mind, readers are urged to use individual judgment in making treatment decisions, recognizing the best interests of the patient and his/her own knowledge and understanding of these issues. The material in *Bouncebacks!* is not intended to substitute for the advice of a qualified attorney or other professional. You should consult a qualified professional for advice about your specific situation. Readers are cautioned to use their own judgment in making decisions on the issues covered in this book because there are on-going changes in these matters. The publisher, authors, reviewers, contributors, and editors disclaim any liability, loss or damage as a result, directly or indirectly, from using or applying any of the contents of *Bouncebacks!*

PRINTED IN THE UNITED STATES OF AMERICA

ISBN 978-1-890018-79-5

HOW DO WE LEARN FROM BOUNCEBACK CASES?

Michael Weinstock

Is there still an opportunity to learn from cases after we know the outcome? Cue your PEER review committee, hospital administrator, or plaintiff attorney: "Of course this case should have been handled differently, look at all those red flags!" But on the front line in a busy emergency department, we know the truth; when surfing in a sea of normalcy, what seems clear to a Monday morning quarterback is not quite as obvious when you are getting rushed out of the pocket during Sunday's game.

Should we just resign ourselves to the practice of defensive medicine, as many of our peers have admitted doing?[1] We are notoriously poor at gauging patient expectations,[2] and making matters worse, modifying our current "best practice" to improve perceived patient satisfaction has been shown to increase mortality by 26%.[3]

We are searching for the "sweet spot" of advocating for a patient's best long-term health, while protecting our own long-term career! Herein lies our message; not extraneous testing, but a more thorough history, recognition of abnormal vital signs, further explanation of abnormal findings, an expanded pediatric-specific differential diagnosis, and a medical decision-making note explaining our though process ... in short, an evaluation reflected in the documentation which tells a cohesive story from beginning to end.

Framing the problem

Wears and Nemeth suggest an approach which is opposite than seems logical: "We do not learn much by asking why the way a practitioner framed a problem turned out to be wrong. We do learn when we discover why that framing seemed so reasonable at the time."[4]

While reading through these 28 stories, by walking in the footsteps of the initial provider, we can see why an evaluation which initially seems reasonable, may sometimes fail to localize the correct diagnosis and therapy. Our goal is to prompt the reader to say, "Yeah, I would have handled this case the same way," then to show how recognition of subtle findings or consideration of a pediatric-specific differential, may have changed the outcome of these young patients.

Meta-cognition and CDRs

Pat Croskerry, a Canadian emergency physician, has defined cognitive dispositions to respond (CDRs), perhaps better defined as "decision-making short cuts." These CDRs help us to function in the rapidly changing work environment of a busy ED. They typically work well, allowing us to rapidly recognize and intervene in high acuity patients and to quickly disposition low acuity patients,[5] but can also lead us astray.

Five common CDRs:

1. Anchoring bias
    - Fixation on a specific feature of the presentation too early in the diagnostic process
    - The provider's thought process becomes *anchored* to that feature
    - Subsequently obtained superior data is not considered

2. Availability bias
   - Tendency for diagnoses to be judged more likely if they occur frequently
   - Common things are common (available)
   - Similar to the "playing the odds" bias
3. Diagnosis momentum
   - A previous diagnosis becomes established without adequate evidence
   - The initial diagnosis gathers momentum with each subsequent provider and serves to suppress further thinking
   - Examples: Otitis media, sinusitis
4. Triage cuing
   - Placing undue or insufficient concern on a complaint/patient based on the triage assessment
   - Example: Triage chief complaint of "Flu symptoms" versus provider history of "headache and fever"
5. Zebra retreat
   - A rare diagnosis figures prominently in the differential, but the provider retreats resulting in a missed or delayed diagnosis
   - Lack of courage of convictions

Is there a way to know when these "decision making short cuts," which normally serve us so well, are misleading? Enter a term, which has received less attention; Meta-cognition, defined as the highest level of cognitive functioning. This occurs when we make a decision to monitor our own decision-making.

Meta-cognition speaks to two main processes in our evaluation of ED patients:

- Do we understand how we make decisions?
- Do we realize when these decisions are prone to error?

Frequency of bouncebacks and pediatric bouncebacks

The rate for emergency medicine bouncebacks within 72 hours is around 3%.[6-8] Whereas many pediatric specific return visits are without a clear medical need,[9] and poor access to follow up care or fear of disease progression are primary motivators of ED returns.[10] After ED discharge, 2.6% of patients are admitted within 7 days.[11] How about the next level of concern, death after ED discharge? David Sklar looked at almost 400,000 patients and found 35 who died from a possible medical error within 7 days of their initial ED visit. Of these, 71% had unexplained tachycardia and 85% had abnormal vital signs on ED discharge.[12] With such a low rate, 1/10,000, it is easy to let our guard down, but considering the almost 175,000 patients we will each see in our careers, vigilance to red flags is essential.

The *Bouncebacks!* series philosophy: Picking the cases for this book

For the first book of this series, *Bouncebacks!* (2006), most of the cases were found by the book authors, then national experts were asked to write commentary about the presenting complaint and final diagnosis, all within the context of the case. The second book, *Bouncebacks! Medical and Legal* (2011) was comprised of cases which went to trial or settlement. It was structured as one fictional day in the life of an emergency physician who reported to their shift, saw 10 "well-appearing" patients, only to subsequently find 10 letters arrive in the mail! These cases were found through court records and appeals decisions; actual ED documentation and deposition and trial testimony were supplied by the attorneys who tried the cases. Each chapter is set up like an episode of the TV show *Law and Order*; first the medical, then the legal.

In contradistinction, many of the cases of *Bouncebacks! Pediatrics* were written by authors who actually cared for these patients. This created a familiarity with the initial presentation and/or bounceback. Commentary often includes a very personal discussion of their discovery of the bounceback, and how an adverse outcome affected them personally; sometimes to the point of marital discord and consideration of suicide. What feelings should we have upon recognizing a child we cared for 24 hours ago is being rushed back to the trauma bay or learning that a parent we spoke with only hours ago will no longer be woken on Christmas morning by their 5-year-old?

Chapter layout for *Bouncebacks! Pediatrics*

Chapter authors range from nationally renowned pediatric emergency medicine attendings and residents to general emergency medicine attendings and residents, both from academic centers and the community. Each of the following "stories" reflects the author's insight and experience. These are patients that any of us could see in any emergency department on any given day.

Many of the cases start with the patient's story and in keeping with the *Bouncebacks!* tradition, all include the physician's actual documentation. Next is a discussion of the risk management/ patient safety features of the initial encounter, either told by the book authors, chapter author, or in the colorful manner of Greg Henry, past president of the American College of Emergency Physicians (ACEP) and arguably the foremost physician medical-legal authority in the country, having been an expert in over 2,400 medical-legal cases. After the condensed description of the return visit (or visits!), the chapter author provides a referenced discussion of the presentation and final diagnosis, all within the context of the case.

Just as the patients are all different, the chapters vary based on the presentation of the patient and the creativity of the author. Illustrations provide a clue to the final diagnosis or a visual reminder of important lessons to take away.

Before the first case, we include two "orienting" chapters; a top 10 list of pediatric pearls by Madeline Matar Joseph and legal insights by Kevin Klauer. Heeding these lessons would have resulted in different outcomes in many of the subsequently presented patients…

A personal note:

The career we have chosen is intense. We are entrusted with society's ultimate responsibility, the care of its children. This accountability shines through with the documentation reproduced on these pages, demonstrating how even a thoughtful and experienced physician can be fooled by subtle findings, how a compassionate physician can be misled by a well-appearing child, and how an anxious parent or ill-informed care giver can lead us astray with demands for testing or when they confuse "association" with "causation."

I have found that as much as I am saddened by the death of a patient, I am often most affected by the reaction of the parents and family. Who cannot relate to this most ultimate of loss? Early in my career, I cared for a young child who arrived in full arrest and expired in the emergency department. When I walked out of the room after trying to console the parents, a nurse approached to ask if *I* was OK, a possibility I had not considered. Pondering why she would ask about *me* after such a tragic loss, I realized that she knew I had two children at home of a similar age. A shudder ran up my spine; sometimes we don't realize we are seeing ourselves in the eyes of strangers.

Greg Henry tells a similar story, of a young child he cared for in traumatic arrest, not realizing its affect on him until a few days later when he grabbed his own young child who was running toward the street. His wife emerged from the house to see him holding his son tight and sobbing, the effects of his futile efforts several days previous only now manifesting themselves.

Summary:

We would like to thank the authors who have opened themselves up by sharing their stories; for helping us to expand our differential diagnosis in an age-specific fashion, to better appreciate subtlety, and to trust in a parent's concern.

Greg Henry's statement in the foreword of the first Bouncebacks! book was applicable for the second, and remains prescient for the third:

> *"The smart doctor is not one who learns from his own mistakes, it is one who learns from the mistakes of others. Here's hoping that this book is read by a lot of smart doctors."*

Michael Weinstock
March 2015

www.embouncebacks.com

References

1. Studdert DM, et al. Defensive medicine among high-risk specialist physicians in a volatile malpractice environment. JAMA. 2005;293:2609–17.
2. Ong S, et al. Antibiotic use for emergency department patients with upper respiratory infections: prescribing practices, patient expectations, and patient satisfaction. Ann Emerg Med. 2007;50:213–20.
3. Fenton J, et al. The cost of satisfaction. A national study of patient satisfaction, health care utilization, expenditures, and mortality. Arch Intern Med. 2012;172(5):405–11.
4. Wears RL, Nemeth CP. Replacing hindsight with insight: toward better understanding of diagnostic failures. Ann Emerg Med. 2007;49:206–9.
5. Croskerry P. Achieving quality in clinical decision making: cognitive strategies and detection of bias. Acad Emerg Med. 2002;9:1184–204.
6. Wilkins PS, Beckett MW. Audit of unexpected return visits to an accident and emergency department. Arch Emerg Med. 1992;9(4):352–6.
7. O'Dwyer F, Bodiwala GG. Unscheduled return visits by patients to the accident and emergency department. Arch Emerg Med. 1991;8(3):196–200.
8. Pierce JM, Kellermann AL, Oster C. "Bounces": an analysis of short-term return visits to a public hospital emergency department. Ann Emerg Med. 1990;19(7):752–7. (over 30,000 patients studied)
9. Zimmer DR, et al. Repeat pediatric visits to a general emergency department. Ann Emerg Med. 1996;28(5):467–73.
10. Rising, KL, et al. Return visits to the emergency department: the patient perspective. Ann Emerg Med. 2014; DOI:10.1016/j.annemergmed.2014.07.015.
11. Gabayan GZ, et al. Factors associated with short-term bounce-back admissions after emergency department discharge. Ann Emerg Med. 2013;62(2):136–44.
12. Sklar DP, Crandall CS, Loeliger E, et al. Unanticipated death after discharge home from the emergency department. Annals Emerg Med. 2007:49(6);735–45.

About the Authors

Michael B. Weinstock, MD

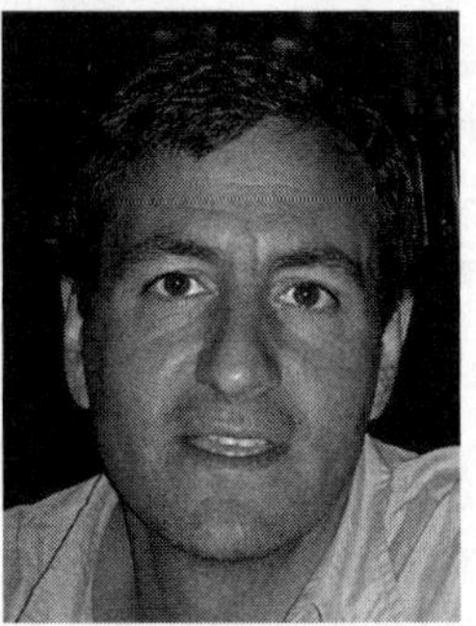

Michael comes from a long line of physicians; his father is an ophthalmologist, both his grandfathers were general surgeons, and his great grandfather was a barber-surgeon in Russia (the guy you didn't want to be referred to!) Michael obtained his bachelor's degree with a major in economics from Northwestern University and his medical degree from The Ohio State University College of Medicine. In 1995, he completed his residency at Riverside Methodist Hospital in Columbus, Ohio.

Michael is a Professor of Emergency Medicine, adjunct in the Department of Emergency Medicine at The Ohio State University, Chairman and Director of Medical Education in the Emergency Department at Mt. Carmel St. Ann's, and Medical Director in The Ohio Dominican University PA studies program.

He is risk management section editor of Emergency Medicine Reviews and Perspectives (EM RAP), a CME program with international circulation to over 15,000 physicians, and editor-in-chief for Urgent Care Reviews and Perspectives (UC RAP) to be released in March 2015. He has lectured nationally on issues such as risk management and patient safety and has published multiple papers in peer-reviewed journals.

In 2006 he authored *Bouncebacks! Emergency Department Cases: ED Returns* and in 2011 *Bouncebacks: Medical and Legal* with reviews in Annals of Emergency Medicine, Archives of Emergency Medicine and JAMA. In 2014 he authored *The Resident's Guide to Ambulatory Care, 7th edition*, a book started while in residency, now with sales of almost 35,000 copies.

Early in his career, while working as a full time Emergency Physician, Michael spent 12 years as a Clinical Assistant Professor in the Infectious Diseases Clinic at The Ohio State University caring for patients with HIV/AIDS and working as a clinical trials sub-investigator. He has practiced medicine on both a local and global scale, including volunteer medical work in Papua New Guinea, Nepal, and the West Indies.

In March 2014 he received an award for Outstanding Contributions to the Field of Emergency Medicine from the University of Maryland Emergency Medicine residency program.

Michael is married to Beth, a family physician, and they have a growing family, including four energetic children: Olivia (15), Eli (14), Theo (10), and Annie (7). In addition to medicine, other passions include skiing, backpacking, traveling and writing. He is a singer/song writer, guitar and harmonica player and leader of *The Big Rockin' Blues Band*.

Michael B. Weinstock, MD
Professor of Emergency Medicine, Adjunct
The Ohio State University College of Medicine,
Emergency Department Chairman and Director of Medical Education
Mt. Carmel St. Ann's Dept. of Emergency Medicine,
Medical director, The Ohio Dominican University PA studies program
Columbus, Ohio

About the Authors

Kevin M. Klauer, DO, EJD, FACEP

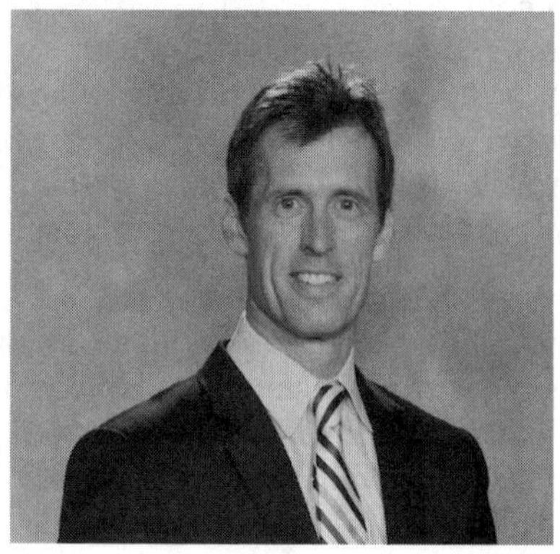

Dr. Klauer is the Chief Medical Officer, Emergency Medicine, Chief Risk Officer and Executive Director of the Patient Safety Organization for TeamHealth. He is an Assistant Clinical Professor at Michigan State University College of Osteopathic Medicine. Dr. Klauer serves as the Medical Editor-in-Chief for ACEP Now, ACEP's monthly publication, and as former Editor-in-Chief for Emergency Physicians Monthly publication. He is the Co-Author of two risk management books: Emergency Medicine Bouncebacks: Medical and Legal and Risk Management and the Emergency Department: Executive Leadership for Protecting Patients and Hospitals. Dr. Klauer also serves as the American College of Emergency Physicians Council Speaker. He received the ACEP National Faculty Teaching Award in 2001 and the Emergency Medicine Resident's Association Robert Dougherty ACEP/ Emergency Medicine Foundation Teaching Fellowship. In 2014, he was the recipient of the American College of Emergency Physicians Honorable Mention Outstanding Speaker of the Year Award and was recognized by the Ohio Chapter of ACEP with the Bill Hall Award for service. Dr. Klauer earned his Executive JD, with honors, from Concord Law School in 2011.

Madeline Matar Joseph, MD, FAAP, FACEP

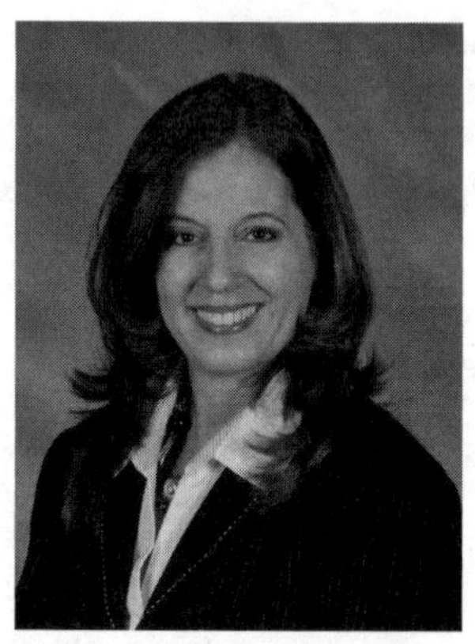

Madeline Matar Joseph, M.D., FAAP, FACEP is a Professor of Emergency Medicine and Pediatrics at the University of Florida College of Medicine-Jacksonville. Dr. Joseph is the Assistant Chair of Pediatrics, and Division Chief and Medical Director of the Pediatric Emergency Medicine in the Emergency Medicine Department. She completed her pediatric residency training at the University of Florida Health Science Center in Jacksonville in 1992 and her pediatric emergency medicine fellowship at the Children's Hospital of Birmingham in Alabama in 1994. Dr. Joseph joined the faculty at UF Emergency Medicine Department-Jacksonville in 1994. During her tenure at UF, she was the director of the pediatric emergency medicine fellowship program (1996–2005) and since 2005 she has been the division chief and medical director of the Pediatric ED.

Over the last two decades, Dr. Joseph has been an active member of numerous national committees at both the American College of Emergency Physicians (ACEP) and the American Academy of Pediatrics Section on Emergency Medicine to advance the emergent care for children. Dr. Joseph was elected to be the Secretary of the ACEP Pediatric Section (2004–

2005), Chair-Elect (2005–2006), and Chair (2006–2007). Dr. Joseph won many awards during her service on the ACEP Pediatric Section, including the 2007 and 2008 Outstanding Newsletter Awards and the 2007 Promoting Section Membership Award. Dr. Joseph is a reviewer of numerous pediatrics and emergency medicine journals, including the journal of Academic Emergency Medicine and serves on the Editorial Board for Pediatric Emergency Medicine Practice. She is one of the co-editors of the book entitled *Pediatric Emergency Medicine Quick Glance*. Dr. Joseph is the author of over 70 publications and book chapters in various pediatric emergency medicine topics, including injury prevention, asthma, sports concussion and recently pediatric obesity.

In addition to her love of her profession, Dr. Joseph cherishes her growing family with her husband Michael. Their three children Andrew (21), Christine (18), and Matthew (13), keep them busy! Madeline's interests include traveling, hiking, taking family trips (Soccer World Cup in Brazil last year), and watching children's soccer games.

Gregory L. Henry, MD, FACEP

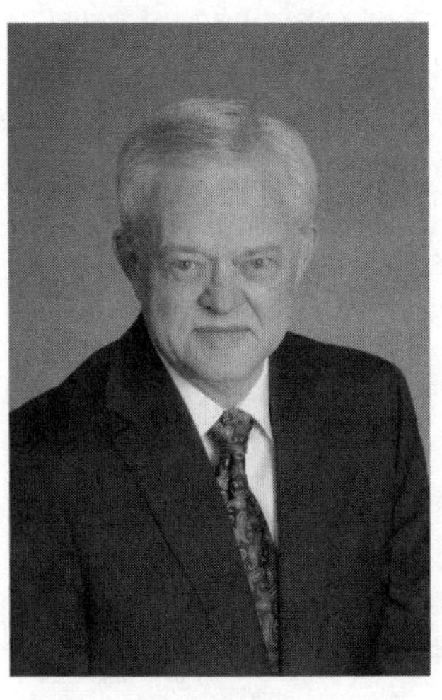

Gregory L. Henry, MD, FACEP, is Clinical Professor in the Department of Emergency Medicine at the University of Michigan Medical School in Ann Arbor, Michigan. Dr. Henry is a past President of the American College of Emergency Physicians, and he is a member of the American Medical Association. He is the former President and Managing Officer of two emergency medicine malpractice insurance companies.

Dr. Henry is a consultant reviewer for five emergency medicine journals, including the Annals of Emergency Medicine and he is on the Editorial Board of ED Management. He is the author of multiple books on neurologic disease and risk management in emergency medicine, as well as over 75 text book chapters and numerous articles on emergency care. Dr. Henry has lectured at over 100 residency programs in emergency medicine and to over 250,000 emergency physicians as various meetings.

His contributions are legend and he has a keen interest in improving patient care and risk management as well as neurologic disease. His expertise in the field of risk management is pre-eminent in the field. He has reviewed over 2,400 malpractice cases and has served as a risk management consultant for numerous physician groups and hospitals.

Dedication, Thanks, Acknowledgements

To my grandfathers: Michael B. Weinstock, MD, a general surgeon who served in WWII, who I never had the opportunity to meet, and Samuel Reinglass, MD, a general surgeon in Canton Ohio, my hometown, whose dedication and service to his patients continues to serve as a role model and inspiration.

Michael

Thank you to my loving family members who drive me in pursuit of excellence. With your inspiration, I hope to leave a small, but recognizable imprint on the world around us.

Kevin

To my supportive husband, family, parents and friends for their love to allow me to pursue dreams out of my comfort zone! My precious children Andrew, Christine and Matthew are always in my heart and inspire me to care for other children to the best of my abilities. I dedicate this book to the many clinicians who serve our children and adolescents seeking care in the Emergency Department. I hope the *Bouncebacks! Pediatrics* book will facilitate safe and optimal emergent care of our children.

Madeline

To all those close to me. Home is that place that when you have to go there, they have to take you in.

Greg

We would like to also thank the many people who contributed, reviewed, encouraged and inspired us. Thanks to David Schumick for the cover design and Hannah Schumick for her illustrations of the characters and situations presented in the cases. To Mike, Will and Kate from Anadem Publishing for the editing and layout.

Michael, Kevin, Madeline and Greg

Table of Contents & Contributors

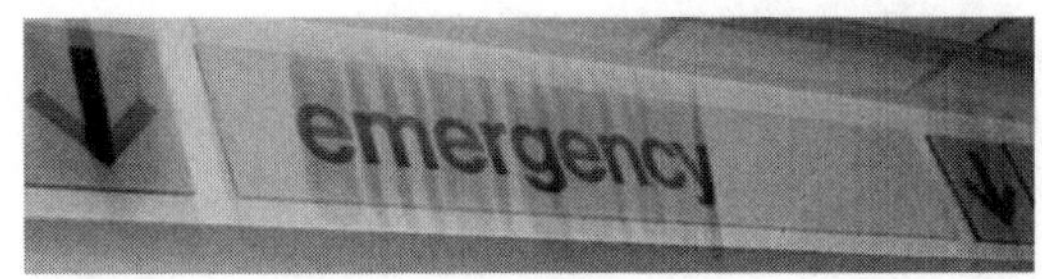

"Children Are Not Just Small Adults"

The Top 10 Tips and Tricks on Pediatric Specific Evaluation and Management

Madeline Matar Joseph, MD, FAAP, FACEP

Professor of Emergency Medicine and Pediatrics
University of Florida College of Medicine–Jacksonville

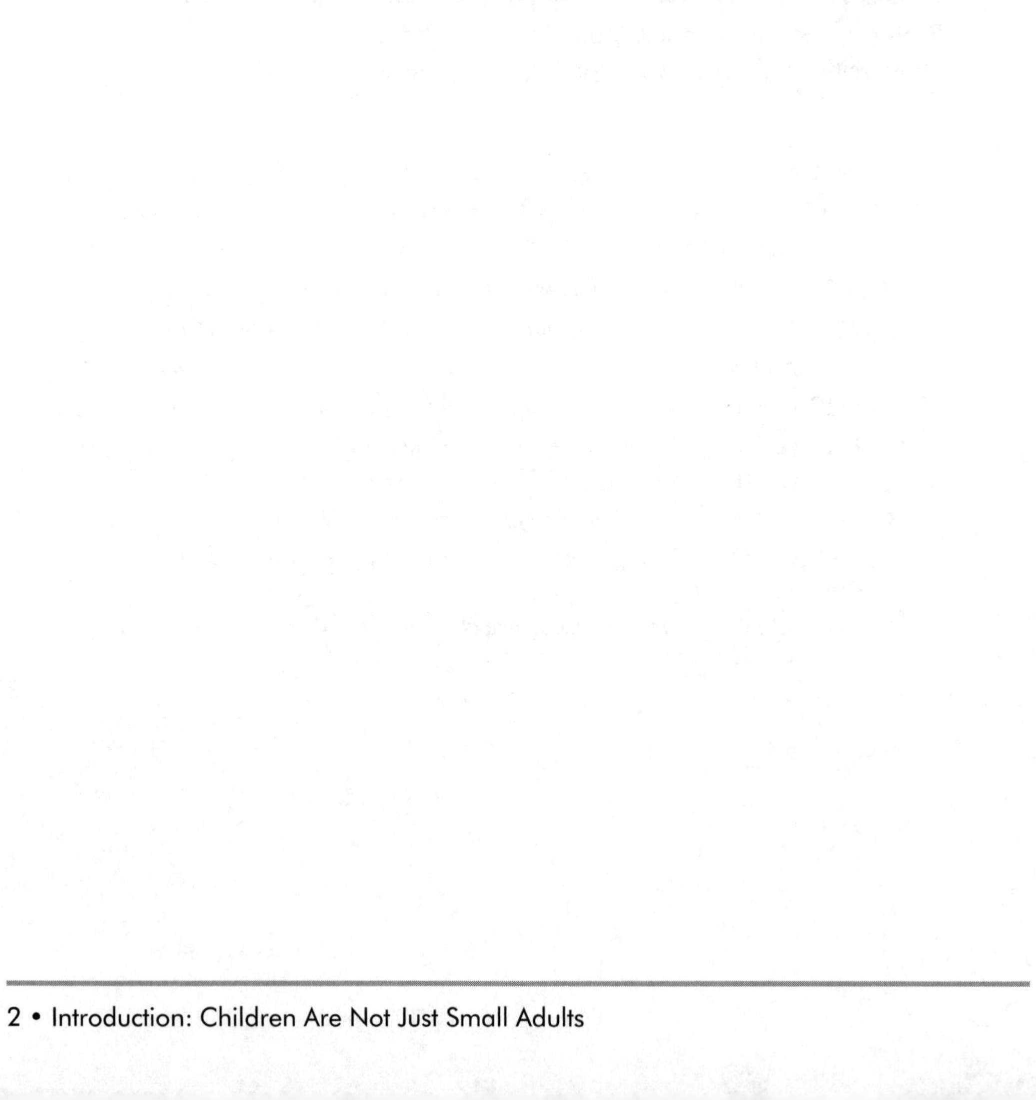

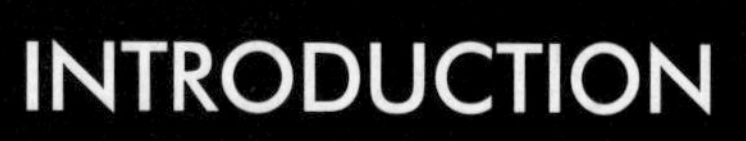

INTRODUCTION

"CHILDREN ARE NOT JUST SMALL ADULTS"

The Top 10 Tips and Tricks on Pediatric Specific Evaluation and Management

Caring for children in the emergency department is rewarding, as most respond quickly to treatment; consider the initially lethargic toddler with high fever and dehydration who is now running around after IV fluids and ibuprofen! But beware—these same presenting symptoms can occur in life-threatening disease. Woe to the physician who wastes valuable time on anti-pyretics during "cold and flu" season in a patient with bacterial meningitis or on anti-emetics in patients with "intussusception" in the midst of viral gastroenteritis season. These are the times when vigilance, recognition of a high risk presentation, and observation of a child's behavior are so important.

Though the evaluation of children follows the same progression as adults—history, exam, testing—there are unique age-based aspects which need to be respected. The following "Top 10 list" will help with the age-specific evaluation and management of children. There are multiple cases in this book where employing these techniques may have saved a child's life.

CLINICAL TIP 1—*Obtaining a history in a pre-verbal child*

Whereas most adults will be able to give a cognizant history, pre-verbal children are unable to describe the actual location, character, and onset of their symptoms. That is why neonatal appendicitis has been reported to have an 82% perforation rate and 28% mortality rate.[1] Tips for obtaining a reliable history include:

- Involve parents: Ask each parent independently about the history.
- Involve caregivers: If they are not in the emergency department, have the parent call them and hand you the phone. They may know more than a parent who has been working all day and then returns home to find an ill child.
- If an event such as a seizure or a fall occurred, try to find witnesses to the event. Call the school or the day care. Speak with the medics before they leave the ED.
- Ask the parents about birth history particularly when taking care of infants.
- Research old charts, looking at previous visits for past medical and surgical histories, medications, or prior evaluation for abuse.

CLINICAL TIP 2—*Performing a good exam on a screaming infant or uncooperative toddler*

Have you even thrown up your arms in frustration trying to perform an abdominal exam on a screaming infant? The following techniques may be helpful:

- Observe the child from across the room for work of breathing (accessory muscle use, nasal flaring), activity level (interactive, good eye contact), muscle tone (sitting on their own, use of all extremities).
- If the child looks ill, pay special attention to how they position themselves:

- o Lying down completely still is very unusual for a child and could indicate an acute abdomen.
  - o Sitting upright, and slightly forward with dyspnea could indicate an asthma exacerbation, retro-pharyngeal abscess, or epiglottitis.
- Talk to the parents first and make occasional eye contact with the toddler to gain their trust.
- Examine the child on parent's lap instead of the exam table.
- Get down on their level, even if they are on the floor playing with a toy. Do not tower!
- Examine tender areas such as ears or injured extremities last.
- Be honest, so you do not lose your credibility. If something is going to hurt, tell in a calm manner.
- Explain what you are doing in children's terms.
- Distraction is a great tool! Be creative with smart phone apps, pictures, or by jingling car keys.

CLINICAL TIP 3—*What to do with the inconsolable baby*

The crying baby represents a challenge to the emergency physician with causes stemming from more serious etiologies such as meningitis and intracranial bleeding from non-accidental trauma to common minor illnesses. History should include information on maternal infection during pregnancy (we still lose newborns to group B strep meningitis), HIV, GC and chlamydia. Inquire about sleep history (is the baby sleeping too much or too little because he is crying all night), feeding (poor feeding is never a good sign), urination (number of urinations in 24 hours, quantity, and last urination) and stooling.

The cry: Pitch and intensity:

- A loud cry is somewhat reassuring
- A weak/listless cry may indicate a seriously ill child
- A high pitched, screeching cry could indicate a painful source such as increased intracranial pressure (ICP) as seen in meningitis or intracranial bleeding

Areas to consider in the physical examination as painful sources are:

- Cornea: Foreign body or corneal abrasion: infant's nails are very sharp and some parents are scared to cut them
- Fundi: Retinal hemorrhages (consider non-accidental trauma)
- Ears: Otitis media or externa, foreign bodies
- Abdomen/Rectal: Anal fissure or trauma; intussusception
- Genitalia: Inguinal hernia, hair tourniquet, scrotal edema (testicular torsion)
- Digits: Hair tourniquet
- Extremities: Immobile extremity (fracture or neurological deficit from intracranial or cervical injuries)
- Metabolic: Urine tox for cocaine
- General: Newborns may be septic without a fever; in fact hypothermia is an even more ominous sign of sepsis. Unexplained tachycardia or tachypnea may be an early sign for sepsis, dehydration, and metabolic acidosis.

CLINICAL TIP 4—*Unique pediatric considerations in emergency airway management*

Anatomic and physiologic differences between children and adults must be considered when managing airway:

- The position of the larynx in infants and children is more cephalad than in adults, creating a more acute angle between the glottic opening and the base of the tongue. The epiglottis is large and floppy, covering more of the glottic aperture.
- The proportionally larger occiput in infants and younger children causes varying degrees of neck flexion in the supine position and may interfere with visualizing the glottic opening during laryngoscopy. Placing a towel roll under the shoulders will improve airway alignment.
- The relatively large tongue in infants and young children can lead to inadequate displacement impacting visualization during direct laryngoscopy. Traditional teaching is that a straight blade can help control the tongue as a curved blade (Mac blade) placed in the vallecula may not elevate the epiglottis as effectively as in adults (because of a weaker hyoepiglottic ligament). A just released head to head study suggests both blades may be equally effective.[2]
- The short pediatric trachea predisposes to right mainstem bronchus intubation or inadvertent extubation. This can occur at the time of intubation, or during unintentional head movement.[3] The trachea increases in length with age (about 5 cm in neonates to 12 cm in adults).
- In adults, the vocal cords comprise the narrowest portion of the airway. In children, the cricoid ring is the narrowest portion. Recent data suggest anatomic narrowing may be greatest at the vocal cords though the elliptical cross sectional shape of the subglottis and the non-distensible cricoid cartilage.[4] This narrowing can create an effective anatomic seal without the need for a cuffed ETT, but …
- A cuffed tube may be preferable to uncuffed tube in certain circumstances such as poor lung compliance, high airway resistance, or a large glottic air leak. Special attention should be paid to tube size, position, and cuff inflation pressure.[5] Using cuffed tubes has led to a reduced need for ETT exchanges and no increase in post-extubation morbidity when compared to un-cuffed tubes.[6]
- Infants and young children may have a pronounced vagal response to laryngoscopy or airway suctioning. Because hypoxia potentiates the risk for bradycardia, efforts to maintain oxygenation before and during endotracheal intubation should be maximized.

CLINICAL TIP 5—*When to suspect meningitis in an immunized patient*

Since the introduction of the *Haemophilus influenza* type B (HIB) and pneumococcal conjugated vaccines in 1990 and 2000, bacterial meningitis has declined dramatically in all age groups except infants < 2 months of age.[7]

Under 1 month of age, the most frequent organisms are:

1. Group B streptococcus (39%)
2. Gram-negative bacilli (32%)
3. *Streptococcus pneumoniae* (14%)
4. *Neisseria meningitides* (12%)

Of note, *Streptococcus pneumoniae* and *Neisseria meningitides* are the most common causes of bacterial meningitis in infants and children older than one month of age.

In infants, manifestations of meningitis may include fever/hypothermia, poor feeding, vomiting, diarrhea, lethargy, restlessness, irritability, bulging fontanel, seizures, jaundice or respiratory distress.[8] A bulging fontanel is neither sensitive nor specific for bacterial meningitis. In one study, it was present in 20% of infants with meningitis, but also in 13% of infants with normal CSF.[9]

In older children, the presentation of meningitis is similar to adults; both variable and non-specific. The classic triad of fever, neck stiffness and mental status change is only present in 44% of cases and even fewer in younger children. In older children, meningitis can present with any combination of fever, headache, photophobia, nausea, vomiting, confusion, or lethargy.

Predisposing factors to bacterial meningitis include:

- Recent infection such as respiratory or otic infection
- Penetrating head trauma-CSF otorrhea or CSF rhinorrhea
- Anatomical defects including dermal sinus, urinary tract anomaly
- Recent VP shunt placement
- Recent travel to areas with endemic meningococcal disease such as Africa
- Recent exposure to someone with meningococcal or HIB meningitis

Tips and tricks:

1. Children who require a CT before LP include:
    - o Altered mental status (to rule out bleeding from non-accidental trauma or mass)
    - o Focal neurologic signs
    - o Papilledema
    - o Focal seizure
    - o Risk for brain abscess: congenital heart diseases: R to L shunt, immune compromised patients
2. If the patient seems unstable for the LP (due to respiratory concerns or hemodynamic instability), do not delay the administration of antimicrobial. Early treatment improves the prognosis of bacterial meningitis and herpes encephalitis.
3. Blood cultures prior to administration of antibiotics are positive in 50% of patients with bacterial meningitis.[8]
4. In children who were treated with antibiotics before the LP was obtained, increased CSF cell count, elevated CSF protein and/or decreased CSF glucose usually are sufficient to make the diagnosis of meningitis.

CLINICAL TIP 6—*Tips for performing a lumbar puncture (LP)*

- Topical anesthetics anesthetize the skin but not the subcutaneous tissue. Use LMX4 (4% lidocaine cream) which takes 20–30 minutes in place of EMLA (that takes an hour to work). You can place the cream on the back while you are obtaining the consent.
- Some emergency physicians are concerned about losing landmarks if they infiltrate with lidocaine in infants, but studies demonstrate that such practice does not interfere with

obtaining CSF and even suggest that use of a local anesthetic make obtaining CSF twice as likely.[10, 11]

- Offer sucrose for analgesia to infants < 6 months (definitely < 2 months). It is shown to be safe and effective when used to reduce procedural pain associated with venipuncture, heal stick and IM injection. A combination of oral sucrose and local anesthetic is better for pain control of LP.
- Best position for LP:
  - ➢ Choose your helper wisely (half of the success goes to the holder!): Careful positioning is required in order to accurately identify landmarks and successfully perform the LP. Children should be observed for adequate respiratory function throughout the procedure.
  - ➢ The lateral recumbent position is used most frequently. The neck is flexed and knees drawn upward by the assistant. A recent study found that neck flexion did not significantly change the inter-spinous space as determined by U/S measurement.[12]
  - ➢ A sitting position may be preferred in children who have the potential for developing respiratory compromise because of hyper-flexion of the neck in the lateral recumbent position. In addition, this position may improve flow of CSF in very small infants < 2 weeks of age. In a recent study,[13] the subarachnoid space width at the site of LP in infants did not change when measured by U/S between 3 positions: flat lateral decubitus, 45-degree tilt, and sitting. An increase in LP success rate with sitting or tilt position could be due to other factors such as increased CSF pressure, increased inter-spinous space widening, or improved identification of landmarks.[13]
- What to do if you hit bone? If bony resistance is felt immediately, this is probably due to puncture over the posterior spinous process. Withdraw the needle to the subcutaneous tissue, confirm that the spine is not rotated, re-palpate to confirm that the puncture site is in the midline and ensure adequate flexion of the spine. Redirect the needle more sharply cephadal.
- What to do if you are in the right space but no CSF is coming out (a dry tap)?
  - o Rotate the spinal needle by 90 degrees
  - o Pull the needle back to subcutaneous tissue and redirect
  - o Replace the stylet and advance the needle slightly
  - o Reattempt the procedure at a different site with a new needle

CLINICAL TIP 7—*Bronchiolitis—RSV Tips and Tricks*

Despite much anticipation of the newly published clinical practice guidelines for the diagnosis and management of bronchiolitis, I suffered a great disappointment; none of the treatments change the course of the disease, or decrease the rate of hospitalization.[14] Despite that, there are some action statements that could help us manage this common disease.

- Bronchiolitis is a clinical diagnosis which starts as an upper respiratory infection (URI) and is followed by lower airway disease with signs and symptoms including tachypnea, wheezing and increased respiratory effort (grunting, nasal flaring, and intercostal and/or subcostal retractions).
- Labs and x-rays should not be obtained routinely.
- The course of bronchiolitis is variable and dynamic ranging from transient events, such as apnea to progressive respiratory distress from lower airway obstruction.

- History should note mental status, feeding and hydration.
- Risk factors for severe disease should be assessed:
  - Age< 12 weeks
  - Prematurity
  - Underlying cardio-pulmonary disease: CHD, Chronic lung disease
  - Immune deficiency
- When managing patients with acute bronchiolitis, suction appropriately, count respiratory rate for an entire minute, and do serial exams as the course of the illness is variable.
- Albuterol is no longer recommended in the treatment of bronchiolitis. In the previous iteration of the guideline, a trial of β-agonists was included as an option. However, given the greater strength of the evidence demonstrating no benefit, and that there is no well-established way to determine an "objective method of response" to bronchodilators in bronchiolitis, this option has been removed. Note: children with severe disease and respiratory failure were excluded from these trials, so these recommendations cannot be generalized to all situations.
- Epinephrine should not be used in children hospitalized for bronchiolitis, except potentially as a rescue agent in severe disease, although further studies are needed.
- Clinicians should not administer systemic corticosteroids to infants with a diagnosis of bronchiolitis in any setting, including the ED. It is difficult to fight the temptation since steroids work so well for asthma and croup. A comprehensive systematic review and large multicenter randomized trials provide clear evidence that corticosteroids alone do not provide significant benefit to children with bronchiolitis. Evidence for potential benefit of combined corticosteroid and agents with both β- and α-agonist activity is at best tentative,[15,16] and additional large trials are needed to clarify whether this therapy is effective. Although there is no evidence of short-term adverse effects from corticosteroid therapy, other than prolonged viral shedding, there is inadequate evidence to be certain of safety. First, do no harm!
- Clinicians should not administer antibacterial medications unless there is a concomitant bacterial infection, or a strong clinical suspicion of one.

CLINICAL TIP 8—*Management of pneumonia in children*

In 2011, the Pediatric Infectious Diseases Society and the Infectious Diseases Society of America developed evidence-based guidelines for the management of community-acquired pneumonia (CAP) in infants and children older than 3 months.[17]

Indications for hospitalization:

- Infants who are younger than 2 months or premature (due to the risk of apnea).[18]
- Hypoxia
- Dehydration
- Toxic-appearing children require resuscitation and respiratory support.
- Presence of an effusion/empyema on chest radiograph.

Therapy for pneumonia:

- Most infants with respiratory syncytial virus (RSV) pneumonia do not require antimicrobials. Serious infections with this organism usually occur in infants with underlying lung disease.

- The vast majority of children diagnosed with pneumonia in the outpatient setting are treated with oral antibiotics. High-dose amoxicillin (80–90 mg/Kg/day) is used as a first-line agent for children with uncomplicated CAP, which provides coverage for S pneumoniae.
- Second- or third-generation cephalosporins and macrolide antibiotics such as azithromycin are acceptable alternatives but should not be used as first-line agents because of lower systemic absorption of the cephalosporins and pneumococcal resistance to macrolides.
- Macrolide antibiotics are useful in school-aged children because they cover the most common bacteriologic and atypical agents (Mycoplasma, Chlamydophila, Legionella).
- Hospitalized patients can be safely treated with narrow-spectrum agents such as ampicillin, as this is the mainstay of current guidelines for pediatric CAP.[19, 20]
- Children who are toxic appearing should receive antibiotic therapy that includes vancomycin (particularly in areas where penicillin-resistant pneumococci and methicillin-resistant S aureus [MRSA] are prevalent) along with a second- or third-generation cephalosporin.
- Influenza A pneumonia that is particularly severe or when it occurs in a high-risk patient may be treated with zanamivir or oseltamivir. Complete recommendations are available from the CDC.

CLINICAL TIP 9—*Recognition and management of testicular torsion*

Testicular torsion is an acute urologic emergency. Timely communication with the patient, caregivers and consultants is crucial to avoid delays in care as well as potential litigation.

Critical actions:

- If testicular torsion is suspected, early urologic consultation is mandatory since definitive treatment is surgery for detorsion and orchiopexy.
- Establish positive rapport with the family by stating that you will treat the patient's pain immediately as well as addressing the etiology.
- Perform Color Doppler US (bedside and in the radiology suite) to demonstrate arterial blood flow to the testicle. The US will also provide information about scrotal anatomy and other testicular disorders.
- Attempt manual detorsion.
- Perform "real time" documentation of the time of your encounter with the patient and the time you contacted the consultant.

CLINICAL TIP 10—*How to recognize child abuse in the ED*

General

- Child abuse is a widely common and often underreported problem.[21]
- Between 1.3% and 15% of childhood injuries that result in emergency department visits are caused by abuse.[22]
- Child abuse occurs at every socioeconomic level, across ethnic and cultural lines, within all religions and at all levels of education.
- The detection and diagnosis of child physical abuse depends on the clinician's ability to recognize suspicious injuries, conduct a careful and complete physical examination with judicious use of auxiliary tests, and consider whether the caregivers' explanation is

supported by the characteristics of the injury or injuries and the child's developmental capabilities.
- Abused children are 25% more likely to experience teen pregnancy, and abused teens are less likely to practice safe sex, putting them at greater risk for STIs.[23]
- Children with abusive head or abdominal injuries are more likely to die or become incapacitated than are children with head or abdominal injuries caused by accidents. The typical progressison is an escalation of violence.[24-26]
- Neglect is the most frequent form of child abuse and most frequent cause of abuse-related death (60–75%). Toddlers with failure to thrive may have thin hair and appear apathetic.

Evaluation for neglect
- If child looks small for age.
- If there is a suspicion of inadequate supervision: History of "accidents" and repetitive injuries.
- Inadequate medical care: Extensive dental caries, neglected wound care.
- Note: an infant falling off the bed is neglect as the parent placed infant in a dangerous situation.

Evaluation for physical abuse-history
Elements in the history that are concerning for intentional trauma include:

1. No explanation or vague explanation for a significant injury.
2. Significant changes in the explanation for the injury from one provider to another or different explanations by different caregivers.
3. An explanation that is inconsistent with the pattern, time, or severity of the injury.
4. An explanation that is inconsistent with the child's physical and/or developmental milestones.

- Short falls may result in bruising; however, more significant types of head trauma, including skull fractures, are exceedingly uncommon.[27,28]
- In patients presenting to the ED with a diagnosis of a life-threatening event (ALTE), child abuse should be considered in the differential, and patients should have a thorough physical examination, including a fundoscopic exam. Consider obtaining a chest x-ray to exclude rib fractures.[29]

Evaluation for physical abuse-exam
Because abusive caregivers are rarely informative regarding the injuries that have been inflicted, special care should be taken for appropriate immobilization of the cervical spine and extremities during the child examination until diagnostic radiographs or imaging can be performed.[30]

Skin Injuries
Location, size, and shape of any bruises, lacerations, burns, bites, or other skin injuries should be documented. Obscure sites for inflicted injuries include the ears, especially the posterior aspects, the neck and angle of the jaw, scalp, and the frenula of the lip and tongue. In contrast to accidental injuries, inflicted injuries tend to occur on surfaces away from bony prominences, such as the neck, head, buttocks, trunk, hands, and upper arms.[31,32]

Bruises in Abuse		
Location	Locations such as inner thighs and other protected areas not likely from accident	1. Assess for mechanics of how injury could occur 2. Check if overlying bones.
Magnitude	Numerous bruising particularly if the patient is not cruising yet	1. Ask about bleeding diseases in family/child. 2. Count the number of bruises—don't use terms such as "many" 3. Photo-documentation is essential
Pattern	Crisp lines are usually the result of high velocity impacts. There may be distinguishable marks such as loops, or other patterns that are abuse	1. Check the entire body.

Burns

a. Categories of burns and abuse (may be multiple)
   - o Physical abuse (e.g., immersion burns, iron burn)
   - o Neglect (e.g., iron left on floor)
   - o Medical neglect (e.g. delay in getting care for substantial burn)
   - o Torture (e.g., multiple cigarette lighter burns)

b. A child as young as 10 months may climb into a bathtub, falling in head first; they don't land perfectly in a sitting position!

c. With pre-existing water, the addition of hot water probably will not be enough to burn and will cause a child to cry out in pain and attempt to exit the tub before a significant burn occurs.

d. The absence of a pain history is worrisome for abuse.

Fractures

Posterior or lateral rib fractures or multiple rib fractures are especially predictive of abusive trauma due to the forceful squeezing of the chest.[33, 34] Cardiopulmonary resuscitation, whether performed by experienced or inexperienced individuals, is an unlikely cause of rib fractures[35] or retinal hemorrhages.

Many fractures may not be clinically detectable. Therefore, a negative clinical examination should not preclude the need for a skeletal radiologic survey when inflicted trauma is suspected, particularly in children younger than 2 years. Non accidental injuries should be distinguished from other diseases that can manifest with multiple fractures, such as Osteogenesis Imperfecta (OI), a rare congenital disorder that typically presents with bone fragility. Other associated findings are common and include deep-blue sclera, ligamentous laxity, osteopenia, wormian skull bones, dentinogenesis imperfecta, positive family history, and hearing loss.

Abdominal injuries

Abdominal bruising is often not seen, even with severe blows to the abdomen. Do not rely on bruising to suspect abdominal injuries in abused children.[36] Liver and pancreatic enzyme tests are helpful in screening children for abdominal trauma, especially when the child presents with acute symptoms or shortly after the incident has occurred. With suspicion, an abdominal/pelvic CT should be performed.

Reporting

- Mandatory reporting: All 50 states have laws requiring physicians to report suspected (not confirmed!) child neglect/abuse to child protective services.
- Most states provide immunity from legal liability for reporters in good faith.

References

1. Karaman A, Cavusoglu YH, Karaman I, et al. Seven cases of neonatal appendicitis with a review of the English language literature of the last century. Pediatr Surg Int. 2003;19:707–709).
2. Passi, Y et al. Comparison of the laryngoscopy views with the size 1 Miller and Macintosh laryngoscope blades lifting the epiglottis or the base of the tongue in infants and children <2 yr of age. Br J Anaesth. 2014;113(5):869–74.
3. Weiss M, Knirsch W, Kretschmar O, et al. Tracheal tube-tip displacement in children during head-neck movement—a radiological assessment. Br J Anaesth. 2006;96:486.
4. Dalal PG, Murray D, Messner AH, et al. Pediatric laryngeal dimensions: an age-based analysis. Anesth Analg. 2009;108:1475.
5. Deakers TW, Reynolds G, Stretton M, Newth CJ. Cuffed endotracheal tubes in pediatric intensive care. J Pediatr. 1994;125:5–62.
6. Kleinman ME, Chameides L, Schexnayder SM, et al. Part 14: pediatric advanced life support: 2010 American Heart Association Guidelines for Cardiopulmonary Resuscitation and Emergency Cardiovascular Care. Circulation. 2010;122:S876.
7. Thigpen MC, Whitney CG, Messonnier NE, et al. Bacterial meningitis in the United States, 1998–2007. N Engl J Med. 2011;364(21):2016–25.
8. Curtis S, Stobart K, Vandermeer B, et al. Clinical features suggestive of meningitis in children: a systematic review of prospective data. Pediatrics. 2010;126:952.
9. Levy M, Wong E, Fried D. Diseases that mimic meningitis. Analysis of 650 lumbar punctures. Clin Pediatr. 1990;29:254.
10. Kaur G, Gupta P, Kumar A. A randomized trial of eutectic mixture of local anesthetics during lumbar puncture in newborns. Arch Pediatr Adolesc Med. 2003;157:1065.
11. Baxter AL, Fisher RG, Burke BL, et al. Lidocaine for lumbar punctures. A help not a hindrance. Arch Pediatr Adolesc Med. 2006;117: 876.
12. Abo A, Chen L, Johnston P, et al. Positioning for lumbar puncture in children evaluated by bedside ultrasound. Pediatrics. 2010;125:e1149.
13. Lo MD, Parisi MT, Brown JC, et al. Sitting or tilt position for infant lumbar puncture does not increase ultrasound measurements of lumbar subarachnoid space width. Pediatr Emerg Care. 2013;29(5):588–91.
14. Ralston SL, Lieberthal AS, Meissner HC, et al. Clinical practice guideline: the diagnosis, management, and prevention of bronchiolitis. Pediatrics. 2014;134:e1474–e1502.
15. Hartling L, Fernandes RM, Bialy L, et al. Steroids and bronchodilators for acute bronchiolitis in the first two years of life: systematic review and meta-analysis. BMJ. 2011;342:d1714
16. Wainwright C, Altamirano L, Cheney M, et al. A multicenter, randomized, double- blind, controlled trial of nebulized epinephrine in infants with acute bronchiolitis. N Engl J Med. 2003;349(1):27–35.

17. Bradley JS, Byington CL, Shah SS, et al. The management of community-acquired pneumonia in infants and children older than 3 months of age: clinical practice guidelines by the pediatric infectious diseases society and the infectious diseases society of America. Clin Infect Dis. 2011;53(7):e25–76.
18. Willwerth BM, Harper MB, Greenes DS. Identifying hospitalized infants who have bronchiolitis and are at high risk for apnea. Ann Emerg Med. 2006;48(4):441–7.
19. Williams DJ, Hall M, Shah SS, et al. Narrow vs broad-spectrum antimicrobial therapy for children hospitalized with pneumonia. Pediatrics. 2013;132(5):e1141–8.
20. Bradley JS, Byington CL, Shah SS, et al. The management of community-acquired pneumonia in infants and children older than 3 months of age: clinical practice guidelines by the Pediatric Infectious diseases Society and the Infectious Diseases Society of America. Clin Infect Dis. 2011;53(7):e25–76.
21. United States Government Accountability Office. Child maltreatment: strengthening national data on child fatalities could aid in prevention (GAO-11-599, 2011). http://www.gao.gov/new.items/d11599.pdf
22. Pless IB, Sibald AD, Smith MA, Russell MD. A reappraisal of the frequency of child abuse seen in pediatric emergency rooms. Child Abuse Negl. 1987;11:193–200.
23. Long-term consequences of child abuse and neglect. Child Welfare Information Gateway. Washington, DC:U.S. Department of Health and Human Services, 2006. http://www.childwelfare.gov/pubs/factsheets/long_term_consequences.cfm
24. Reece RM, Sege R. Childhood head injuries: accidental or inflicted. Arch Pediatr Adolesc Med. 2000;154:11–5.
25. Feldman KW, Bethel R, Shugeman RP, et al. The cause of infant and toddler subdural hemorrhage: a prospective study. Pediatrics. 2001;108:636–46.
26. Canty TG Sr, Canty TG Jr, Brown C. Injuries of the gastrointestinal tract from blunt trauma in children: a 12-year experience at a designated pediatric trauma center. J Trauma. 1999;46:234–40.
27. Warrington SA, Wright CM. ALSPAC Study Team. Accidents and resulting injuries in premobile infants: data from the ALSPAC study. Arch Dis Child. 2001;85:104–7.
28. Johnson K, Fischer T, Chapman S, et al. Accidental head injuries in children under 5 years of age. Clin Radiol. 2005;60:464–8.
29. Parker K, Pitetti R. Mortality and child abuse in children presenting with apparent life-threatening events. Pediatr Emerg Care. 2011;27(7):591–5.
30. Kellogg ND. Evaluation of Suspected Child Physical Abuse. Pediatrics. 2007;119;1232.
31. Maguire S, Mann MK, Sibert J, et al. Are there patterns of bruising in childhood which are diagnostic or suggestive of abuse? A systematic review. Arch Dis Child. 2005;90:182–6.
32. Sugar N, Taylor J, Feldman K. Puget Sound Pediatric Research Network. Bruises in infants and toddlers: those who don't cruise rarely bruise. Arch Pediatr Adolesc Med. 1999;153:399–403.
33. Bulloch B, Schubert CJ, Brophy PB, Jet al. Cause and clinical characteristics of rib fractures in infants. Pediatrics. 2000;105(4):1232–41. Available at: www.pediatrics. org/cgi/content/full/105/4/e480.
34. Barness KA, Cha ES, Bensard DD, et al. The positive predictive value of rib fractures as an indicator of nonaccidental trauma in children. J Trauma. 2003;54:1107–10.

35. Spevak MR, Kleinman PK, Belanger PL, et al. Cardiopulmonary resuscitation and rib fractures in infants: a postmortem radiologic-pathologic study. JAMA. 1994;272:617–8.
36. Thompson S. Accidental or inflicted? Evaluating cutaneous, skeletal, and abdominal trauma in children. Pediatr Ann. 2005;34:372–81.

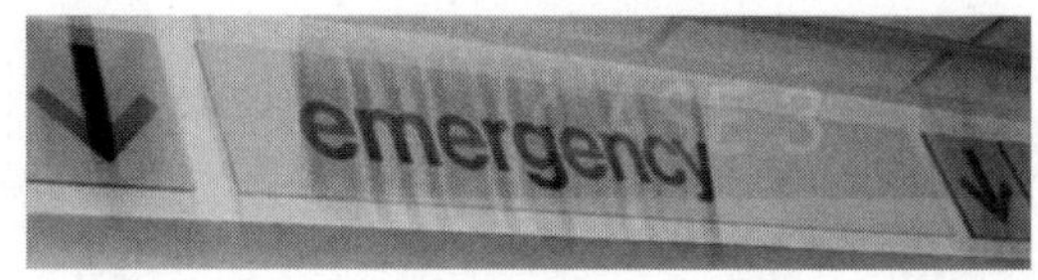

PEDIATRIC MALPRACTICE IS NOT "CHILD SIZED"

Kevin M. Klauer, DO, EJD, FACEP

Assistant Clinical Professor, Michigan State University College of Osteopathic Medicine
Chief Medical Officer, Chief Risk Officer, TEAMHealth
Executive Director, TEAMHealth Patient Safety Organization
Editor in Chief, ACEP Now
Speaker, ACEP Council

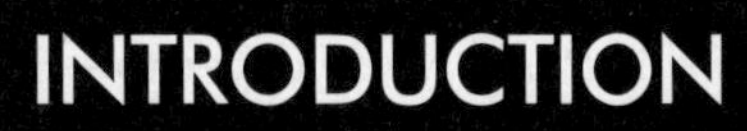

INTRODUCTION

PEDIATRIC MALPRACTICE IS NOT "CHILD SIZED"

Liability associated with pediatric patients is definitely not child-sized. Quite the contrary, negligence often carries with it disproportionate risk. The life expectancy of a child is far greater than that of an adult, thus, the special or economic damages can be substantial when the cost of convalescent and ongoing care is calculated. Pediatric patients often make very sympathetic plaintiffs in the eyes of the juror equating to potential astronomical economic damages for a lifetime of ongoing care. Complicating matters, the statute of limitations may be exaggerated and extended (tolled) beyond the limitations for cases involving adult claimants.

The "Discovery of harm" rule is critical to the concept of the pediatric statutes of limitations; the injured party has the right to file a claim upon *discovery* of the alleged injury. The statute of limitations does not begin until the individual becomes aware of the injury or should have reasonably known the injury has occurred. Any delay must be reasonable, based on the individual circumstances. In addition, for minors, the limitations are tolled or delayed until the age of majority, at which time the former minor can now reasonably recognize and "discover" the injury and its implications on his or her quality of life.

A listing of statutes of limitation by state is provided by the National Conference of State Legislatures at http://www.ncsl.org/research/financial-services-and-commerce/medical-liability-malpractice-statutes-of-limitation.aspx[1]

Necessary Elements of a Lawsuit (Tort of Negligence)

The elements required for a negligence lawsuit are no different for children than for adults.

1. Duty to treat
2. Breach of the standard of care in carrying out that duty
3. Causation (direct and proximate)
4. Damages

Duty to treat

In an emergency department, duty is typically not contestable; it is established upon your arrival to work and the patient's arrival for treatment.

Standard of care

That duty, or duty of care, carries with it the standard of care; the degree of diligence, prudence or caution required of the individual owing the duty of care for another. In ordinary negligence, the "Reasonable person" standard is utilized. In other words, what a reasonable individual, with similar training in similar circumstances, would do. Often, physicians assume that duty of care refers to medical care. However, this is a broad term applied to the tort of negligence, beyond professional liability for alleged medical malpractice. A duty of care is owed to those we encounter in all aspects of our lives.

For instance, if someone is driving a car and runs a red light and injures a pedestrian, the same elements would be required in a lawsuit alleging negligence. Did the driver owe a duty to the pedestrian? Yes. Did the driver act as a reasonable driver in similar circumstances would? Maybe. Are there any circumstances where running the red light would be reasonable? What? Deliberating the facts of the case is the only way to know for certain. One might say that running a red light is negligence per se, however, would it matter to a jury, that the driver ran the red light because they had suffered a stroke or if this was the only course of action to avoid a child who ran out into the street? Establishing whether the duty of care was provided (the standard of care met) can get complicated very quickly and are matters of fact, as opposed to law, that are left for jurors to decide.

Causation (direct and proximate)

Causation is, perhaps, the most complex of the required elements. In order for the defendant to be found negligent, their alleged negligence must be the direct (actual or factual) and proximate (legal) cause of plaintiff's injury or damages. Actual causation means that "But for" the actions of the defendant, the injury would not have occurred.

Proximate cause, or the legal cause, considers that the alleged negligence must be the primary cause of the injury. In other words, the chain of causation from direct causation to the injury must not be interrupted by a superseding event, which would relieve the defendant, or alleged tortfeasor, of negligence.

Example: A 2-year old boy is evaluated for a minor head injury and discharged (mildly confused) after a radiology report of a normal CT scan of the brain. The child dies two hours later from an epidural hematoma. Is the act of discharging the patient negligent? A plaintiff's argument would be that the act of discharging the patient is the direct (actual) cause of the patient's injury, in this case death. "But for" discharging the patient, he would have survived.

However, is discharging the patient also the proximate (legal) cause of the patient's death? If no further facts were known, a strong argument would be made that if the act of discharging the patient is the direct cause of the patient's death, then it must also be the proximate (legal) cause and the requirement for causation has been met. However, if the radiologist misread the CT scan, but reported a negative result to the emergency department, a strong argument could be made that the radiologist's negligent interpretation supersedes that of the discharging physician, thus, breaking the chain of causation. Therefore, despite the argument that discharging the patient may be the direct or actual cause of the patient's death, it is not the proximate cause. This is the basis of a proximate cause defense.

Damages

Damages are required for a lawsuit alleging negligence. The plaintiff must have experienced damages of some kind, secondary to the alleged negligence, resulting from an act of commission or omission, of the defendant(s). So, even if a defendant was admittedly negligent, without damages, there is no case. Although a bit of an oversimplification, two types of damages are routinely considered in cases of alleged medical malpractice: Special and General.

Special damages, economic damages, are quantifiable losses suffered by the plaintiff. Such damages may include, but are not limited to:

- Medical expenses (immediate and ongoing)
- Lost income (past and future)
- Anatomical loss (e.g., necrosed testicle from misdiagnosed torsion).

General damages, or non-economic damages, include non-monetary losses including, but not limited to:

- Pain and suffering
- Loss of companionship
- Loss of consortium (benefits of a family relationship)
- Disfigurement
- Loss of function.

Emergency medicine malpractice

The risk climate in emergency medicine isn't a favorable one for a variety of reasons, including the complexity of the cases, volume of patients seen and operational and workflow challenges. The American Society of Health Care Risk Management publishes their benchmark analysis each year. Based on the 2013 report, claims frequency was reported to be 1 case per 26,809 ED visits, with twice as many settling for expenses than paying indemnity to the plaintiff.[2] Claims frequency has been fairly consistent since 2006[2]. Claims severity, based on the average amount of indemnity paid per claim, has been slowly increasing from $150,000 in 2006 to $163,000 in 2013.[2]

Diederich Healthcare published data from their 2013 medical malpractice payout analysis, noting that $3.6 billion was paid for 12,142 claims in the United States in 2012 (1 every 43 minutes), a reduction of 3.4% compared to 2011.[3] From a geographical perspective, they reported that five states were responsible for 48% of the payments: New York, Pennsylvania, California, New Jersey and Florida, respectively.[3]

In their 2014 analysis, they reported a 4.7% increase in total payments ($168 million more than in 2012), but New York experienced a $73 million decrease.[4] They note that the last time payments were at this level was in 2009.[4] Indemnity payments from judgments (trial) reduced from 5% in 2012 to 3% in 2013. The overwhelming number of successful plaintiff cases end in settlement, as opposed to courtroom verdicts.

Pediatric malpractice

There is limited data specifically regarding pediatric emergency department claims. However, the information that is available appears to support current experience. For instance, Selbst, et al., reported that in a 16-year closed claims database, lawsuits involving children in U.S. emergency departments or urgent care centers were settled 93% of the time, with indemnity paid in 30% of those cases. Of those tried in court, 80% resulted in a defense verdict,[5] similar to adult malpractice.[7]

Outcome of Claims (%)	
Settled after litigation began	47
Settled before litigation	29
Case dropped	9
Settled by court	7 (dismissed by action of court)
Judgment for defendant	6
Judgment for plaintiff	1
Mediation	1

Selbst SM, et al. Epidemiology and etiology of malpractice lawsuits involving children in US emergency departments and urgent care centers. Pediatr Emerg Care. 2005;21(3)165–9. Table 5. Copyright© 2005 Lippincott Williams & Wilkins. Used with permission.

The most common diagnoses in pediatric malpractice claims are:

- Meningitis
- Appendicitis
- Arm fracture
- Testicular torsion

Diagnoses associated with death were more likely from pneumonia and meningitis (both less likely now secondary to advances in immunization strategies for S. pneumoniae and H. Influenzae).[5] Diagnoses vary by age group:

Most Common Diagnoses Involved in Malpractice Claims (by Age Group)			
	First	**Second**	**Third**
0–2 y	Meningitis	Impaired neonate	Pneumonia
3–5 y	Fracture	Meningitis	Appendicitis
6–11 y	Fracture	Appendicitis	Meningitis
12–17 y	Fracture	Appendicitis	Testicular torsion

Selbst SM, et al. Epidemiology and etiology of malpractice lawsuits involving children in US emergency departments and urgent care centers. Pediatr Emerg Care. 2005;21(3)165–9. Table 3. Copyright© 2005 Lippincott Williams & Wilkins. Used with permission.

Causes of pediatric "midadventures" were predominately diagnostic, accounting for 39% of claims. When "no medical error" was found, indemnity was only paid in 0.4% of the cases (18 of 391 cases) for a total of $1.1 million.

Top 10 Misadventures		
	Number of claims, N = 2132	% Total Claims
Diagnostic error	832	39
No medical error	391	18
Improper performance of procedure	386	18
Failure to supervise other staff	120	6
Resuscitation/procedure not done	95	4
Delay in treatment	84	4
Medication error	63	3
Failure to admit to hospital	57	3
Failure to consult/refer	53	3
Failure to respond appropriately	51	2

Selbst SM, et al. Epidemiology and etiology of malpractice lawsuits involving children in US emergency departments and urgent care centers. Pediatr Emerg Care. 2005;21(3)165–9. Table 4. Copyright© 2005 Lippincott Williams & Wilkins. Used with permission.

An excellent closed claims analysis was published in *Pediatrics* in 2008, which identified general pediatric risk, including the most common clinical entities resulting in lawsuits.[6]

- Most Prevalent in Order of Frequency
  1. Brain-damaged infant
  2. Meningitis
  3. Routine infant or child health check
  4. Respiratory problems in newborns
  5. Appendicitis
  6. Pneumonia
  7. Specified nonteratogenic anomalies
  8. Premature birth
  9. Birth
  10. Asthma
- Most Prevalent Caused by Error in Diagnosis
  1. Meningitis
  2. Appendicitis
  3. Specified nonteratogenic anomalies
  4. Pneumonia
  5. Brain-damaged infant

Summary

The risk management climate in pediatric Emergency Medicine is challenging, however, understanding the common high-risk entities and possessing a fundamental knowledge of the current legal landscape may help providers navigate the best care for their patients while limiting risk to themselves and other stakeholders.

Whereas our last book (*Bouncebacks! Medical and Legal*) contained cases that all went to trial or settlement, very few of the cases in *Bouncebacks! Pediatrics* resulted in legal action. As you read the following chapters, consider which of these patients had high risk features including an incomplete history or abnormal vitals and left the ED with diagnostic uncertainty.

Our primary goal is to provide medical care which maximizes patient safety, but keeping an eye toward a potential legal action, in some ways "keeps us honest." The aim is to hit the "sweet spot" of a safe patient evaluation without overtesting, while transcending standard of care for *excellence* in care.

References

1. National Conference of State Legislatures; http://www.ncsl.org/research/financial-services-and-commerce/medical-liability-malpractice-statutes-of-limitation.aspx. Accessed December 10, 2014.
2. 2013 Hospital and Physician Professional Liability: Benchmark Analysis; October 2013.
3. 2013 Medical Malpractice Payout Analysis. Diederich Healthcare; http://www.diederichhealthcare.com/the-standard/2013-medical-malpractice-payout-analysis/ Accessed October 12, 2013.
4. 2014 Medical Malpractice Payout Analysis. Diederich Healthcare; http://www.diederichhealthcare.com/the-standard/2014-medical-malpractice-payout-analysis/ Accessed November 11, 2014.
5. Selbst SM, et al. Epidemiology and etiology of malpractice lawsuits involving children in US emergency departments and urgent care centers. Pediatr Emerg Care. 2005; 21(3):165–9.
6. Gary N. McAbee, et al. Medical diagnoses commonly associated with pediatric malpractice lawsuits in the United States. Pediatrics. 2008;122;e1282–e1286.
7. Brown TW, et al. An epidemiologic study of closed emergency department malpractice claims in a national database of physician malpractice insurers. Acad Emerg Med. 2010;17(5):553–60.

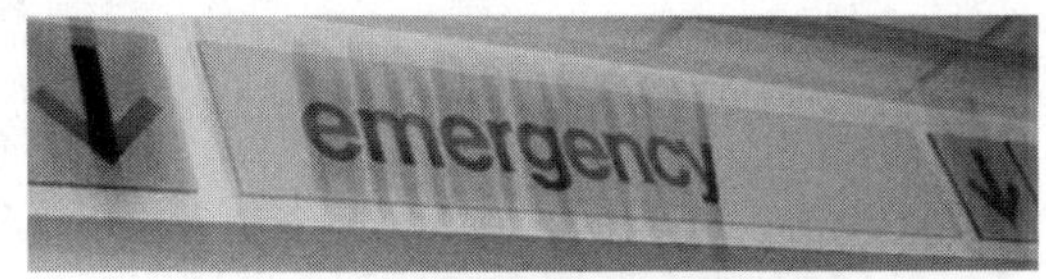

CASE 1

10-YEAR-OLD BOY WITH FEVER AND HEADACHE

Joseph Ravera, MD
Fellow In Pediatric Emergency Medicine
Harbor-UCLA Medical Center

Marianne Gausche-Hill, MD, FACEP, FAAP
Professor of Clinical Medicine, David Geffen School of Medicine at UCLA
Vice Chair and Chief of the Division of Pediatric Emergency Medicine
Director Pediatric Emergency Medicine and EMS Fellowships
Harbor-UCLA Medical Center, Department of Emergency Medicine

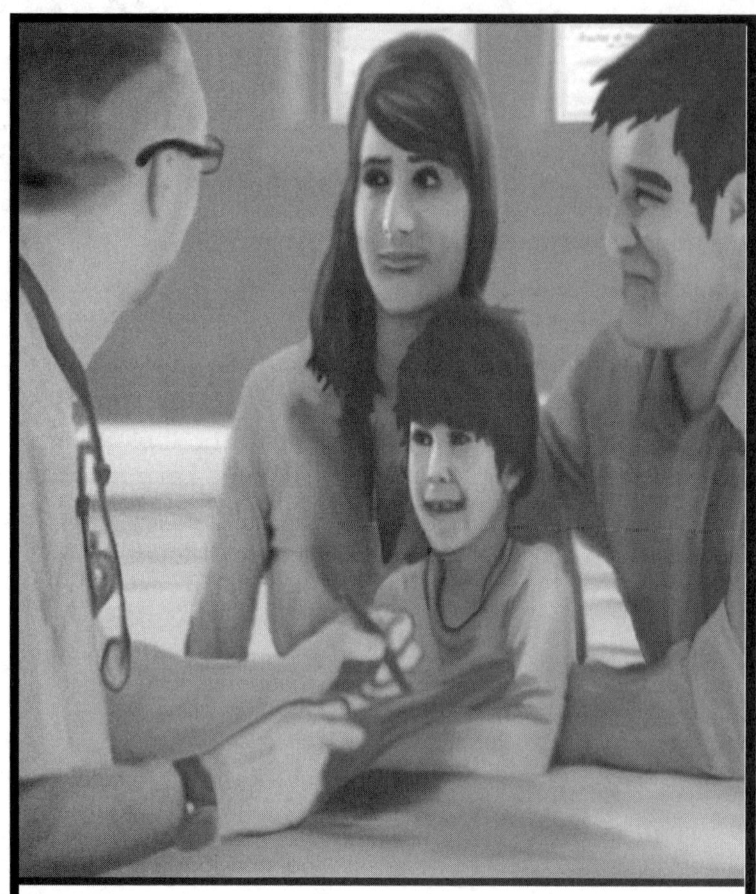

"The spinal tap was negative, he has a viral syndrome."

CASE 1

10-YEAR-OLD BOY WITH FEVER AND HEADACHE

PART 1—MEDICAL

I. The Doctor's Version (the following is the actual documentation of the provider)

Date: October 2, 2009
Time: 10:03
Chief Complaint: Fever and headache
Nurse note: He says he has had a headache and a fever beginning today. Triaged as Category 3; alert and appropriate, but somewhat sleepy. Pain scale is 5/10.

HPI: Pt complains of a HA and a fever which started this morning. He feels sleepy and states he did not sleep well the previous night because he was worried about his friend who was recently hospitalized with meningitis and is in an ICU. He cannot remember the name of the hospital where his friend is in the ICU. Mother states that her son often gets headaches with fever but this time it seems more severe. Denies trauma or other family members ill. He denies photophobia, difficulty moving his neck, nausea or vomiting, runny nose, cough, chest complaints, abdominal pain, dysuria, flank or back pain, or rash.

PAST MEDICAL HISTORY:
NKDA
PMH: Asthma, uses albuterol sporadically. No previous hospitalizations
Social History: In fourth grade, good student, lives with Mom, Dad and younger brother.

VITAL SIGNS

Time	Temp	Pulse	Resp	Syst	Diast	Sat	Weight
17:05	102.2F	130	22	110	80	99%	36

Constitutional: Alert and well developed preadolescent, cap refill < 2 seconds
Mental Status/Psychiatric: Alert and oriented, appears anxious; states he is worried he has what his friend has.
Head & Neck: Anicteric. Neck is supple without meningismus. No LAN. Throat without erythema or exudate.
Pupils: PERRL. EOMs full conjunctiva clear
Chest: Clear to auscultation and equal breath sounds bilaterally.
Cardiac: S1, S2 without murmur, rub, or gallop.
Abdomen: Abdominal exam is benign, nondistended, nontender. No hepatosplenomegaly.

GU: No swelling or erythema. Testes descended. Uncircumcised.
Extremities: Without rash or petechiae
Neuro: Cranial and cerebellar function normal. Motor and sensation intact.

ED COURSE:
10:30: Ibuprofen 360 mg PO, IV Normal Saline 720 mL bolus (20 ml/kg).
Testing:

- CBC, CHEM 10, Blood Culture, UA and Cx
- CXR
- CSF protein, glucose, cell count, gm stain and cx

10:45: Consent for lumbar puncture (LP) obtained from Mother. During the LP the boy became anxious and agitated and had to be held in position. Fluid is clear without xanthochromia.
11:00: Mother alerted staff of a rash on the legs after procedure. I did go into the room and re-examined pt. There are some ill-defined pink macular patches on lower legs consistent with pt being held for the LP. Pt sleeping comfortably
11:30 (Test results): WBC count 4,000, diff 7% bands and otherwise normal. Plt nl. Chem 10 normal. CXR WNL per rad. UA WNL. CSF: No WBC cells, protein and glucose nl., gm stain neg for organisms

MDM: Recheck temp at 38 degrees and pulse decreased to 120 bpm. Headache improved after LP. Clinical picture not consistent with bacterial meningitis.

DIAGNOSIS: Viral syndrome and headache.

12:00 - Disposition: Return to ED if the headache became more severe or associated with nausea and vomiting. F/U with PMD for a recheck in 2 days. OTC ibuprofen or acetaminophen prn for headache.

➢**Author's personal note (MW):** I first heard about this case from Marianne after the "all-LA" (Los Angeles) emergency medicine conference a few years ago. She was sitting in the second row and approached me as the conference ended about a bounceback case which had gone bad. I initially thought that it was an interesting case, but had minimal teaching value. The provider was vigilant and pursued a diagnosis to the point of performing a lumbar puncture ... so what more could have been done? What lessons could be learned from such a thorough evaluation?

What a far way this case has come, now the lead chapter. When I read through the actual evaluation and documentation, I recognized that this case exemplified our goal; to inspire the reader to transcend a legal *standard of care* for a patient-centered *excellence* in care. It is a case which is neither esoteric nor obvious, one which many of us could say, "Yeah. I would have done the same thing."

This case highlights three primary lessons we hope to portray in this *Bouncebacks!* volume:

- Recognition of the high risk patient
- The importance of a thorough history
- An expanded pediatric-specific differential diagnosis

So what *was* the diagnosis? Was the provider correct? We'll give you a clue: they were right about one thing; the patient did not have meningitis …

II.The Errors—Risk Management/Patient Safety Issues

Risk management/patient safety issue #1:

Error: Inadequate history (part 1)

Discussion: The patient's chief complaint was headache, but there was very little history of the actual headache, such as onset, exacerbating factors, duration, character, and associated or neurologic symptoms. The nurse documented pain scale of 5/10, which at least described the *severity* of the headache. The description of the second complaint of fever was similarly thin; duration, response to therapy, associated symptoms. There was a nice review of systems (ROS) but an inadequate history of *present* illness.

✔ **Teaching point:** The history of present illness should focus on a description of the chief complaint as well as pertinent negatives.

Risk management/patient safety issue #2:

Error: Inadequate history (part 2)

Discussion: Arguably the most important aspect of this encounter was to learn the diagnosis of the patient's friend. Even thought he could not remember the name of the hospital, a call could have been placed to the family or friends who may have known of the diagnosis or name of the hospital. A history of a friend with "meningitis" is quite different than a history of a friend with "meningitis" who is in an *ICU*. Trying to obtain information from others is often an exercise in futility, but sometimes-essential data is uncovered; consider bystanders to a seizure, drug overdose, suicide attempt, syncopal episode, or child abuse/neglect.

✔ **Teaching point:** Exposure history needs to be investigated when symptoms could be from a serious illness.

Risk management/patient safety issue #3:

Error: Failure to consider a differential diagnosis that includes possible life threatening diagnoses.

Discussion: Although the emergency physicians considered meningitis in the differential, they failed to consider other life threatening disease such as sepsis. The patient's tachycardia and fever without an alternate diagnosis were concerning. A serum lactate may have been helpful. This patient was treated and discharged in under 2 hours, even with an LP, clearly an anomaly in most ED's! Consideration could have been given to a more prolonged period of observation.

✔ **Teaching point:** A high risk patient evaluation often requires a multifaceted approach

Risk management/patient safety issue #4:

Error: Failure to appreciate the significance of a low WBC and bandemia.

Discussion: The physicians in this case rationalized that the low WBC and bandemia were due to viral illness, although the patient did not have typical viral signs and symptoms. Although nonspecific, elevated WBCs are easily recognized as a cause for concern, a WBC count <5,000 also indicates the potential for serious illness and is part of the criteria for sepsis.

✔ **Teaching point:** Leukopenia may indicate serious infection.

Risk management/patient safety issue #5:

Error: Attributing a new physical exam finding to a benign cause.

Discussion: The patient had a new finding of rash, which in the context of a patient exposed to meningitis, required a more detailed description and explanation. Documentation of the distribution of the rash is important to know; was it in the shape of the hand that was holding him or more generalized? Removing the shoes to see if the rash involved the soles, or if it was symmetric, and if it blanched with pressure would have been helpful. Of note, a petechial rash due to straining/vomiting would typically appear around the eyes or at least above the nipple line and not on the lower extremities. In infants, the rash might start in the genital areas. Was a longer period of observation required after the discovery of a new rash?

✔ **Teaching point:** Sometimes a random question from a concerned parent can be a clue to the diagnosis.

Risk management/patient safety issue #6:

Error: Failure to appreciate the significance of the elevated heart rate as a sign of sepsis.

Discussion: The physician attributed the elevated heart rate to fever. Although the patient received fluid resuscitation and an antipyretic, the heart rate remained elevated. This should have prompted consideration of a thorough reassessment and an expanded differential.

✔ **Teaching point:** An elevated heart rate may be the sole clue to systemic inflammatory response (SIRS) and/or possible sepsis.

III. Greg Henry Comments

"I fully recognize that I'm an old man and lack sophistication"

A child with altered mental status and a friend "somewhere in the ICU" with meningitis sounds to me like someone who needs treatment. I would have empirically, long before a gram stain or culture was back, started this child on medication. The classic "kids close together" meningitis at this age is meningococcal meningitis.

There is precious little evidence to suggest that steroids actually change the morbidity or mortality. I think its use is up in the air. Similarly, the use of anti-viral medications is all over the map. Does giving Acyclovir really cause much harm? Probably not; I would have included it.

As a side note, 10 year olds feel pain just as adults do; there is no contraindication to giving mild sedation such as ketamine or versed when doing a lumbar puncture. The mother feels better, the patient feels better, and I feel better.

I fully recognize that I'm an old man and lack sophistication. I have seen meningococcemia go from 2 petechial lesions to damn-near dead in hours. Meningococcemia is a bad actor; a full court press should have been undertaken. The last teenager I saw die with this disease had been at the hospital a total of 3 hours.

IV. The Bounceback

The patient is discharged around noon and goes home and falls asleep. Later that afternoon, at 1730, the hospital ED staff receives this message from the squad box:

EMS: "This is medic 18 – we are enroute with an unresponsive 10-year-old male. Pt is limp and has agonal respirations and a thready pulse. Bag-mask ventilation in progress. IO is being place for fluid resuscitation"

ED: "Bed placement on arrival, medic 18. We are awaiting your arrival"

- On presentation in the ED, staff recognizes the patient as the same 10-year-old child who had been seen earlier with fever and HA
- Hx: Pt is unresponsive. IO in place. Parents not yet arrived.
- PE: The patchy pink macular rash noted earlier is now purpuric.
- ED course:
  - o IV ATB started upon arrival: Ceftriaxone and vancomycin
  - o Aggressive fluid resuscitation is initiated. BP remains low. Pt receives multiple additional 20ml/kg boluses of IVF without improvement
  - o Dopamine is started and rapidly increased without success
  - o Pt. goes into cardiac arrest.
  - o Multiple rounds of ALS are attempted without success and the pt is pronounced dead
- The next day results from the blood and CSF cultures return. Both grow *Neisseria meningitides.*

FINAL DIAGNOSIS: Meningococcemia, overwhelming sepsis

PART 2—ANALYSIS

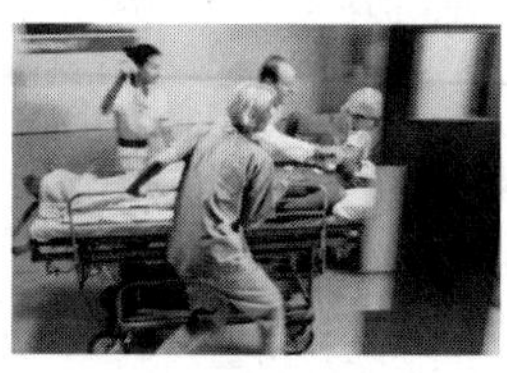

EVALUATION OF PATIENTS EXPOSED TO SERIOUS ILLNESS—MENINGOCOCCEMIA

Joseph Ravera, MD

Fellow In Pediatric Emergency Medicine
Harbor-UCLA Medical Center

Marianne Gausche-Hill, MD, FACEP, FAAP

Professor of Clinical Medicine , David Geffen School of Medicine at UCLA
Vice Chair and Chief of the Division of Pediatric Emergency Medicine
Director Pediatric Emergency Medicine and EMS Fellowships
Harbor-UCLA Medical Center, Department of Emergency Medicine

Epidemiology

Meningococcemia is the type of disease that keeps emergency physicians and pediatricians up at night. It is rare in developed countries (0.53 per 100,000) but what it lacks in commonality, it makes up for with virulence with a case fatality rate of 11%, and a 28% cognitive impairment rate.[1,2] What makes this disease particularly insidious is that the initial symptoms of malaise, fever, headaches and myalgias, mimic the ubiquitous "viral syndrome," which is several orders of magnitude more common.[3] Suffice to say, this is a disease that the average emergency physician may come across only once a decade, but given the potential serious outcome, we need to remain vigilant.

In our case, the emergency physician (EP) was presented with a patient who appeared well, but had concerning symptoms (fever and headache), recent exposure to a friend who was currently in the ICU with meningitis, and no alternative diagnosis. This is a strong epidemiologic risk factor. Other risk factors include:

- Close quartering
- Known immunodeficiency
- Asplenia[3, 4]

In this case, the risk factor was volunteered by the patient and family, but many families may not understand the importance of recent exposure. Asking the question of "are any of your friends in the hospital with similar symptoms" (think carbon monoxide exposure, food poisoning, drug overdose/exposure) can be an effective screening tool when evaluating the patient with "viral syndrome."

Evaluation for meningococcal disease

It was clear that the emergency physicians thought about the potential of a serious bacterial disease, including meningococcal meningitis as evidenced by the work up, which included a lumbar puncture. But there was a cognitive error in reliance on laboratory testing to exclude the diagnosis of invasive meningococcal disease. Unfortunately, classic risk stratification for children with fever is ineffective in screening for meningococcal disease.[1,4] One review of 296 meningococcemia cases in children <21 years of age demonstrated a median WBC of 16,100 with a range of 1,400-40,000.[1] This variability demonstrates that physicians should not rely solely on a WBC as a "rule in" or "rule out" test with invasive meningococcal disease.[1] In that same review, only 58% of the children had meningococcal meningitis. In our case, the negative LP ruled out other forms of meningitis, but did not rule out invasive meningococcal disease, including meningococcal sepsis.

Lessons from this case

When analyzing any case retrospectively it's always hard to separate the outcome from the decision-making. The fact that this child ended up dying of meningococcemia makes the clinical decision seem obvious, but if he actually had a viral syndrome as the providers thought, it would have been quickly forgotten as one of the tens of thousands of "viral syndromes" we each see in our careers.

Meningococcal disease occurs in outbreaks. Our patient's risk was multiple folds higher because of his exposure. The absence of meningitis in cases of invasive meningococcal disease is a poor prognostic sign, and in our case, the exclusion as evidenced by a normal lumbar puncture was misinterpreted by the emergency physicians as a lack of serious bacterial disease. The patient's symptoms combined with his exposure put him at a high risk for invasive meningococcal disease and consideration of admission with IV antibiotics and follow up cultures.

With these points in mind, consider this synopsis: A child with exposure to meningitis presents with fever, headache, myalgias, and in the ED develops a rash. His work up is negative for meningitis and he "appears well" after IV fluids and antipyretics. The two key learning points from this scenario:

1. The work up did not rule out the diagnosis of other invasive meningococcal disease.
2. The epidemiologic risk factor should not have been minimized.[4]

✔ Teaching points:

1. It is critically important to take a careful history when life-threatening disease is suspected.
2. Exposure to another patient with critical illness is an important risk factor for meningococcal disease.
3. Labs cannot reliably screen nor rule out serious invasive meningococcal disease.
4. The lack of meningitis is a poor prognostic sign and does not exclude the possibility of meningococcemia.

References

1. Stovall SH, Schutze GE. Meningococcal infections in children from Arkansas. Pediatr Infect Dis J. 2002;21(5):366–70.
2. Cohn AC, MacNeil JR, Harrison LH, et al. Changes in Neisseria meningitidis disease epidemiology in the United States, 1998–2007: implications for prevention of meningococcal disease. Clin Infect Dis. 2010;50(2):184–91.
3. Campsall PA, Laupland KB, Niven DJ. Severe meningococcal infection: a review of epidemiology, diagnosis, and management. Crit Care Clin. 2013;29(3):393–409.
4. Brigham KS, Sandora TJ: Neisseria meningitides: Epidemiology, treatment, and prevention in adolescents. Curr Opin Pediatr. 2009;21:437–43.

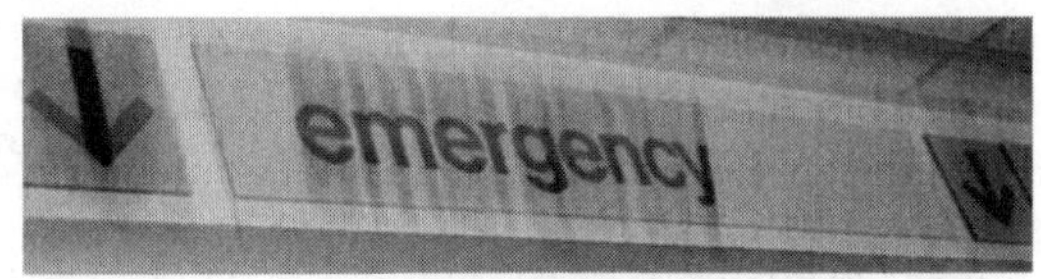

CASE 2

5-YEAR-OLD BOY WITH VOMITING

Emily Fontane, MD, FAAP, FACEP
Associate Professor
Emergency Medicine/Pediatrics
University Florida College of Medicine—Jacksonville

Heide Valdes, MD
Pediatric Emergency Medicine Fellow
University Florida College of Medicine—Jacksonville

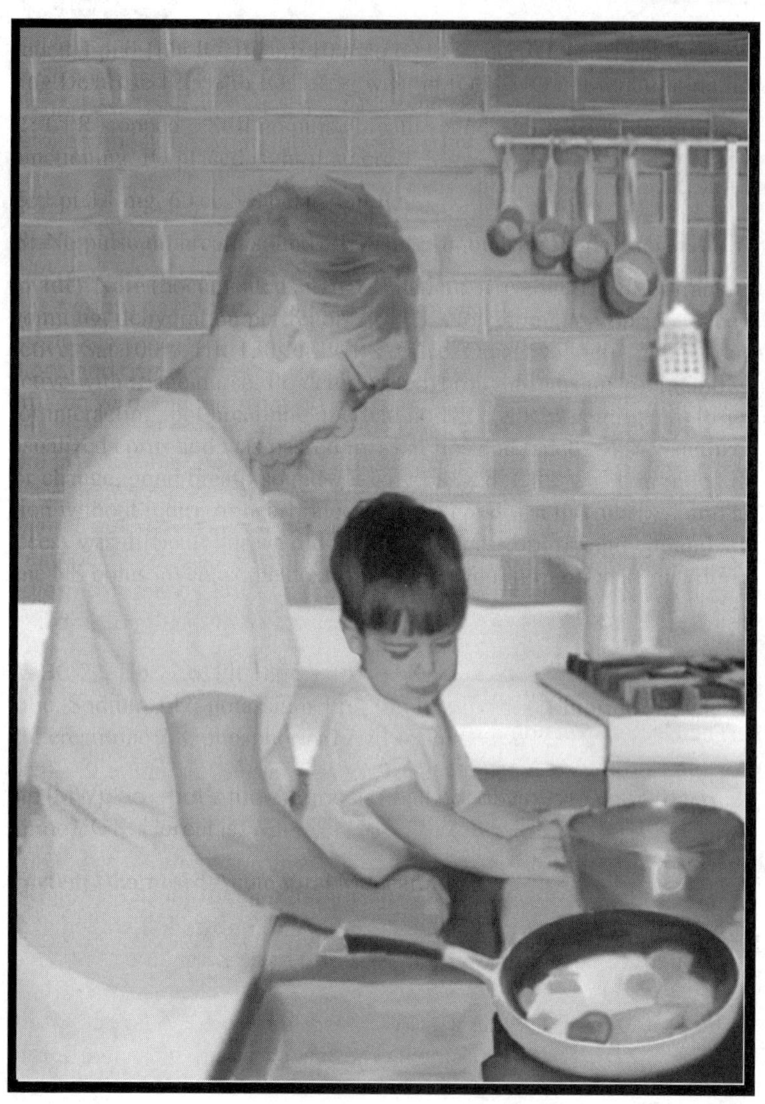

CASE 2

5-YEAR-OLD BOY WITH VOMITING

PART 1—MEDICAL

I. The Patient's Story

Jordan is a 5-year-old boy who lives with his single mother, a busy public defender, in South Carolina. His maternal grandmother works as a custodian in NYC and has a 4th grade education; she comes to visit Jordan every summer. On August 25, Jordan's grandmother wakes at 8:00 am to make scrambled eggs and cheese. Half an hour later, Jordan begins to vomit, experiencing 2 additional episodes over the next several hours. Jordan's mother is working on a high-profile case and his grandmother does not want to disturb her, so she takes him to the emergency department to be checked for food poisoning. Although the emergency room appears crowded, Jordan is promptly triaged and examined by an emergency physician at 11:17 AM.

II. The Doctor's Version (the following is the actual documentation of the provider)

Date: August 25, at 11:10 AM
Chief Complaint: Vomiting
Triage Note: Grandmother says the patient started vomiting food about 8:45 am after eating eggs and cheese. The grandmother is concerned the patient may have "food poisoning." No diarrhea. No cough or runny nose. The patient is awake and alert. He clings to grandmother during vital signs assessment. Lungs clear.

HPI: (Per emergency physician, Dr. Henry Watson) Triage note reviewed. Three episodes of non-bilious, non-bloody emesis over the last 2 hours starting one-half hour after eating eggs and cheese, toast, and orange juice. Vomiting not associated with coughing. No diarrhea or other URI symptoms reported. Patient denies stomachache. He has urinated once today. He has not eaten or been offered any liquids since his symptoms began. No medications were given for his symptoms prior to arrival. Jordan was previously in good health. His immunizations are up to date.

PAST MEDICAL HISTORY:
Allergies: none
Medications: none
PMH/PSH: Appendectomy
Social History: Lives with mother, grandmother and two dogs. Attends day camp once a week.
ROS: No recent trauma or urinary symptoms, otherwise negative.

EXAM:

VITAL SIGNS					
Temp (F)	RR	HR	BP	Sat	Weight
98.7 F oral	24	135	112/58	99% room air	18.8 kg

Constitutional: Alert and well developed. Appears tired but in no acute distress. Clings to caregiver.
HEENT: Unremarkable EENT. Mucous membranes are moist.
Neck: Supple without lymphadenopathy.
Heart: Regular rhythm without murmur. Capillary refill is < 3 seconds.
Lungs: Clear in all fields. No accessory muscle use.
Abdomen: A well-healed midline scar is present, audible BS, mild diffuse discomfort to palpation, no guarding or rebound, and no masses.
Back: No tenderness.
GU: Exam deferred.
Skin: Warm and dry without rash.
Extremities: Unremarkable.
Neurological: Alert and oriented to caregiver and examiner, normal cranial nerves and motor functions.

ORDERS:
12:55 – Phenergan oral solution 18.75 mg PO. PO challenge. Discharge to home with Phenergan prescription.

MDM (12:58): Confirmed the caregiver cooked breakfast thoroughly and ate the same breakfast. She denies any symptoms. She says, "Jordan's appendix was taken out." Reassured caregiver "food poisoning" unlikely since food properly cooked. Appendicitis ruled out. Discussed diagnosis and plan to treat symptoms. Use Phenergan at home as needed, to follow up in 3 to 5 days with patient's PCP and to return for worsening.

13:30 – (Per RN): Grandmother says patient had an episode of vomiting which she cleaned up. She says he drank electrolyte solution "too quickly." Patient awake and alert. Appears tired. Follow up and return instructions given. Grandmother acknowledges these instructions.

DIAGNOSIS: Gastroenteritis

DISPOSITION: Discharged home with caregiver. Condition Rx for Phenergan 18.75 mg PO every 4 to 6 hours PRN vomiting. Return to ED for any worsening. Discharge instructions for gastroenteritis

III. The Errors—Risk Management/Patient Safety Issues

Chapter author's note: There is a Sherlock Holmes quote (Sir Arthur Conan Doyle's "A Scandal in Bohemia") that comes to mind: "You *see* but you do not *observe*."

Risk management/patient safety issue #1:

Error: No attempt to contact Jordan's mother; no request for Jordan's medical record.

Discussion: A consent to treat (unless there is an emergency) needs to be obtained, even if it is phone consent. However, such consent should not delay the EMTALA mandated medical screening examination, as the federal statute takes precedence over the state statute, which requires parental or guardian consent. Children are often brought to the emergency department by a caregiver who is not the legal guardian and who may not be familiar with all details of the medical history. There was no documentation that an attempt was made to secure and review Jordan's medical records. If it had been, the record would have revealed that Jordan was hospitalized for appendicitis with perforation and peritonitis 3 months prior to his most recent visit. He had an extended length of stay due to a complicated surgical course. His discharge diagnosis was appendicitis with perforation and peritonitis.

✔ **Teaching point:** Important information may be obtained by contacting the legal guardian/ parent and reviewing previous medical records.

Risk management/patient safety issue #2:

Error: Missed red flag (vertical abdominal incision for appendicitis).

Discussion: Most appendectomies are done via laparoscopy or right lower quadrant incision. A vertical scar for an appendectomy could have tipped-off the physician that Jordan had had a complicated appendicitis.

✔ **Teaching point:** A seemingly insignificant finding on physical exam viewed in the context of the entire clinical picture may be the clue that solves the riddle and changes the outcome.

Risk management/patient safety issue #3:

Error: Inadequate examination.

Discussion: A GU examination is essential in all pediatric male patients with vomiting to evaluate for testicular torsion and incarcerated hernia. The notation under the GU physical exam section simply says "deferred."

✔ **Teaching point:** GU exams are not optional in children with vomiting.

Risk management/patient safety issue #4:

Error: Inadequate communication across providers.

Discussion: Medical providers involved in the care of patients have a responsibility to communicate clearly and effectively with one another. In Jordan's case, the triage nurse, emergency physician, medication nurse and Jordan's grandmother all fell short. The triage nurse should have told the emergency physician about Jordan's 4th episode of vomiting. The physician should have reviewed the entire emergency medicine chart, including nurse notes. The grandmother should have provided contact info for the mother.

✔ **Teaching point:** Clear communication between healthcare providers saves lives.

Risk management/patient safety issue #5:

Error: Prescribing a sedating anti-emetic with potential to mask worsening or evolving disease process.

Discussion: Label warnings by the FDA for careful use of Phenergan in children were published in national journals in 2000 due to sedation effects and a decreased respiratory drive in children.[19] The use of Phenergan in children as an anti-emetic has declined since the generic form of Zofran (ondansetron) was introduced in 2006.[17-21] Zofran has been shown to have a better side-effect profile. In this case, the use of a sedating anti-emetic for home use may have made Jordan sleepy, interfering with his ability to report worsening symptoms.

✔ **Teaching point:** Common, and potentially dangerous, medication effects should be considered and disclosed for all medications prescribed.

Risk management/patient safety issue #6:

Error: Failure to observe and re-examine patient.

Discussion: Arguably, the highest yielding procedure performed by the emergency physician is the serial assessment, but there was no documentation of a repeat exam. The one reassessment by the nurse, just before discharge, was not reassuring. A short observation period may have also helped the emergency team gather more information about Jordan's disease process.

Even with the amount of time he was there, he did vomit again, so, he was not "improved;" however, the doctor was not aware this had occurred. With a definitive diagnosis of gastroenteritis, continued vomiting would be expected. Unfortunately, this chart did not reflect a firm diagnosis of gastroenteritis due to the absence of diarrhea. Why diagnose "gastroenteritis" when we are able to more accurately diagnose "vomiting?"

The last note written about the patient's status before discharge is that he was "tired." What does this mean? Is he dehydrated, sleepy from the Phenergan, or is there something more serious brewing? With this uncertainty, observation, continued rehydration and a recheck may have been the safest approach.[22-23]

✔ **Teaching point:** Observation and re-examination may allow recognition of disease progression.

Risk management/patient safety issue #7:

Error: Failure to consider worse case diagnosis and narrowing the differential diagnoses too prematurely.

Discussion: One of the most memorable medical school teachings is the differential diagnosis. Physicians are wise to remain wary of the non-specific single-symptom chief complaint. The list of reasons for vomiting is long, and life-threatening diseases should be ruled out by an excellent history, physical examination and diagnostics when indicated.

✔ **Teaching point:** If you don't consider a disease, you will never diagnose it.

Risk management/patient safety issue #8:

Error: Failure to recognize or repeat abnormal VS.

Discussion: Jordan's HR is abnormal; a pulse of 135 in a 5-year-old should be considered abnormal until proven otherwise. Rechecking the vitals prior to discharge represent our last chance to get it right.

✔ **Teaching point:** Recheck vitals prior to discharge.

IV. The Bounceback

August 25 - the same day as ED discharge

- 20:30—Jordan's grandmother puts Jordan to bed after his second dose of Phenergan. He has refused any fluids and has become quite sleepy.
- 23:55 – Jordan's mother returns home and speaks with the grandmother about his condition. When she goes into Jordan's room to check on him she finds green vomit on his pillow. She tries to arouse him, but he is unresponsive. She calls 911.
- 23:59—EMS personnel quickly arrive to find an unresponsive 5-year-old boy with a "rapid, weak" pulse and a "tight" abdomen. EMS providers place Jordan on a stretcher. Jordan has "a high temperature." They place an oxygen mask on Jordan's face. An attempt to place an IV in his arm is unsuccessful so an interosseous line (IO) is placed.
- EMS starts a fluid bolus, check his blood sugar, and transports him emergently to the same emergency department. Jordan's distraught mother and grandmother are allowed to ride along.
- Enroute to the ED, Jordan loses his pulse and stops breathing. Chest compressions are started and oxygenation is provided by bag-valve-mask (BVM).
- On arrival to the emergency department, EMS providers are actively providing chest compressions and BVM breaths. CPR is continued and monitoring is initiated.
- Heart rhythm shows pulseless electrical activity (PEA).
- Pt is intubated and chest compressions are continued. ALS medications are administered.
- 02:17—After prolonged code without response, resuscitation efforts are discontinued. Patient is pronounced dead.
- Jordan's grandmother is frantic and has to be admitted for chest pain.

August 27 – Autopsy reveals intra-abdominal adhesions causing small bowel obstruction, small bowel perforation, peritonitis, acute pulmonary and hepatic congestion. Toxicology is negative except for promethazine at therapeutic levels.

CAUSE OF DEATH: Severe septic shock with multi-organ system failure.

FOLLOW UP: The family files a suit against the ED physician and the hospital. The case is eventually settled.

PART 2—THE ANALYSIS

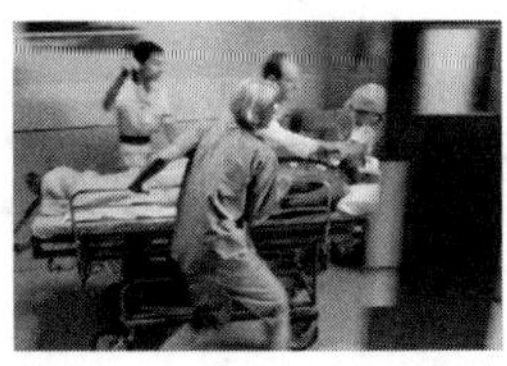

EVALUATION OF VOMITING, DIAGNOSIS OF SMALL BOWEL OBSTRUCTION

Emily Fontane, MD, FAAP, FACEP
Associate Professor
Emergency Medicine/Pediatrics
University Florida College of Medicine—Jacksonville

Heide Valdes, MD
Pediatric Emergency Medicine Fellow
University Florida College of Medicine—Jacksonville

Evaluation of vomiting

Vomiting is a highly specific physical event that results in the rapid, forceful evacuation of gastric contents in retrograde fashion from the stomach up to and out of the mouth.[1,2] Vomiting is a non-specific symptom that is commonly associated with gastrointestinal viral infections in children beyond infancy but can be associated with more serious conditions including bowel obstruction.[1,2]

The differential diagnosis of vomiting in the pediatric population is vast and includes infectious etiologies, anatomical abnormalities, and metabolic disorders. Vomiting may be caused by an adverse reaction to food or medications.[1,2]

Vomiting

Neonate (<1 month)	Infant (>1-12 months)	Toddler (>1-4 years)	Child (4-12 years)	Teenager (13-19 years)
GER or GERD	GER or GERD	Gastroenteritis	Gastroenteritis	Gastroenteritis
Feeding intolerance	Acute otitis media	Urinary tract infection	Pharyngitis	Peptic ulcer disease
Pyloric stenosis	Protein intolerance	Pharyngitis	Post infectious gastroparesis	Cyclic vomiting
Meconium ileus	Gastroenteritis	GERD	Eosinophilic esophagitis	Eosinophilic esophagitis
Congenital atresia or webs	Pyloric stenosis	Eosinophilic esophagitis	Appendicitis	Pregnancy
Malrotation with midgut volvulus	Intussusception	Celiac disease	Celiac disease	Poisoning/toxic ingestion
Necrotizing enterocolitis	UTI	Intracranial lesion	Pancreatitis	Migraine
Metabolic disorders (inborn errors of metabolism)	Malrotation with midgut volvulus	Malrotation	IBD	Diabetic ketoacidosis
Hirschsprung's disease	Intracranial lesion	Poisoning/toxic ingestion	Trauma (duodenal hematoma)	Rumination syndrome
Protein intolerance	Metabolic disorders	Adrenal insufficiency	Poisoning/toxic ingestion	Drug abuse
Infection (UTI or meningitis)	Child abuse Munchausen syndrome by proxy			Appendicitis Gallstone Pancreatitis Bulimia IBD

IBD=inflammatory bowel disease; GER=gastro-esophageal reflux; GERD=gastro-esophageal reflux disease; UTI=urinary tract infection.

Parashette KR, Croffie J. Vomiting. Pediatr in Rev. 2013;34:307–21. Copyright © 2013, American Academy of Pediatrics. Used with permission.

Pediatric appendicitis and vital sign rechecks

Misdiagnosed appendicitis is the 4th cause of self-reported medical error among academic, pediatric physicians after misdiagnosis of medication side effects, infections and psychiatric disorders.[3] Fear of missing appendicitis is a constant source of anguish for pediatric EM providers. It is notoriously difficult to diagnose in young children.[4-7] The inflamed appendix can rupture within 12 hours of pain onset leaving a very narrow window for errors.[5] A physician may sigh with relief when told that his pediatric patient with vomiting has had an appendectomy, but this only excludes one diagnosis.

One of the biggest challenges a provider faces when caring for pediatric patients, especially in the emergency setting, is the interpretation of vital signs. Normal vital signs change with increasing age and have a wider acceptable range with decreasing age (AHA, PALS). The heart rate and vascular resistance will increase with circulatory insufficiency while a normal blood pressure may be falsely reassuring. Jordan's heart rate in triage is abnormal, a repeat check before discharge may have assisted in an accurate diagnosis.

Bowel obstruction in children

Bowel obstruction in children Jordan's age is most commonly due to intussusception.[4,6,7] Less common causes include adhesive bowel obstruction. Authors of a 1997 review of conventional appendectomies in children noted that patients with complicated appendicitis (perforated appendicitis) and open appendectomy had a 3.8% likelihood of adhesive small bowel obstruction within 4–6 years.[8] Another study of 1,105 appendectomies in children revealed that adhesive small bowel obstruction was related to a perforated appendicitis and not the surgical approach.[9] In this study, the mean time from appendectomy to the development of intestinal obstruction was between 2 weeks and 2.5 months, not far from Jonathan's timeline. Complicated appendicitis, including appendicitis associated with perforation, is associated with a higher rate of post-operative complications including adhesive bowel obstruction.[10-13] Complicated appendicitis and post-operative complications are associated with young age.[24]

An article published in the Journal of The Royal Society of Medicine in 2010 showed that adhesive bowel obstruction can occur years after surgery.[14] The authors found that for children younger than 5 years of age the readmission rate directly attributable to adhesions was 4% within 4 years after abdominal surgery.[14] Review of the records showed that Jordan's mother was advised by his surgeon that there would be a risk of adhesions and bowel obstruction. Jordan's grandmother was not aware of this information.

An emergency physician must be vigilant when a caregiver brings a young patient to the ED, as the caregiver may not possess a complete knowledge of the patient's medical history. It is the emergency physician's responsibility to document the historian's relationship to the young patient, and to contact the legal guardian.[14]

The anti-emetic of choice in children: Ondansetron (Zofran)

Since the approval of generic Zofran (ondansetron) in 2006, it has become the preferred anti-emetic for use in children. However, a meta-analysis published in 2008 revealed that Phenergan (promethazine) was the most common anti-emetic prescribed by emergency physicians to children with AGE (acute gastroenteritis) in the US.[18] Phenergan has sedating properties and has been implicated in several respiratory fatalities in children.[19] Its use is discouraged in children less than 2 years old, and caution is advised when using it in children older than 2 years old.

Chapter Summary

Jordan's case occurred at a facility that did not have an electronic medical record (EMR), making it more difficult to review old records. If they had been obtained, it would have shown that Jordan's appendicitis was initially missed and that he was noted to have perforation at surgery, necessitating an open laparotomy. His lengthy post-operative hospital course was complicated by fever, a second surgery for a "wash out," and need for prolonged IV antibiotics, increasing his risk of a subsequent SBO.

➤Author's note (MW):

Would a different outcome have occurred if the provider had recognized the sentinel clue of a large abdominal scar (indicating a complex previous appendectomy)? This case is a classic "bouncebacks" case; a speck of sand in the ocean, a blade of grass in central park ... several episodes of vomiting in a nation of 5-year-olds with gastroenteritis. There was a mystery brewing and the importance of a subtle clue was not fully appreciated. If recognized, would it have prompted the provider to obtain old records, discuss the history with the mother, prolong the ED observation, repeat the abdominal exam, recheck the vitals and consider small bowel obstruction as a cause of isolated vomiting? We will never know.

References

1. Parashette KR, Croffie J. Vomiting. Pediatr in Rev. 2013;34:307–21.
2. QuigleyEMM,Hasler WL, Parkman HP.AGA technical review on nausea and vomiting. Gastroenterology. 2001;120(1): 263–286.
3. Singh H, Thomas EJ, Wilson T, et al. Errors of diagnosis in pediatric practice: a multisite survey. Pediatrics. 2010;126:70–9.
4. Shah S. An update on common gastrointestinal emergencies. Emerg Med Clin N Am. 2013;31:755–93.
5. Bansal S, Banever, GT, Karrer FM, et al. Appendicitis in children less than 5 years old: influence of age on presentation and outcome. Am J Surg. 2012;204:1031–5.
6. van Heurn LW, Pakarinen MP, Wester T. Contemporary management of abdominal surgical emergencies in infants and children. BJS. 2014;101:e24–33.
7. Kim JS. Acute abdominal pain in children. Pediatr Gastroenterol Hepatol Nutr. 2013;164:219–24.
8. Ahlberg G, Bergdahl S, Rutqvist J, et al. Mechanical small-bowel obstruction after conventional appendectomy in children. Eur J Pediatr Surg. 1997;7:13–5.

9. Tsao KJ, St Peter SD, Valusek PA, et al. Adhesive small bowel obstruction after appendectomy in children: comparison between the laparoscopic and open approach. J Pediatr Surg. 2007;42:939–42.
10. Grant HW, Parker MC, Wilson MS, et al. Adhesions after abdominal surgery in children. J Pediatr Surg. 2008;43:152–6.
11. Ikeda H, Ishimaru Y, Takayasu H, et al. Laparoscopic versus open appendectomy in children with uncomplicated and complicated appendicitis. J Pediatr Surg. 2004;39:1680–5.
12. Wang X, Zhang W, Yang X, et al. Complicated appendicitis in children: is laparoscopic appendectomy appropriate? A comparative study with the open appendectomy—our experience. J Pediatr Surg. 2009;44:1924–7.
13. Markar SR, Blackburn S, Cobb R, et al. Laparoscopic versus open appendectomy for complicated and uncomplicated appendicitis in children. J Gastrointest Surg. 2012;16:1993–2004.
14. Rajab TK, Ahmad UM, Kelly E. Implications of late complications from adhesions for preoperative informed consent. J R Soc Med. 2010;103:317–21.
15. Selbst SM. Treating minors without their parents. Pediatr Emerg Care. 1985;1:168–73.
16. Kwon KT, Rudkin SE, Langdorf MI. Antiemetic use in pediatric gastroenteritis: a national survey of emergency physicians, pediatricians, and pediatric emergency physicians. Clin Pediatr. 2002;41:641–52.
17. Leung AK, Robson WL. Acute gastroenteritis in children: role of anti-emetic medication for gastroenteritis-related vomiting. Paediatr Drugs. 2007;9:175–84.
18. Pfeil N, Uhlig U, Kostev K, et al. Antiemetic medications in children with presumed infectious gastroenteritis—pharmacoepidemiology in Europe and Northern America. J Pediatr. 2008;153:659–62.
19. Starke PR, Weaver J, Chowdhury BA. Boxed warning added to promethazine labeling for pediatric use. N Eng J Med. 2005;352:2653.
20. Manteuffel J. Use of antiemetics in children with acute gastroenteritis: are they safe and effective? J Emerg Trauma Shock. 2009;21:3–5.
21. Patanwala AE, Amini R, Hays DP, Rosen P. Antiemetic therapy for nausea and vomiting in the emergency department. J Emerg Med. 2010;39:330–336.
22. Mace SE. Pediatric observation medicine. Emerg Med Clin North Am. 2001;19:239–54.
23. Wai S, Ma L, Kim E, Adekunle-Ojo A. The utility of the emergency department observation unit for children with abdominal pain. Pediatr Emerg Care. 2013;29:574–8.
24. Johnson KA, Svirbely JR, Sriram MG et al. Automated medical algorithms: issues for medical errors. J Am Med Inform Assoc. 2002;9:s56–7.

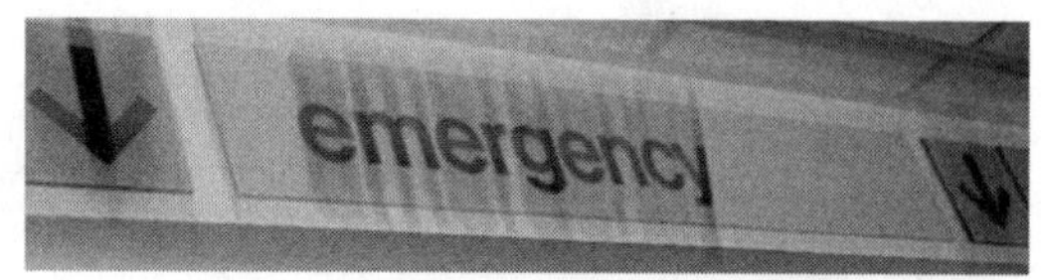

CASE 3

14-YEAR-OLD WITH VOMITING AND BUMPS ON TONGUE

Ariel Cohen, DO, PGY 3
Department of Emergency Medicine
Case Western Reserve University
MetroHealth Medical Center/Cleveland Clinic

PART 1—MEDICAL

PART 2—THE ANALYSIS

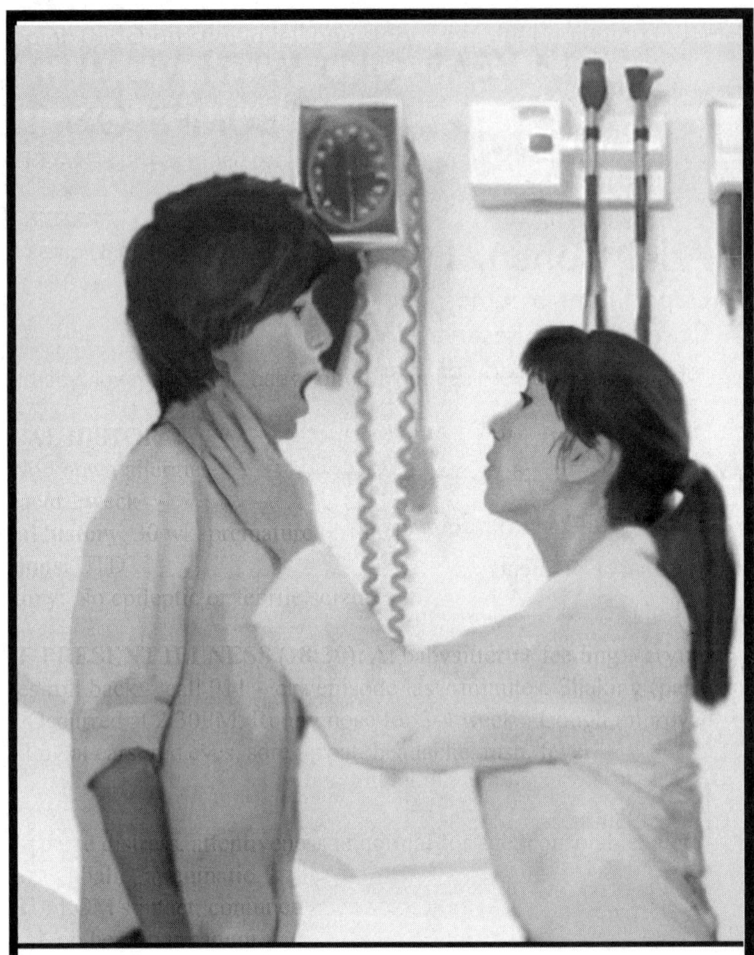

"My mouth is so dry it's hard for me to answer your questions"

CASE 3

14-YEAR-OLD WITH VOMITING AND BUMPS ON TONGUE

PART 1—MEDICAL

I. The Doctor's Version (the following is the actual documentation of the provider)

Date: July 5, 2013 19:05

Chief complaint: Vomiting, bumps on tongue

Nurse note:
Nausea/vomiting: onset last night; vomit x 1 today.
Symptom of mouth/tongue/lip: onset "this past week"; bumps are painful.
Weak: "my mouth is dry."

HISTORY OF PRESENT ILLNESS – (Per physician, Dr. X):

14 year old male here for vomiting, mouth dry and trouble breathing and feels like he has heartburn
Sx started yesterday.
No fevers. No diarrhea.
+ cough. No RN/congestion.
No other pain.

History obtained from the family

REVIEW OF SYSTEMS:
Greater than 10 ROS have been reviewed and are negative except as noted in HPI and/or below.

Constitutional: no weight loss, no fevers, no chills
Skin: no rashes
Eyes: no vision changes
Ears/Nose/Throat: no rhinorrhea, no sore throat
Respiratory: no cough, no shortness of breath
Cardiovascular: no chest pain
Genitourinary: no urinary symptoms, no hematuria
Musculoskeletal: no joint swelling, no deformity, no myalgias
Neurologic: no weakness, no numbness, no other neuro symptoms
Psychiatric: no depression, no hallucinations
Hematologic/Lymphatic/Immunologic: no history of bleeding disorders, no recurrent infections
Endocrine: no history of diabetes

PAST MEDICAL HISTORY:

Allergies: NKDA
Medications: None
PMH: denies
Social History: never had any immunizations
Family History: No family history on file. No sick contacts.

EXAM:

VITAL SIGNS							
Time	Temp(F)	Rt	Pulse	Resp	Syst	Diast	SpO2
19:46	97.7	Oral	92	17	111	76	100%RA

General Appearance: awake, alert, no distress, oriented to time, place and person
Skin: warm, well perfused with no diaphoresis/rash
Head: normocepahlic, atraumatic
Eyes: conjunctivae not injected / corneas clear. PERRL
Nose/sinuses: no sinus TTP or rhinorrhea noted
Oropharynx: symmetric posterior OP without exudate/erythema. Tongue w/ yellowish white plaque. Moist mucous membranes
Neck: supple, no lymphadenopathy
Back: no CVAT
Lungs: clear to auscultation, breath sounds equal and symmetric bilaterally, no wheezes/rales or rhonchi. No signs of respiratory distress
Heart: regular rate and rhythm. Normal S1 and S2. No murmurs, clicks or gallops
Abdomen: soft, mild epigastric ttp, neg murphy's sign. No ttp over mcburney's point
Extremities: moves all extremities. No deformities, edema, or skin discoloration, normal peripheral perfusion/pulses
Neuro: awake and normally oriented. Grossly intact/symmetric motor and sensation to light touch
Psych: normal affect

ED COURSE:

21:42 – Ondansetron (Zofran) 4 mg oral, aluminum & magnesium hydroxide-simethicone (Maalox ES) oral suspension, lidocaine (Xylocaine viscous) 2% soln (10mL mouth/throat)
PO fluids tolerated in the ED

Medical decision making (MDM): The patient was reexamined and abdomen remains soft with no rebound or guarding noted. The patient has tolerated PO in the ED and no immediate life-threatening or surgical process has been identified. The patient has been instructed as to proper follow up and has been educated about abdominal pain regarding warning signs and when to come back to the ED, including but not limited to: fevers, vomiting with inability tolerate PO fluids, worsening or new abdominal pain or any new symptoms previously not present (i.e. GI bleeding, diarrhea, or bilious or bloody emesis). The patient verbalized understanding. Appropriate discharge instructions were also provided in written form.

DIAGNOSIS: 1. Gastritis 2. Leukoplakia of tongue

DISPOSITION (22:08): Patient was discharged home by the ED physician
Condition upon discharge - Stable.
Rx for famotidine (Pepcid) 20mg qday; promethazine (Phenergan) 25mg tid prn nausea
Follow up with PCP for further evaluation and reexamination. Return to ER if symptoms change.

II. Greg Henry Comments

"I wish they all smelled like the acetone off my grandmother's fruit cake"

No matter how sophisticated we become, the diagnosis of such a patient is difficult. On the above visit, there is only one finding that sticks out—thrush. Why would a 14-year-old have thrush? This could be a result of antibiotic use or inhaled steroids for asthma, neither of which occurred in this case. It can be the result of suppression of the immune system or undiagnosed AIDS, which is not supported in the history. I have seen this child; I wish they all smelled like the acetone off my grandmother's fruit cake, but that is not the case.

III. The Bounceback

ED visit #2 – July 6, 2013 – (One day after initial ED visit)

- 23:10 – Arrives by car. Mom has pt in to triage window stating pt lethargic, not talking, eyes rolling back
- 23:13 – rushed to high acuity room, resident immediately in room. Quick H&P done while vitals obtained
- **HPI:** Since this morning the pt has had ongoing chest and abdominal burning and generalized body pain. Took pepcid this AM without improvement. Throughout day became progressively more lethargic to point of becoming unresponsive. Also not making sense with speaking and seeing things not there.
- **ROS:** +12lb wt loss past week, anorexia; no fever or diarrhea,, no polyuria or polydipsia
- **Vitals:** Temp 96.8, pulse 148, resp 26, BP 127/52, SpO2 98% on RA; GCS 8 (E2 = open to pain, V2 = moans to pain, M4 = withdraws to pain); MM dry; no acetone on breath; tachycardic; kussmaul breathing
- 23:15 – Gluc >600; two 18g IV's and labs obtained, 1L fluid bolus initiated, ECG: sinus tach
- 23:45 – pulse 133, resp 37, BP 140/76, 100% on 2L NC; 1L IVF given
- 00:04 – Physician report called to PICU, insulin gtt started in consultation with PICU
- **Labs:** (00:21)
  - ABG: pH 6.874, pCO2 26, Base Excess -31.8; HCO3 5.
  - CBC WBC 33.3; H/H 16.6 / 52, bands 12
  - Metabolic: Gluc 942, Na 132, K 7.1, Cl 98, HCO3 5, BUN 44, Cr 2.5, AG 36, Mag 4.1, Phos 9.0
- 00:58 – Transferred to PICU

Final ED diagnosis:

1. DKA
2. Severe electrolyte derangements
3. Acute Renal Failure

HOSPITAL COURSE

- Hospital day #1: best GCS 11 (E4, V2, M 5), awake, not following commands, varies between making no sound and speech not comprehensible, labs tending in right direction but still tachycardic, tachypneic, eyes sunken, mouth dry
  - o Managed with two bag system: NS w/ 20 meq KCl and D5NS w/ 20 meq KCl
  - o Serum osm: 369 (01:30) →364 (05:00) →352 (07:00) → 338 (11:00) → 334 (15:00) → 328 (18:00)
  - o BMP: (06:43) gluc 387, Na 144, K 6.1, Cl 120, HCO3 7, BUN 40, Cr 1.8, AG 23
  - o UA: pro 30, gluc >500, ketones 80, blood large, squams 3-5
  - o CBC: WBC 20.5; H/H 16.8/50.8, bands 20
  - o CT head for fluctuating GCS and prolonged AMS = no intracranial abnormalities
- Hospital day #2: GCS varying between 12-15; EEG with generalized encephalopathy; difficulty transitioning off IVF and insulin gtt and too altered to tolerate PO
  - o Serum osm: 329 (02:00) →326 (06:00) → 320 (10:00) → 308 (13:00)
  - o BMP: (06:00) gluc 329, Na 146, K 3.6, Cl 119, HCO3 15, BUN 16, Cr 1.06, AG 16
- Hospital day #3: alert, tolerating PO, on subQ insulin, transferred to floor
- Hospital day #4: discharged, mental status back to baseline, no deficits

FINAL DIAGNOSIS: Diabetic ketoacidosis (DKA); Acute kidney injury (AKI); new onset diabetes mellitus (DM)

IV. Greg Henry Comments—Part 2

We went through a 15-year period of time where we believed that fluids caused cerebral edema. This was the source of much consternation and multiple lawsuits some of which I was involved as an expert. No one understands cerebral edema in these children. There is no evidence to suggest that withholding fluids is a good idea; the standard 20mg per kg bolus is still a reasonable place to start. Thankfully, the current literature has refined our ignorance.

PART 2—THE ANALYSIS

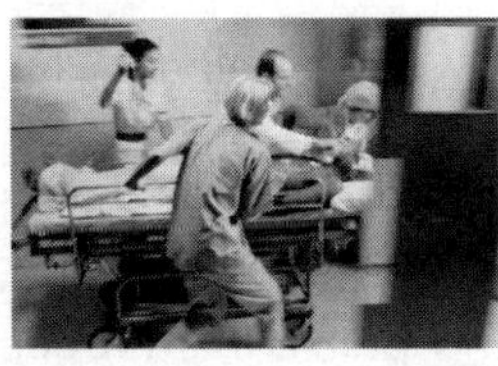

DIAGNOSIS AND MANAGEMENT OF PEDIATRIC DKA

Ariel Cohen, DO, PGY 3

Department of Emergency Medicine
Case Western Reserve University
MetroHealth Medical Center/Cleveland Clinic

Diagnosis of diabetes and DKA

Emergency physicians are no strangers to diabetes. Yet, as familiar as we are with management of complications, catching new-onset diabetes before it reaches the severity of DKA remains difficult. The diagnosis depends simply on a bedside glucose test, but we need to first suspect it.

On a medical school test, the etiology of the triad below is easy, but these symptoms are not frequently served to the provider on a plate, instead mixed with other misleading symptoms such as abdominal pain, dizziness, weight loss, and fatigue.

- Polyuria,
- Polydipsia,
- Polyphagia

Herein lies the first caveats of identifying new-onset diabetes early; there is a consistently recognizable cluster of symptoms that are usually present weeks before patients develop DKA, but parents are not aware that these symptoms should be of concern and they are more difficult to notice in younger children.[5, 10, 33, 41] Sometimes the patient is brought in for a more "concerning" symptom and the diabetic symptoms are overlooked.[24, 25, 37] Of note, once the mother in this case had been asked about polydipsia and polyuria a few times, she did recall her son had had these symptoms. We as providers are less aware of the infrequently offered, yet specific symptoms of diabetes, nocturia/enuresis and thrush.[15, 26, 28, 34, 38, 39] While it might be difficult to elicit the symptom of polyuria, parents tend to be more aware of enuresis/ nocturia, which is secondary to polyuria.

In this bounceback, an overlooked symptom was present; thrush. When patients present to the ED in DKA, candidiasis, oral and perineal, is often found to have been present on a prior PCP visit.[1, 3, 24, 25, 36] In this case, we have an adolescent male complaining of a dry mouth and painful bumps on his tongue and is noted to have yellowish white plaques. The plaques of leukoplakia are bright white and more often found on the buccal mucosa, gums and sides of the tongue and like thrush, do not easily rub off. While Candida is common in infants and adolescent females (because their estrogenized vaginal mucosa is rich in glycogen), young females and adolescent boys should not be predisposed, and thus, a diagnosis of thrush or stomatitis should prompt concern for diabetes,[26,34] though it is rare for candidiasis to be the first, isolated sign of diabetes. Another nonspecific but potentially concerning symptom is blurred vision.[22]

If the clinician does not diagnose diabetes upon initial presentation, sometimes there is still the opportunity to diagnose DKA in its early stages, before it becomes severe. The patient in this case presented with the ALL of the vague yet classic symptoms for early DKA: Abdominal pain, nausea, vomiting, anorexia. The most common misdiagnosis of these symptoms is gastroenteritis, yet patients in DKA do not have diarrhea. The abdominal pain is often vague in nature and diffuse, however, multiple case studies demonstrate that the pain is not associated with any real intra-abdominal pathology.[9,31] Severity of the pain may be related to the degree of acidosis.[35]

Lab abnormalities in DKA: CBC and lipase

1. **CBC:** Leukocytosis is common in DKA; it is likely due to stress and possibly from elevated levels of cortisol and norepinephrine. WBC counts are typically in the 10,000–15,000 range. Counts over 25,000 may indicate infection.[10,11,19] Differentiating the acute from the non-acute abdomen by using an elevated WBC count remains difficult.
2. **Potassium:** Potassium may be elevated from insulin deficiency, hypertonicity and academia. Caution in patients with low potassium as this indicates severe total body deficiency. These patients should have aggressive replacement and cardiac monitoring for cardiac dysrhythmias.[19] Insulin therapy should be delayed until potassium is replaced.
3. **Lipase:** Common "belly labs" also include lipase +/- amylase. Amylase and lipase are often non-specifically elevated in DKA. Amylase elevation is correlated with pH and serum osmolality, and lipase elevation is correlated with serum osmolality, however, neither correlates with GI symptoms or pancreatic imaging studies. The diagnosis of acute pancreatitis not be solely based on levels even three times upper limit of normal.[43]

Back to our case

Armed with this new knowledge, could this child's outcome have been different? Our patient had abdominal pain *plus* oral symptoms. As the above studies show, the first crucial piece to making the diagnosis is to be cognizant of the multiple symptoms and have a heightened awareness for the subtle signs of diabetes and DKA. Should one more minute have been spent investigating this young man's oral complaints, it would have likely revealed that these lesions did not develop in relationship to the emesis. Even the triage note documents the timeline of symptoms as distinct from one another. The oral symptoms preceded the emesis, which could have alerted the physician to look for a more unifying explanation of the symptoms instead of the seemingly unrelated diagnoses of gastritis and leukoplakia.

Treatment of DKA

Let's start with defining "severe" DKA, as defined by blood pH. There is slight variance in the exact pH value depending on the source. A conservative definition for severe DKA:[42]

- pH < 7.1
- HCO3 is in the range of $<5 \mathrm{mmol/L}$

Note: Either an ABG or VBG is acceptable; on average, pH differs by a 0.03 unit difference and HCO3 by 1.3mmol units.

From one perspective, regardless of severity, treatment can be condensed to 4 major tenets:

1. Fluid
2. Electrolyte replacement
3. Insulin
4. Address any underlying infection

So, what's the big deal with severity? Any ED doc can answer such a simple question: "Dispo." ... duh! In most hospitals, patients on an insulin drip can only go to an ICU or stepdown unit. Of note, an insulin drip is recommended for moderate and severe disease:

- The insulin drip dose, 0.1mg/kg/hr, does not change based on severity.
- An insulin bolus prior to the drip is not recommended in pediatrics.[29]
- Insulin should not be started prior to the first set of electrolytes due to the risk of hypokalemia.[2]

Ongoing ED DKA management and cerebral edema

For those who have to manage these patients for more than a few hours in the ED, if glucose is not decreasing by 50–75mg/h, the insulin infusion may be doubled every hour until a steady glucose decline at this rate is achieved, although the hydration status should be assessed first. [18, 19] Severe DKA should concern you for two additional reasons: these kids are very sick and also, if your colleagues upstairs have not read the literature recently, you may be blamed for inducing the dreaded...drum roll please...*cerebral edema*. So, not all comers with DKA are the same, and treating severe DKA is not so cut and dry.

Our patient had severe DKA with an altered mental state. What is different about the treatment of severe DKA? For children in mild to moderate DKA, there is no rush to treat. This is in contradistinction to children with severe DKA; they are at risk for shock, and time is of the essence. What varies in the rush to treat is *how* to replace fluid and electrolytes. This topic continues to come under scrutiny in the literature despite advances in medicine in the past 30 years, because the morbidity and mortality has not significantly changed.[6, 21, 27]

Management of DKA with IVF and insulin

First, fluid resuscitate the child, addressing cardiovascular compromise.[29] Recommendations vary between LR and NS as well as 10mg/kg and 20mg/kg boluses. Boluses are repeated until the patient is hemodynamically stable, but some have also suggested not exceeding 50mg/kg in the first 4 hours of the resuscitation. From here, recommendations become even more variable, with some continuing NS, some switching to 0.45% NS, and rates between 1.5 and 2x maintenance or rates based on calculated total deficit and replacement spread out over 24 to 48 hours. It is recommended that you choose a guideline to follow and stick to it. In our patient, once the glucose was around 200–300, the two bag system was employed, for easy titration of glucose as it gets in the lower ranges, since insulin often needs to be continued until the bicarb is above 15 or the anion gap has closed. Administration of supplemental bicarb is not recommended.[12]

Allowing blood glucose to drop to hypoglycemic levels is a common mistake that may be dangerous in and of itself and usually results in a rebound ketosis derived by counter-regulatory hormones. Rebound ketosis necessitates a longer duration of treatment. The other hazard is that rapid correction of hyperglycemia and hyperosmolarity may shift water rapidly to the hyperosmolar intracellular space and may induce cerebral edema.

Cerebral edema—fluids, osmolality, pH—what does the recent literature show?

One of the commonly used tables for diagnostic criteria, Kitabchi 2004, includes a few more variables than are required for diagnosis of DKA: serum osmolality and mental status.[17, 18] For some time, it has been thought that serum osmolality affects mental status (regardless of the presence of cerebral edema) and needs to be tightly controlled. But interestingly enough, osmolality in DKA is variable, yet there is a consistent change in mental status related to severity of disease, which is defined by pH. This raises the question, is cerebral edema also related to pH?

In house, our patient's serum osmolality was followed until close to normal, with the goal to lower it no more than 2 mOsm/hour. The concern was that rapid changes in osmolality cause cerebral edema. Support for this comes from papers and reference books that cite 2 studies, from 1981 and 1997 that showed a correlation between serum osmolality and altered mental status. These papers go on to recommend a decrease in serum osmolality of <3 mOsm/kg/hour.[7, 16, 17] They also advise that if the patient is stuporous or in a coma, and the osmolality is <320mOsm/kg, one should consider other causes of the mental status change.[9] This is the extent of recommendations related to osmolality, even in more recent literature.

Most current recommendations advise cautious fluid administration precisely because of this concern, stating that aggressive fluid administration *may* cause cerebral edema. For something so critical, fluid recommendations remain consistent yet vague and recommendations for following serum osmolality are highly variable. How can something so important not be consistently advised in reference material?

As noted, serum osmolality is variable at all disease severity levels. Suffice it to say that using serum osmolality as a guide is starting to sound fishy. And indeed, more recent studies confirm this. The consensus in most recent literature is that the pathophysiology of cerebral edema in DKA is not precisely known and seems to be multifactorial.[20, 40] Current knowledge is best summarized by an article in Emergency Medicine Journal 2004:[4]: "Considering the inconclusive nature of the current literature, no treatment strategies can be definitively recommended. Some studies have suggested that vigorous hydration leading to rapid changes in osmolality may be associated with cerebral edema, but they have insufficient methodology to suggest a causal relation. Other large trials do not show any relation between hydration treatment and cerebral edema." Studies since this review continue to confirm this position, but have now consistently shown there are consistent risk factors for the development of cerebral edema.

Children who are at risk for presenting in DKA are also the ones at risk for cerebral edema: younger with new onset diabetes and a longer duration of symptoms and hence presenting more ill, (meaning in DKA and of those in DKA, more severe). Well-established risk factors for cerebral edema [8, 12, 13, 14, 16, 44] include:

- new onset diabetes,
- <5 yo,
- longer duration of sxs,
- more severe acidosis,
- higher potassium,
- lower bicarb,
- high serum urea nitrogen
- hypocapnia after adjusting for acidosis.

Looking at age as a risk factor, one thing to note—cerebral edema is rare in adults; so just being a child puts you at risk, which is compounded at<5yo. You also might notice that many of the risk factors are related. When severely acidotic, the potassium is higher, and the bicarb is lower (and this is reflected in Kitabchi's diagnostic table).[17, 18] In addition, this describes a sicker child to begin with: more acidotic and dehydrated, hence these risk associations may reflect the greater likelihood of severe DKA. Just as these are risk factors, recent studies consistently also find that lower pH and younger age (versus plasma sodium, corrected sodium and osmolality) were the only independent determinants of impaired conscious level.[8]

While multiple recent studies, controlling for DKA severity, have not found an association between fluid administration (hypotonic solutions at rates and volumes that exceed recommendations) or serum osmolality (initial value or changes during treatment) and cerebral edema, the literature also continues to suggest that there are risk factors associated with treatment, including administration of insulin in the first hour of fluid replacement, attenuated rise of corrected serum sodium during treatment, and the use of bicarbonate.[44] The evidence that cerebral edema is primarily iatrogenic is not compelling. One other finding that lends support to this belief is that there are multiple reports of symptomatic cerebral edema in children before the initiation of therapy.[12] Intubation and hyperventilation, which is considered by clinicians when cerebral edema develops, is associated with worse outcomes.

Diagnosis of cerebral edema

The best treatment is to catch cerebral edema early. The first thing to know about diagnosis is, it is *clinical* (up to 40% of initial brain imaging is normal). Second, abnormal neurological signs are common in kids with DKA, but they don't all have cerebral edema or need therapy. Third, GCS score is insensitive, as demonstrated by the fact that children have had clinically relevant signs of neurological compromise (e.g., incontinence, vomiting, headache, heart rate deceleration), despite minimal or no changes in their Glasgow coma scale rating. Given this, Muir et al. in 2004 developed a model for early detection.

Diagnosis of cerebral edema—Muir 2004

Diagnostic Criteria

- Abnormal motor or verbal response to pain
- Decorticate or Decerebrate posture
- Cranial Nerve Palsy (especially III, IV, or VI)
- Abnormal neurologic respiratory pattern (grunting, Cheyne-Stokes, tachypnea, apnea etc)

Major Criteria

- Altered mentation / fluctuating level of consciousness
- Heart rate decelerations (decline of more than 20 bpm) not due to improved hydration or sleep
- Age-inappropriate incontinence

Minor Criteria

- Vomiting
- Headache
- Lethargy or being not easily aroused from sleep
- Diastolic BP < 90 mmHg
- Age < 5 yrs

Having either 1 Diagnostic Criterion, 2 Major Criteria, or 1 Major and 2 Minor criteria lead to 92% sensitivity and 96% specificity for recognition of CE early enough for intervention, which translates to an NNT of 6.[23, 32]

Emergent management of cerebral edema

Once you've decided to treat for cerebral edema, besides elevating the head of the bed to 30 degrees, you have two options:

1. Mannitol: 1g/kg over 20 minutes and may be repeated as needed in 1–2 hours
2. Hypertonic saline: 5–10 ml/kg 3% saline (consider with caution)

Lastly, cerebral edema by itself is not an indication for intubation; intubation should be reserved for respiratory compromise. If your patient requires intubation, avoid hyperventilation, as this is a significant risk factor for poor outcome.

Chapter Summary

We see this type of patient on a frequent basis, likely in the non-acute area, since he or she is relatively well appearing with no abnormal vitals or highly worrisome complaints. What can we do the next time, to avoid the dreaded greeting from a colleague, "Hey, you remember that patient..." The answer lies in seeking a unified diagnosis for seemingly discordant nonspecific symptoms.

- Ask specifically about polyuria, polydipsia, polyphagia and weight loss.
- Painful oral plaques are classic for Candida. It is not classic for pre-adolescent girls or boys, or even adolescent males to develop this in isolation, thus should raise the clinician's concern as to a more pernicious cause.
- Do not give insulin until electrolytes are known, since hypokalemia is a real risk.
- The optimal rate of glucose decline is 100 mg/dL/h. Do not allow the blood glucose level to fall below 200 mg/dL during the first 4–5 hours of treatment. In this case, the glucose was managed correctly with the blood glucose dropping from 942 mg/dL at 0:04 to 387 mg/dL at 6:43. (<100 mg/dL per hour).
- Bicarbonate is not recommended in any circumstance. It is associated with increased risk for cerebral edema.
- Insulin bolus is not recommended; it is associated with increased risk for cerebral edema.

- Cerebral edema is a *clinical* diagnosis. GCS scores are insensitive for early detection. Consider using diagnostic criteria proposed by Muir, et al.
- Phenergan can cause a decrease in mental status, making the diagnosis of DKA and cerebral edema more difficult.
- Cerebral edema alone is not an indication for intubation. Intubate for respiratory compromise and avoid hyperventilation.

References

1. Ali K, Harnden A, Edge JA. Type 1 diabetes in children. BMJ. 2011;342:d294.
2. Arora S, Cheng D, Wyler B., et al. Prevalence of hypokalemia in ED patients with diabetic ketoacidosis. Amer J Emerg Med. 2012;30(3):481–4.
3. Binita S, Lucchesi M, Amodio J, et al. Atlas of pediatric emergency medicine, 2d ed. New York NY: McGraw-Hill:2013.
4. Brown T B. Cerebral oedema in childhood diabetic ketoacidosis: Is treatment a factor? Emerg Med J. 2004;21(2):141–4.
5. Bui H, To T, Stein R., Fung K, Daneman D. Is diabetic ketoacidosis at disease onset a result of missed diagnosis? J Pediatr. 2012;156(3):472–7.
6. Charfen M, Fernandezfrackelton M. Diabetic ketoacidosis. Emerg Med Clin N Am. 2005;23(3):609–28.
7. Chiasson J, Aris-Jilwan N, Belanger R, et al. Diagnosis and treatment of diabetic ketoacidosis and the hyperglycemic hyperosmolar state. CMAJ. 2003;168(7):859–66.
8. Edge JA, Roy Y, Bergomi A, et al. Conscious level in children with diabetic ketoacidosis is related to severity of acidosis and not to blood glucose concentration. Pediatr Diabetes. 2006;7(1):11–15.
9. Farcy D, Chiu W, Flaxman A, et al. Critical care emergency medicine. New York NY:McGraw-Hill. 2012.
10. Felner EI, White PC. Improving management of diabetic ketoacidosis in children. Pediatrics, 2001;108(3):735–40.
11. Flood RG, Chiang VW. Rate and prediction of infection in children with diabetic ketoacidosis. Am J Emerg Med. 2001;19(4):270–3.
12. Glaser NS, Wootton-Gorges SL, Buonocore MH, et al. Subclinical cerebral edema in children with diabetic ketoacidosis randomized to 2 different rehydration protocols. Pediatrics. 2013;131(1), e73–e80.
13. Glaser NS, Barnes P, Neely EK, et al. Frequency of sub-clinical cerebral edema in children with diabetic ketoacidosis. Pediatr Diabetes. 2006;7(2);75–80.
14. Glaser NS, Barnes P, Neely EK, et al. Correlation of clinical and biochemical findings with diabetic ketoacidosis related cerebral edema in children using magnetic resonance diffusion-weighted imaging. J Pediatr. 2008;153(4), 541–6.e1.
15. Hamilton DV, Mundia S S, Lister J. Mode of presentation of juvenile diabetes. BMJ. 1976;2(6029):211–2.
16. Hoorn EJ, Carlotti AP, Costa LA, et al. Preventing a drop in effective plasma osmolality to minimize the likelihood of cerebral edema during treatment of children with diabetic ketoacidosis. J Pediatr. 2007;150(5):467–73.

17. Jeha, G, Haymond M. (n.d.). Treatment and complications of diabetic ketoacidosis in children. Up To Date. Retrieved 4-20-14, from http://www.uptodate.com/contents/search
18. Kitabchi AE, Umpierrez GE, Murphy MB. American Diabetes Association. Hyperglycemic crises in diabetes. Diabetes Care. 2004;27:S94–S102.
19. Kitabchi AE, Umpierrez GE, Miles JM, et al. Hyperglycemic crises in adult patients with diabetes. Diabetes Care. 2009;32(7), 1335–43.
20. Lawrence SE, Cummings EA, Gaboury I, et al. Population-based study of incidence and risk factors for cerebral edema in pediatric diabetic ketoacidosis. J Pediatr. 2005;146(5):688–92.
21. Mallare JT, Cordice CC, Ryan BA, et al. Identifying risk factors for the development of diabetic ketoacidosis in new onset Type 1 diabetes mellitus. Clin Pediatr. 2003;42(7):591–7.
22. Marx J, Hockberger R. Emergency medicine concepts and clinical practice (8th ed. 2013). London:Elsevier Health Sciences.
23. Muir AB, Quisling RG, Yang MC, Rosenbloom AL. Cerebral Edema in Childhood Diabetic Ketoacidosis: Natural history, radiographic findings, and early identification . Diabetes Care. 2004;27(7):1541–6.
24. Pawlowicz M, Birkholz D, Niedzwiecki M, et al. Difficulties or mistakes in diagnosing type 1 diabetes mellitus in children? The consequences of delayed diagnosis. Endokrynol Diabetol Chor Przemiany Materii Wieku Rozw. 2008;14:7–12.
25. Pawlowicz M, Birkholz D, Niedzwiecki M, et al. Difficulties or mistakes in diagnosing type 1 diabetes in children? Demographic factors influencing delayed diagnosis. Pediatr Diabetes. 2009;10:542–9.
26. Quinn M, Fleischman A, Rosnder B, Nigrin D, et al. Characteristics at diagnosis of type 1 diabetes in children younger than 6 years. Pediatrics. 2006;148:366–71.
27. Rewers A, Dolan LM, Dabelea D, Williams D, et al. Presence of diabetic ketoacidosis at diagnosis of diabetes mellitus in youth: the search for diabetes in youth study. Pediatrics. 2008;121(5):e1258–e66.
28. Roche EF, Menon A, Gill D, et al. Clinical presentation of type 1 diabetes. Pediatr Diabetes. 2005;6(2):75–8.
29. Rosenbloom AL. The management of diabetic ketoacidosis in children. Diabetes Ther.2010;1(2):103–20.
30. Slovis CM, Mork VG, Slovis RJ, et al. Diabetic ketoacidosis and infection: Leukocyte count and differential as early predictors of serious infection. Am J Emerg Med. 1987;5(1): 1–5.
31. Stewart C. Diabetic emergencies: diagnosis and management of hyperglycemic disorders. Emerg Med Pract. 2004;6, 1–24.
32. Strange GR. Pediatric emergency medicine (3rd ed. 2009). New York NY: McGraw Hill Medical.
33. Ting W, Huang C, Lo F, et al. Clinical and laboratory characteristics of type 1 diabetes in children and adolescents: experience from a medical center. Acta Paediatr Taiwan. 2007;48:119–24.
34. Tintinalli JE. Tintinalli's emergency medicine manual (7th ed. 2012). New York NY: McGraw-Hill Medical.

35. Umpierrez G, Freire AX. Abdominal pain in patients with hyperglycemic crises. J Critical Care. 2002;17(1):63–7.
36. Usher-Smith JA, Thompson MJ, Sharp SJ, et al. Factors associated with the presence of diabetic ketoacidosis at diagnosis of diabetes in children and young adults: a systematic review. BMJ, 2011;343(1): d4092. doi: 10.1136/bmj.d4092.
37. Usher-Smith JA, Thompson MJ, Walter FM. "Looking for the needle in the haystack": a qualitative study of the pathway to diagnosis of type 1 diabetes in children. BMJ Open. 2013;3(12):e004068 doi:10.1136/bmjopen-2013-004068.
38. Vanelli M, Chiari G, Ghizzoni L, et al. Effectiveness of a prevention program for diabetic ketoacidosis in children. An 8-year study in schools and private practices. Diabetes Care. 1999;22(1):7–9.
39. Vanelli M, Chiari G, Lacava S, Iovane B. Campaign for diabetic ketoacidosis prevention still effective 8 years later. Diabetes Care. 2007;30(4):e12.
40. White PC, Dickson BA. Low morbidity and mortality in children with diabetic ketoacidosis treated with isotonic fluids. J Pediatr. 2013;163(3):761–6.
41. Wolfsdorf J. Diabetic ketoacidosis in infants, children, and adolescents: a consensus statement from the American Diabetes Association. Diabetes Care. 2006;29(5):1150–9.
42. Wolfsdorf J, Craig ME, Daneman D, et al. Diabetic ketoacidosis in children and adolescents with diabetes. Pediatr Diabetes. 2009;10:118–33.
43. Yadav D, Nair S, Norkus E, et al. Elevation of amylase and lipase in diabetic ketoacidosis (DKA) is related to metabolic derangements. Gastroenterology. 2000;118(4):DOI:http://dx.doi.org/10.1016/S0016-5085(00)80448-5.
44. Glaser N, et al. the Pediatric Emergency Medicine Collaborative Research Committee of the American Academy of Pediatrics Risk factors for cerebral edema in children with diabetic ketoacidosis. N Engl J Med. 2001;344: 264–9.

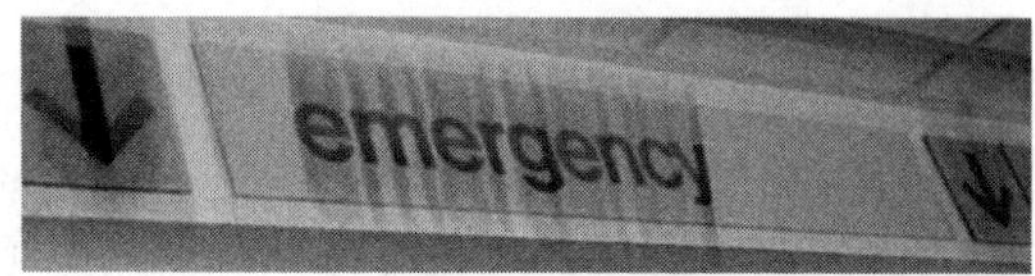

CASE 4

18-MONTH-OLD CHILD WITH FEVER AND VOMITING

Annalise Sorrentino, MD, FACEP, FAAP

Professor of pediatric emergency medicine
Division of Emergency Medicine, University of Alabama, Birmingham
Assistant Dean of students, University of Alabama School of Medicine

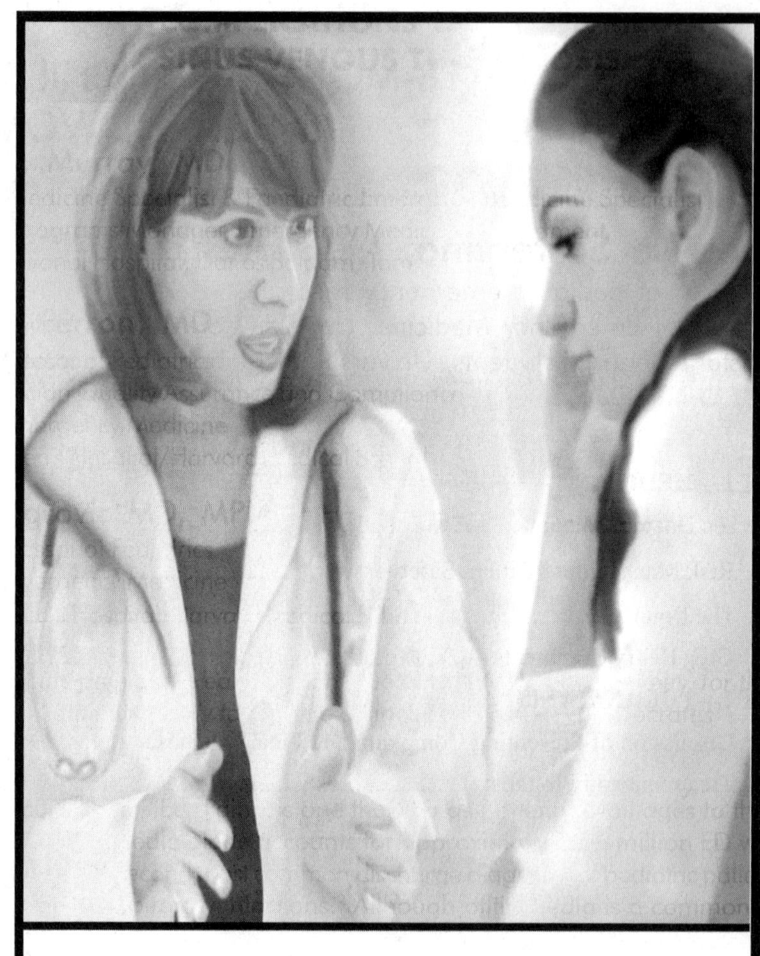

"Remember that kid you saw?"

CASE 4

18-MONTH-OLD CHILD WITH FEVER AND VOMITING

PART 1—MEDICAL

I. The Doctor's Version (the following is the actual documentation of the provider)

Date: Sunday, 8/24/2008

Chief Complaint: Fever and vomiting

Nurse note: 21:03: Dad states that the patient has vomited three times today and has been acting really lethargic. Mom states that the patient has had a fever of 100 today. No diarrhea. Normal wet diapers. Decreased appetite, but drinking well. Intervention (21:37): Ibuprofen 110 mg given per standing orders/guidelines.

HISTORY OF PRESENT ILLNESS (23:16): Presenting problem started 1-2 days ago. Father and mother are the source of the history. Temperature was between 101-102. Febrile over the past 24 hours. No history of chills or sweats. Child is having true episodes of vomiting and not just "spitting up." Nondescript vomitus without blood. No ill contacts with similar GI symptoms. No history of blood in bowel movement. No history to suggest a urinary problem. Does not seem to be urinating more frequently. No history of significant rash or skin eruption. No history to suggest any alteration or decrease in normal activity. Child is taking fluids well. Fair appetite, eating but not normal. No runny nose or cough. No history to suggest earache.

PMH: No significant PMH/PSH. Child was a full term, normal gestation, normal weight with no complications at birth.
ROS: Except as noted, all other ROS negative.

VITAL SIGNS

Time	Temp(F)	Pulse	Resp	Syst	Diast
21:33	100.6(R)	123	43	73	52

PHYSICAL EXAM (23:16):

General: Not ill appearing. No apparent distress. Mental development appears appropriate for age. Hydration status: well hydrated. Accompanied by mother and father.

Neurological: Alert nontoxic child. Interacts well with environment and examiner. Age appropriate behavior. Normal tone. Good body control. Age appropriate movement. Pupils equal round and reactive to light.

ENT: TM's clear. Moist mucous membranes without petechiae or inflammation. Normal posterior pharynx without inflammation, exudate, or drainage.

Pulmonary: Nonlabored respiratory rate and effort. Normal breath sounds bilaterally. No evidence of stridor. No cough. Patient is on room air.

Cardiac: Regular cardiac rate and rhythm. No audible murmur or rub. Brisk capillary refill.

Abdomen: Soft, non-tender abdomen. No abdominal masses, asymmetry or organomegaly.

TESTING: Urine: Microscopic: WBC: 5-6, RBC: 1-2, No bacteria/No yeast/Epithelial cells: 4+

ED COURSE: Oral rehydration solution taken (Amount not documented)

RECHECK VITAL SIGNS

Time	Temp(F)	Pulse	Resp	Syst	Diast
23:42	100.3(R)	118	24	76	44

DIAGNOSIS: Fever, vomiting

DISPOSITION (23:59): Discharge to home, Continue supportive care with antipyretics and fluids, Follow-up with PMD in A.M. for re-check

II. Risk Management/Patient Safety Issues

Risk management/patient safety issue #1:

Consideration: Minimal exploration of nurse documentation of lethargy.

Discussion: The nurse note stated "patient has been acting really lethargic." A combination of low-grade fever, vomiting and lethargy can indicate an intracranial process including meningitis, encephalitis, subdural hematoma (abuse), tumor or simply be a "red herring." A child with fever, vomiting, and possible lethargy should include a neck exam to evaluate for rigidity and meningeal signs.

✔ **Teaching point:** The physician can disagree with the nurse's assessment, but should indicate that in the note.

Risk management/patient safety issue #2:

Consideration: Specific documentation of patient's level of activity.

Discussion: The physical examination of the child should include the documentation of the general appearance, such as active, playful, engaged. The documentation in this case of "mental development appropriate for age" is not adequately descriptive, especially when the nurse documented lethargy!

✔ **Teaching point:** A lot of things need to go right for a patient to be running around and smiling, if this is the appearance of the patient, document it.

Risk management/patient safety issue #3:

Consideration: Further testing.

Discussion: Urine testing can assess for multiple diagnoses including dehydration (urine specific gravity and ketonuria) and DKA (glycosuria). UTI is unlikely in an 18-month-old infant presenting with low-grade fever and vomiting particularly if he is circumcised (which was not mentioned in the examination of this patient).

✔ **Teaching point:** The lowly urine dip yields a tremendous amount of information.

Risk management/patient safety issue #4:

Consideration: Low blood pressure.

Discussion: Blood pressure: Per the Pediatric Advanced Life Support (PALS) 2012 guidelines, normal blood pressure range for a 2 -year-old male is a systolic pressure of 88–106 mmHg and a diastolic pressure of 42–61 mmHg. The BP is only minimally low, but the physician documents that the patient is "well hydrated." The repeat BP is slightly improved and the pulse is lower. This clinician likely thought dehydration was the cause of the abnormal vital signs. Was it?

✔ **Teaching point:** Caution in patients with unexplained abnormal signs.

➢**Author's Note (MW):** There are some subtle clues which are discussed below, but in the end there is not really much to go on here. The primary learning value of this chapter is an expanded differential.

III. The Bounceback

The next day (14 hours after ED discharge)

14:08 - Incoming Patient Report by private medical doctor (PMD) - Lethargic, appears dry, RR 50, HR 151; being bagged for urine, h/o fever but none now.

14:41 – Triage nurse – Pt. is carried into ED, lethargic, no crying or withdrawal to pain.

- **Vitals -** Temp 98.2F rectally/Pulse 150/Respirations 44/BP unable to obtain.
- Pt develops seizure-like activity in waiting room. Pt. with eyes open and deviated to side, non-responsive. Baby noted to be tense but no jerking motions. Grinding teeth. Poor resp. effort. Doctor immediately notified

MD note: Patient carried by me to bed 12. Multiple RNs and MDs following. Upon arrival at bedside no pulse or breath sounds. Bagging/compressions started

- **15:04:** 4.0 cuffed ETT was placed. IV access attempted – unsuccessful. Interosseous (IO) line attempted left tibia – unsuccessful.
- **15:07:** Hold CPR – No pulse/spontaneous breath sounds. CPR continued. Another attempt at IV unsuccessful. 0.1mg of Epi per ETT.
- **15:09:** IO placed right tibia. Epi 0.1 mg pushed through IO.
- **15:12:** 10Fr OG placed with 20 mL orange liquid obtained. Right IO not functioning. IO placed in left tibia.
- **15:14:** Attempting femoral line. 1mg Epi in ETT.
- **15:17:** Hold CPR – No pulse, no breath sounds. Continue CPR. Dextrose stick (DS) = 43.

- **15:21:** IV access attempted – unsuccessful. Femoral line unsuccessful. 98.1 rectal temp. 1 mg Epi in ETT. 0.2 mg of atropine given per ETT. Left IO not functioning.
- **15:23:** Attempting right femoral line. Unsuccessful with femoral line. IO attempted in right femur.
- **15:30:** IV access still being attempted – unsuccessful. IO placed in left iliac crest
- **15:31:** 60 ml NS pushed in IO. Stop CPR – Check pulse – No pulse/breath sounds. CPR continued. Epi 0.1mg IO. Bicarb 10 meq IO. NS 60cc IO. Fem stick X 3 unsuccessful. Pushing Dextrose 12.5% in IO. 1.25g went in IO but IO not functioning now.
- **15:42:** CPR stopped – Still no pulse/breath sounds. CPR continued. Femoral line dc'd - not functioning. IO placed right iliac crest.
- **15:45:** Epi 0.1 mg, 60 cc NS pushed in IO.
- **15:48:** No pulse no breath sounds. Patient pronounced by physician.

Clinical Provider Note (documented at 16:12) Patient arrived to ER after transfer from PCP – Pt. with vomiting, dehydration per report of PCP. Not acting appropriate, sleepy but sitting up, interactive. Sat 100%, HR 150s at PCP's office. On arrival here, patient remained sleepy but interactive with triage nurse. Pt. deteriorated, brought to exam room and was found to be staring, not interacting, not breathing and had no HR. CPR was initiated. Pt was intubated by me: Visualized cords and was passed to 13 at lips and taped. Mist visualized in tube, good color change, good breath sounds. Easily bagged. CPR was continued throughout resuscitation without return of heart rate. We gave epi down the tube x 4 and atropine x 1. Venous access was difficult but we did obtain IO access briefly and epi and atropine were given, some NS bolus given, some dextrose given. No return of heart rate during resuscitation.

Labs:

- CBC: WBC 22, Hb 12.6, Plt 185
- Metabolic: Sodium 142, potassium 11.4 (no hemolysis), Chloride 99, CO2 8, glucose 25, BUN 29, creatinine 2.8, phosphorus 17.7 (3.9-6.5)

➢**Author's note (MW):** So what's the diagnosis? Still not obvious to you? (because it's *definitely* not obvious to me). OK. Here it is:

- **Post Mortem Diagnosis:** Acute Viral Myocarditis

IV. Greg Henry Comments

"There but for the grace of God go I"

Be honest. In virtually every emergency department in America this child would have gone home and been handled the exact same way. Looking good, minimal temperature, no other findings. The child is taking fluids. The child is not ill appearing. The documentation seems excellent, and I would expect this child to do well.

There is little evidence that we can change the outcome of viral myocarditis; depending on the virus involved and the extent of the inflammation, there is little more to do than supportive care. That being said, just as myocarditis killed this child, this is the kind of death which can kill the spirit of the emergency physician. The death of a young child is always a traumatic event. To suggest that every 18-month-old with a fever get an ECG and a workup for myocarditis is worse. This emergency physician is in the same position all of us would been in: "there but for the grace of God go I."

PART 2—THE ANALYSIS

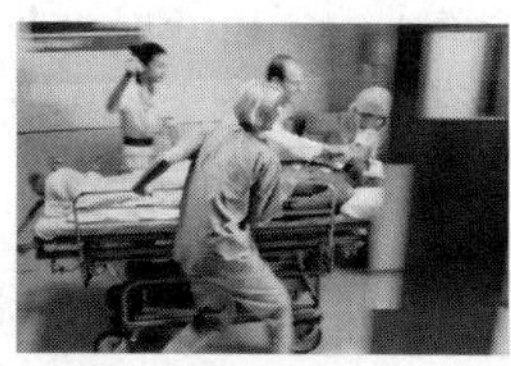

PEDIATRIC MYOCARDITIS—DIAGNOSIS, MANAGEMENT, AND A PERSONAL NOTE

Annalise Sorrentino, MD, FACEP, FAAP

Professor of pediatric emergency medicine
Division of Emergency Medicine, University of Alabama, Birmingham
Assistant Dean of students, University of Alabama School of Medicine

Although rare, acute myocarditis is a potentially life-threatening illness that is challenging to diagnose. Because some children are asymptomatic, the true incidence of myocarditis is unknown, although some have estimated 1 per 100,000 children.[1] A study published in 2012 found that the mean age of patients was 9.2 years (n = 514), with a bimodal peak in infancy and again in mid-teenage years. Males accounted for 64% of the patients and 41% were non-Hispanic whites, with 22% African American and 18% Hispanic.[2]

Etiology and Pathogenesis

Potential causes of myocarditis include toxic, autoimmune, bacterial infection and hypersensitivity,[3] however, the most common cause in the United States is viral infection.[4] Enteroviruses are the most commonly identified, followed by parvovirus B19, human herpes virus 6 (HHV6), influenza, parainfluenza, and adenovirus.[4] There was a growing association with parvovirus B19 and myocarditis, but it was also shown that parvovirus is present in a large percentage of patients who do not develop myocarditis.[5] The damage to the myocytes is due to direct cellular damage as well as immune response of the host.[6]

Based on severity of presentation, myocarditis can be categorized into one of three subsets: acute, fulminant, and chronic. Cases of acute disease may have milder, subclinical disease and go undiagnosed. Fulminant cases tend to present with cardiovascular collapse, but if they survive their initial hemodynamic instability, have a more favorable outcome. Chronic cases can progress to dilated cardiomyopathy.[4]

Clinical Presentation—History and Physical Exam

The clinical presentation of children with myocarditis can range from asymptomatic to cardiopulmonary failure (acute fulminant myocarditis), and has some variability with age.[4,6] It has been implicated in cases of sudden cardiac death in patients with seemingly minor or unrelated prodromal symptoms,[4] much like our patient. Although the history may be very nonspecific, a retrospective look at pediatric patients with myocarditis revealed that the most common presenting symptoms included shortness of breath, vomiting and poor feeding;[6] the complaint of chest pain is seen exclusively in patients older than 10 years of age.[4] Of note, like our unfortunate 18-month-old, 83% of patients are not diagnosed on their first visit to a health care provider.[6]

Signs of cardiac dysfunction such as poor perfusion, weak pulses, hypotension, and tachycardia may be detected on examination.[4] I have always used resting tachycardia as a marker to increase my suspicions, but one study reported that 66% of patients with myocarditis had normal heart rates.

The most common presenting physical category is respiratory, with tachypnea being the most common finding. Gastrointestinal symptoms are found more commonly in those less than 10 years of age, as was the case with our patient, although the symptoms are often those seen with many of the nonspecific viral illnesses encountered in the ED on a regular basis.

Specific cardiac findings are typically found in patients older than 10 years of age.[7] As is often the challenge when caring for young children, they cannot typically communicate their symptoms and will have vague complaints: fussy, lethargic, "not acting right," instead of the chest pain and difficulty breathing that might lead you in a different direction, such as obtaining labs or ECG.

Diagnostic Evaluation

Patients with suspected myocarditis should undergo electrocardiography and chest radiography. ECGs are often abnormal in cases of myocarditis, but a normal tracing does not preclude the diagnosis.

Findings can be highly variable, but most commonly seen are sinus tachycardia:

- with low voltage QRS complexes and
- inverted T waves

Other abnormalities may include:

- ventricular hypertrophy
- nonspecific ST segment changes
- dysrhythmias, heart block
- ischemia patterns.[3, 4]

Chest x-rays are abnormal in 60–90% of cases of myocarditis, and typically demonstrate cardiomegaly and pulmonary venous congestion.[4] If a chest x-ray had been obtained in this patient, it is likely that it would have shown some abnormalities, given the patient's subsequent rapid decline. Hindsight is always 20/20, but even knowing the final diagnosis, I have a difficult time finding a specific reason to have ordered a CXR during the first visit, particularly since he did not have tachypnea or another reason to consider pneumonia. The initial RR was 40 (normal range for 18 month old), which decreased to 24 on repeat examination.

There are no specific laboratory tests for myocarditis. Complete blood counts and inflammatory markers may be helpful, but as with the ECG, normal values do not exclude the diagnosis. Viral serology may be helpful, but will not impact therapy. Troponin T has demonstrated a sensitivity of 71% and a specificity of 86% at a cutoff of > 0.052 ng/mL.[3, 4] One study showed that the most sensitive marker for myocarditis was serum aspartate aminotransferase (AST), with elevated values in 85% of patients with confirmed myocarditis.[7] Creatinine phosokinase–MB isoenzymes (CK-MB) are elevated most commonly when an associated elevation of the ST segments on an electrocardiogram (ECG) is present.

When myocarditis is suspected, echocardiography is typically performed to look for evaluation of left ventricular function and cardiac structure, as well as wall motion abnormalities.[3] It can also help distinguish between fulminant and acute disease as those with fulminant myocarditis have normal left ventricular diastolic dimensions and increased septal thickness, while the opposite is true in acute disease.[4]

Historically, the gold standard for diagnosis of myocarditis has been endomyocardial biopsy with pathologic criteria for diagnosis (Dallas criteria). However, the disease is often patchy, so the sensitivity is low, and the interpretation of the biopsy has been found to have variability among observers.[4] More recently, cardiac MRI (cMRI) has shown promise as a diagnostic tool in myocarditis. Its ability to detect even patchy disease coupled with gadolinium enhancement of affected cells and non-invasive properties make it an increasingly popular alternative. The Lake Louise cMRI criteria are applied to radiographic results with a diagnostic accuracy approaching 80%.[3]

➢**Author's note (MMJ):** Even though the diagnostic accuracy of the cMRI is 80%, there are no firm indications, particularly when patients do not present with classic symptoms, such as chest pain.

Treatment and Prognosis

The treatment of pediatric myocarditis is mainly supportive and aimed at the clinical manifestations. These may include therapies for heart failure and/or arrhythmias. Diuretics, afterload reducers, inotropes and beta-blockers are frequently used. Other therapies that have been investigated include immunomodulators, corticosteroids, and intravenous gamma globulin (IVIG).[8] In some patients with fulminant disease, extracorporeal membrane oxygenation (ECMO) or a ventricular assist device (VAD) may be necessary.

VADs are typically used as a bridge to transplantation, although there was some hope that by using the device, the myocardium could recover and transplant be avoided. Some have quoted a VAD recovery rate of up to 16%, but experience in the United States has shown a < 10% recovery rate. Cardiac transplantation for dilated cardiomyopathy has an overall 10 year survival rate of ~70%, with myocarditis accounting for about 12% of the patients transplanted. However, more recent analysis shows a 2.7 times increased mortality for patients with myocarditis requiring transplant compared to other causes of hypertrophic cardiomyopathy. Those patients also tended to be older and more likely to die of acute rejection.[9]

Since the true incidence of pediatric myocarditis is unknown, outcomes are equally difficult to describe. Some studies have suggested that one-third of patients will recover completely, one-third of patients will die, and one-third of patients will have continued cardiac complications.[5] Another larger case series of 514 patients demonstrated a mortality rate of 7%.[3] Those with fulminant disease tend to have better outcomes if they survive the initial 72 hours.

The Five Most Hated Words ...

I was the treating physician when this child presented on her initial visit to the ED. I remember her and her family very clearly. I remember what room they were in. I remember what nurse was assigned to them. I remember waving to them when they were walking out and thanking me. I also remember that there was something that just didn't feel right. I couldn't put my finger on it, but couldn't come up with anything on history or physical examination that supported that feeling. However, as I was walking through the department the next afternoon and a good friend of mine stopped me and said the five most hated words to any EM physician, "Remember that kid you saw?", I instantly knew who she was talking about.

Decision making in the ED occurs rapidly. As emergency physicians, we pride ourselves on being able to quickly decide if someone is "sick or not-sick." Although we have always known that there is a combination of factors that go into our decisions (primarily experience and evidence, in differing amounts), this is now officially referred to as the dual process theory,[11] describing the interaction between our intuition and our deductive reasoning skills.

Dual process theory is a combination of:

- System 1 diagnostic reasoning (rapid, intuitive, almost completely unconscious, the "gut feeling," gestalt or "blink response") and,
- System 2 diagnostic reasoning (deliberate, intensive, hypothesis driven)[10]

We are good at the System 1 stuff and, not surprisingly, we get better with experience. Most importantly, it can be quite accurate. Supporting the idea of intuition in medicine often goes right against the evidence-based practices we have all been trained to use. You can't teach intuition, but you can teach to acknowledge it. As stated in one paper, "Intuition is far from perfect, but it works."[11] Pay attention to it. Would it have made a difference in this case? I don't know, but I wish it had.

References

1. Allan CK, Fulton DR. Clinical manifestations and diagnosis of myocarditis in children. www.uptodate.com. Accessed 2/13/2014.
2. Ghelani SJ, et al. Demographics, trends, and outcomes in pediatric acute myocarditis in the United States, 2006–2011. Circ Cardiovasc Qual Outcomes. 2012;5:622–7.
3. Canter CE, Simpson KP. Diagnosis and treatment of myocarditis in children in the current era. Circulation. 2014;129:115–28.
4. Durani Y, Giordano K, Goudie BW. Myocarditis and pericarditis in children. Pediatr Clin N Am. 2010;57:1281–303.
5. Yajima T, Knowlton KU. Viral myocarditis from the perspective of the virus. Circulation. 2009;119:2615–24.
6. Levine MC, Klugman D, Teach SJ. Update on myocarditis in children. Curr Opin Pediatr. 2010;22:278–83.
7. Freedman SB, et al. Pediatric myocarditis: emergency department clinical findings and diagnostic evaluation. Pediatrics 2007;120:1278–85.
8. Allan CK, Fulton DR. Treatment and prognosis of myocarditis in children. www.uptodate.com. Accessed 2/13/2014.
9. Canter CE, Simpson KP. Diagnosis and treatment of myocarditis in children in the current era. Circulation. 2014;129:115–28.
10. Wiswell J, Tsao K, Bellolio F, Hess EP, Cabrera D. "Sick" or "not-sick": accuracy of System 1 diagnostic reasoning for the prediction of disposition and acuity in patients presenting to an academic ED. Am J Emerg Med. 2013;31:1448–52.
11. Dhaliwal G. Going with your gut. J Gen Intern Med. 2010;26(2):107–9.

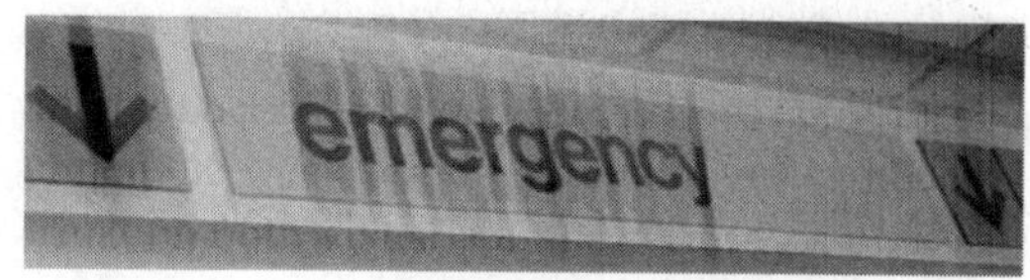

CASE 5

16-WEEK-OLD WITH BLOODY VOMITUS

Patti Robitaille, MD, FACEP
Attending Emergency Physician
Immediate Health Associates
Columbus, Ohio

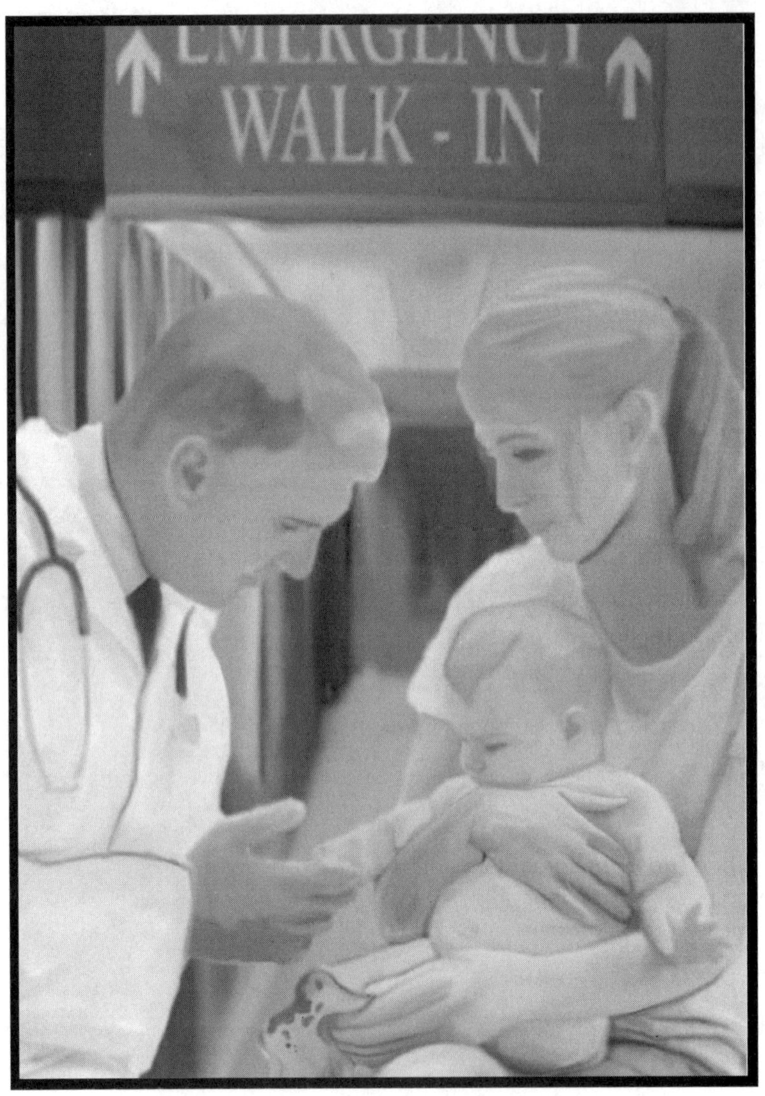
WALK - IN

CASE 5

16-WEEK-OLD WITH BLOODY VOMITUS

PART 1—MEDICAL

I. The Doctor's Version (the following is the actual documentation of the provider)

CHIEF COMPLAINT: Bloody vomitus

VITAL SIGNS									
Time	Temp(F)	Rt	Pulse	Resp	Syst	Diast	Pos	O2 Sat	O2%
09:14	97.8	Ax	127	34	98	0	L	99	RA

TRIAGE (at 09:02): mother states "blood in spit up. baby sitter put paper towel in baby's mouth and it came out with blood. looks like she is gagging". Parents brought patient in with paper towel that has blood on it that patient's mother states came from patient's mouth. Patient does have noted pink-tinged vomit on the collar of her clothing.

PAST MEDICAL HISTORY:
Allergies: No known allergies.
Meds: Axid
Immunizations: The infant/child's immunizations are current
Past medical history: GERD
No significant surgical history.

HISTORY OF PRESENT ILLNESS (documented at 13:51): This child apparently vomited a pinkish fluid today that may have been blood. child has no significant medical or surgical history except when being approximately 10 weeks premature at birth. There is a history of reflux. There have been no black or tarry stools noted at home. His been no diarrhea or nausea or vomiting. No fever, chills, nausea, blood in stools, constipation.

EXAM (documented at 13:52)
General: Well-appearing; active, alert, in no apparent distress.
Head: Normocephalic; atraumatic.
Eyes: PERRL
Ears: TM's normal, no bulging or signs of otitis media, canals normal
Oral: Posterior pharynx is pink without exudates, erythema. there are two areas that may be a source of bleeding one is the frenula and the other is a small area on the mucosa that may have leaked a small amount of blood.

Nose: The nose is normal in appearance without rhinorrhea
Resp: Normal chest excursion with respiration; breath sounds clear and equal bilaterally; no wheezes, retractions, rhonchi, or rales
Card: Regular rhythm, without murmurs, rub or gallop
Abd: Non-distended; non-tender, without rigidity, rebound or guarding
Skin: Warm and dry; no apparent lesions

Orders: CBC (at 10:44 Pt. parents refused blood draw after first attempt was unsuccessful.)

PROGRESS NOTES (documented at 13:53): We attempted a blood draw for a CBC. the parents at this time feel the child is okay and that the lesions in the mouth are the source of the bleeding and want to follow up with her pediatrician and are not interested in any more attempts at a blood draw. I let them go at this time.

DIAGNOSIS (at 10:42): GI Bleed

DISPOSITION: The patient was discharged to Home carried by parent accompanied by parent/guardian. Aftercare instructions for Gastritis/heartburn/peptic ulcer. Pt. released from ED at 10:52.

II. The Errors—Risk Management/Patient Safety Issues

Risk management/patient safety issue #1:

Error: History is not pediatric specific.

Discussion: This is a pediatric patient. Therefore, providers should expand their history to unearth information that was not volunteered.

- Pregnancy history: Was the pregnancy uncomplicated or was there gestational diabetes, pre-eclampsia, preterm labor, or issues?
- Delivery history: Was the patient full-term or an early delivery? Any complications with the delivery? What was the birth weight and what is the current weight?
- Medical history: Any health issues? Surgeries? Are immunizations up-to-date?
- Social history: Is the infant breast-fed or bottle-fed? Smokers in the house? Who are the primary caregivers?

✔ **Teaching point:** Casting a wide net will sometimes yield important information.

Risk management/patient safety issue #2:

Error: Presumption that the patient has no significant medical history.

Discussion: The child has no significant medical or surgical history...except for being approximately 10 weeks premature at birth! This is a significant piece of information, which mandates follow-up questions. Why was the patient premature? Was the patient on a ventilator and how long? How are the family/caregivers responding to the stressors of caring for a premature infant?

✔ **Teaching point:** Concerning data often needs further investigation.

Risk management/patient safety issue #3:

Error: On the physical examination, two potential bleeding sites in the mouth were noted, without additional investigation.

Discussion: The physical examination notes that the frenulum and another small mucosal region might be the source of bleeding. If that is true, there must be some source of oral trauma. Breast or bottle-feeding should not cause a mucosal injury. There was no mention of potential trauma or fall in the triage note, HPI, or progress notes.

✔ **Teaching point:** In non-verbal pediatric patients, it is important to ensure the propsed mechanism explains the injury.

Risk management/patient safety issue #4:

Error: Incomplete hematologic evaluation.

Discussion: Whether a CBC was warranted is debatable. However, once ordered, the hematologic ED evaluation should be complete. The CBC will check for leukemia, anemia, and thrombocytopenia. If you are going down this pathway, consider coagulation studies to rule out bleeding disorders such as hemophilia. Questions regarding excessive maternal bleeding associated with delivery and requiring blood transfusion, bruises, blood in the urine or stool, will further quantify the history. Other testing such a bleeding times, vitamin C levels, vitamin K levels, and histamine levels are usually not available in an ED setting and can be done by the specialist if clinically indicated. Explaining your thought process to the caregivers will help gain their trust.

✔ **Teaching point:** If you initiate an investigation, finish the thought process.

Risk management/patient safety issue #5:

Error: Committing to a GI source of bleeding as a diagnosis.

Discussion: What do we really know about the source of the blood? Blood, from the patient's mouth, is shown on a paper towel and on the collar of the clothing. The blood in the mouth could be from the nose, mouth, lungs, or stomach or even from the mother's nipple (though this patient presumably was at the baby sitters when the blood was found so it is unlikely it is from breast feeding with a cracked nipple). HPI notes "no black or tarry stools", but a rectal exam for occult blood or trauma was not done. It is unlikely that reflux would cause GI bleeding in a neonate. Patients and physicians would all like to have a pinpoint diagnosis in the ED setting; however, it is not always possible. Bottom line: We do not definitively know the source of bleeding is GI.

✔ **Teaching point:** Understand the limitations of an ED evaluation and the ability to make a definitive diagnosis.

Risk management/patient safety issue #6:

Error: The chart does not have a clearly unified story.

Discussion: A chart must flow, from triage to diagnosis. In any medical encounter, the triage and HOPI dictate the exam, followed by the appropriate work-up, then medical decision making, followed by diagnosis and disposition. In this instance, the triage and HOPI concentrate on potential vomiting as the source of blood. The physical exam notes potential bleeding from the frenulum and another mucosal region, as does the progress note. The diagnosis then goes back to "GI bleeding" with aftercare instructions for "gastritis/heartburn/peptic ulcer."

✔ **Teaching point:** This chart should tell one story, from the beginning to the end.

III. The Bounceback: ED return 12 days later to children's hospital

CHIEF COMPLAINT: Eyes rolled back

VITAL SIGNS

Time	Temp(F)	Rt	Pulse	Resp	Syst	Diast	Weight
18:02	98.6	Ax	148	40	108	53	5.9kg
20:42			149	36	93	63	

TRIAGE: Put baby down for nap – baby rolled from back to belly and was unresponsive

PAST MEDICAL HISTORY:

Allergies: No known allergies.
Meds: Prevacid 1 week
Past medical history: 30 wk. premature birth CPAP/Reflux
Immunizations: UTD
Family history: No epileptic or febrile seizures

HISTORY OF PRESENT ILLNESS (18:30): At babysitter → feeding – crying → On back to stomach/eyes roll back – call 911 – cry/episode last? minutes. Shaking (per babysitter) lasted 10 minutes. Occurred at 2:30PM. Runny nose for 3-4 weeks. Cough improved. No n/v/d, earache, pulling at ears, red eyes, sore throat, headache, rash, fever.

EXAM

General: No acute distress, attentiveness is normal for age, consolable, alert
Head: Normocephalic; atraumatic.
Eyes: PERRL, EOM's intact, conjunctiva and lids normal
Ears: Normal, no hemotympanum
Oral: Pharynx normal
Nose: Normal
Neck: Supple, no masses, thyroid normal
Resp: No respiratory distress, breath sounds normal
Card: Regular rate and rhythm, heart sounds normal, strong peripheral pulses
Abd: Nontender, no organomegaly
Ext: Nontender, normal ROM. Discoloration left wrist
Neuro: Cranial nerves normal as tested, no motor or sensory deficit

ORDERS: IV D5.2NS at 24ml/hr

RESULTS: (At 19:20) sent to head CT.
CT results: New and old subdural hematomas
XR results: Negative left wrist XR

MEDICAL DECISION MAKING: Concern for abuse by PMD so sent to ED for evaluation. Abuse concern due to previous injuries at babysitter that cannot be adequately explained.

DIAGNOSIS: Subdural hematoma, alleged physical abuse

DISPOSITION: Admit to neurosurgery and trauma. Report Faxed to floor at 21:55

HOSPITAL COURSE:

General surgery consult: 4 month former premature infant presenting today with unresponsive episode which lasted about 10 minutes, extreme irritability following incident. Child at babysitters during incident. Hx of bruises and cuts with babysitter prior. As per parents, babysitter stated she left infant on back, answered phone, and infant unresponsive eyes rolled back in head." Called EMS, called mom at work. Infant with baby sitter 7A-5P M-Fri for 6 weeks. One prior incident with bruise to left wrist, cut to mouth once also.

Patient admitted to neurosurgery, abuse consult, SS consult, skeletal series, ophtho consult

FINAL DIAGNOSIS: Subdural hematoma secondary to child abuse

IV. Greg Henry Comments

"Maintain a high index of suspicion when the history does not match the physical findings."

Don't get me started on the topic of child abuse, it is too hard. The longer I was in medicine the tougher it got—I'm not really as heartless a guy as they say I am. When the story doesn't sound right, it's not right. In this case, physical exam is everything: no 16-week-old should have a torn frenulum. To dismiss such vomiting as GI bleeding is extremely cavalier. Even if it is GI bleeding, in a 16-week-old, this would require evaluation for a myriad of causes and require aggressive intervention. Maintain a high index of suspicion when the history does not match the physical findings. Child abuse is still alive and well in America.

PART 2—THE ANALYSIS

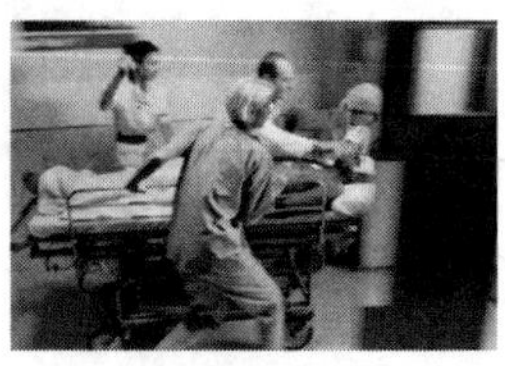

CHILD ABUSE: WHEN TO SUSPECT, HOW TO EXAMINE, TIPS FOR DOCUMENTATION

Patti Robitaille, MD, FACEP
Attending Emergency Physician
Immediate Health Associates
Columbus, Ohio

The differential diagnosis

Our patient is a 16-week-old, born prematurely at 30 weeks, with blood noted in the patient's mouth. What is the etiology of this bleeding? A generic differential diagnosis includes:

1. Trauma
2. Environmental temperature/humidity (dry or cracked lips/oral mucosa)
3. Bleeding dyscrasia from low platelets, hemophilia, VonWillebrand's disease
4. Neonatal leukemias, cancer: neonates with acute myelocytic leukemia (AML) fare much better than those with acute lymphocytic leukemia (ALL). [35]
5. Vitamin K deficiency bleeding (VKDB) of the newborn occurs in the first two weeks of life. The American Academy of Pediatrics has recommended vitamin K 0.5-1mg IM be administered to all newborns.[1]
6. Vitamin C deficiency and an increased histamine level may occur with hyperemesis gravidarum, malnutrition, surgery, or infection, in the pregnant patient. Subdural hemorrhages have been diagnosed by ultrasound, even before labor. Barlow's disease or infantile scurvy can be considered in cases with bruising, broken bones, and subdural hematoma.[2] Some authors advocate the measurement of vitamin C and histamine levels before attributing injuries to shaken baby syndrome.[3]
7. Glutaric acidemia, a genetic disorder due to a missing or decreased functioning enzyme "glutaryl-CoA dehydrogenase" which breaks down certain amino acids, results in acidemia and causes a myriad of symptoms, including cerebral edema and cerebral hemorrhage.[4,5] As a clinically important feature, this genetic disorder does not predispose the patient to fractures.
8. Hemorrhagic pulmonary edema from suffocation or strangulation, with bloody fluid in the mouth.

Oronasal bleeding in infants

A ten year retrospective study reviewing a small number of nasal and oral bleeding cases in children younger than 2 years of age concluded that oronasal bleeding in this age group is rare and should prompt consideration for child abuse as a potential etiology.[6]

Our patient had blood in the mouth without an adequate explanation, and it was attributed to a GI bleed without consideration of forced feeding.

Subdural hematoma in children

Though head injuries in children may occur due to accidental trauma, inflicted head trauma is the most common cause of death in children who are less than one year of age. Of patients with inflicted head trauma, 45% have permanent neurologic damage vs. 5% of those from accidental head trauma.[7]

The history of shaken baby syndrome

John Caffey was initially a primary care pediatrician from 1925–1930, later becoming only the second pediatric radiologist in North America. Caffey established "normal" for pediatric radiographs[8] and later authored a classic article which linked subdural hematomas in children, long bone fractures, and lack of history of trauma or injury.[9] Caffey encouraged follow-up studies, noting, "The presence of unexplained fractures in the long bones (salient fractures) warrants investigation of subdural hematoma. Routine roentgen examination of the long bones in subdural hematoma is necessary for the identification of fractures because many of them are silent clinically." Twenty-five years later, Caffey wrote about intentionally "shaken infants," linking the triad of brain injury, long bone injuries/fractures, and retinal hemorrhages.[10, 11] Caffey ends his paper by proposing a nationwide educational campaign:

> "Guard well your baby's precious head,
> Shake, jerk and slap it never,
> Lest you bruise his brain and twist his mind,
> Or whiplash him dead, forever." [11]

Duhaime, et al., conducted a retrospective study of suspected shaken injuries, along with a biomechanical study, in an effort to replicate the mechanism of injury of shaking. The model had an infant size/weight head, three different neck models, and a padded or metal bar impact surface. Duhaime concluded that these injuries were caused by shaking and blunt impact.[12]

In Ewing-Cobbs, et al.,[7] prospective, longitudinal study of children 0–6 years old who were hospitalized for traumatic brain injury (TBI), comparing between inflicted (abuse) TBI vs. accidental TBI indicated the following:

- 70% of inflicted TBI patients were less than one year old.
- 50% of inflicted TBI patients had no reported history of trauma. In patients with accidental TBI, all had reported history of trauma.
- Subdural hematomas occur in greater frequency with inflicted TBI (80%) than accidental TBI (45%).
- Epidural hematomas (20%) and shear injuries (20%) were only seen in the accidental TBI group.
- Retinal hemorrhages occurred in 70% of inflicted TBI patients, none in the accidental TBI group.
- Subsequent seizures occur more often in the inflicted TBI group (65% vs. 20%).
- Mental deficiency was greater in the inflicted TBI group.
- No difference in motor skills scores in the two groups.

There is a call for standardized definitions, examinations, and the execution of controlled, prospective clinical trials[13,14] and the recognition of the weaknesses of the literature and prior study conclusions, when applied to the world of law.[15,16]

Work up in Patients with Suspected Child Abuse:

History and the physical examination findings determine which laboratory and diagnostic imaging studies are necessary.[36]

1. If a bleeding problem is suspected, a basic bleeding evaluation (CBC, PT, and PTT) may suggest the need for more sophisticated bleeding evaluation and/or hematology consultation.
2. Radiographic studies may include:
   - Noncontrast brain CT—the initial screen for subdural hematoma, subarachnoid hemorrhage, cerebral contusion, cerebral edema, infarction, and white matter changes.
   - Diffusion weighted MRI—may distinguish between acute and chronic cerebral infarction.
   - An initial skeletal survey (Kempe series) will search for occult fractures. Rib fractures and long bone fractures are more prevalent in children with inflicted traumatic injuries, with rib fractures having the highest probability for abuse at 70%. There is a high correlation between multiple fractures and abuse. 80% of inflicted fractures are seen in children who are less than 18 months old.
   - A bone scan will identify subperiosteal hemorrhage and early fracture healing.
   - If a genetic bone disease such as osteogenesis imperfecta (OI) or mineralization defect is suspected, screening calcium, magnesium, phosphorus, and vitamin D levels are indicated. Review of radiographs with a pediatric radiologist is ideal to evaluate bones for signs of poor growth or healing.

     Note: OI should be suspected in the presence of "blue sclera," repeated fractures and short stature.
3. Screening for abdominal injury is recommended in children younger than age 5 years in whom abuse is suspected, even in the absence of symptoms (abdominal pain, vomiting) or clear external evidence of abdominal injury.

Multidisciplinary investigation: When investigating alleged abuse, a multi-disciplinary approach can be used including: [7,17,18,19,20,21,22]

- Pediatrician
- Pediatric neurosurgeon, for management of any intracranial injury
- Pediatric neurologist, for examination and optimization of outcomes
- Orthopedist, for fracture management
- Ophthalmology, for the complete eye examination and confirmation of retinal hemorrhages
- Forensic pathologist, in the case of death, for classification of the timing and mechanism of injury
- Social services, including child protective services
- Police

Incidence of child abuse

Child maltreatment/abuse is under-reported, due to lack of consideration, recognition, and detection. Child maltreatment is divided into four categories:

1. Neglect
2. Physical abuse
3. Emotional abuse
4. Sexual abuse

Neglect is the most common child maltreatment, with physical abuse second. Physical abuse affects all cultures and socio-economic groups. The incidence is similar for male and female children. This risk of abuse increases with age, but fatal and serious injuries are most common under the age of two.[21, 23]

The "Child Abuse Prevention and Treatment Act" was signed by Congress in 1974.[24] The most recent periodic, congressionally mandated data collection by the Fourth National Incidence Study of Child Abuse and Neglect (NIS-4) occurred in 2005–6. It reported 1.25 million children were maltreated: 61% neglected, 26% physically abused, 12% emotionally abused, and 11% sexually abused (children may fall into more than one category).[25]

Risk factors for child abuse:

The World Health Organization has published a comprehensive list of risk factors for child maltreatment.[26] A condensed list of risk factors includes the following:

1. *Risk factors for parents/caregivers*: difficulty bonding with child, caregiver who was maltreated as a child, unaware of typical child development or unrealistic developmental expectations, disciplines with physical punishment, has physical/mental/cognitive health issues, lack of self-control, alcohol/drug abuse, criminal activity, socially isolated, depression or low self-esteem, lack of parenting skills due to age or lack of education, financial difficulties.
2. *Risk factors for the child*: unwanted baby, high needs (prematurity, disabled, chronic illness), cries and difficult to comfort, mental health issues, multiple birth, many siblings, exhibits violence, criminal behavior, self-abuse, animal abuse, aggression towards peers.
3. *Relationship factors*: lack of parent-child bonding, family breakdown, violence in the family, disrespect in the family, isolation in the community, lack of support network, discrimination against the family, involvement in criminal/violent activities in the community.
4. *Community factors*: violence, gender and social inequality, lack of housing, lack of support services, unemployment, poverty, alcohol/drug abuse, lack of institutional policies and programs.
5. *Societal factors*: social/economic/health/education policies that cause a poor standard of living or socioeconomic inequality/instability, and social/cultural norms of violence towards others, demand rigid gender roles, and diminish the status of the child, child pornography/prostitution/labor.

Mandatory reporting for child abuse

Physician, nurses, and health care workers are mandatory reporters of suspected child abuse and neglect, as are school professionals, social workers, mental health professionals, childcare providers, medical examiners/coroners, and law enforcement officers. A report must be made if the reporter "suspects or has a reason to believe that a child has been abused or neglected" or "has knowledge of, or observes a child be subjected to, conditions that should reasonably result in harm to the child." [27]

A report made in "good faith" means that the reporter had actual knowledge or reason to believe that the child was subjected to abuse or neglect. There is immunity, both for mandatory and voluntary reports of child abuse/neglect.[28] There are penalties for the failure to report child abuse/neglect, which vary from state to state, including misdemeanor charges, felony charges, monetary fines, jail terms, or civil liability for any subsequent damages.[29]

The report of child abuse/neglect can be made to Child Protective Services or to law enforcement agencies. Many states have a telephone hotline or internet mechanism for reporting.[30]

Screening for child abuse

A diagnosis cannot be made, if it is not considered in the differential. At this time, we are left to diagnostic consideration, clinical vigilance, appropriate documentation, and reporting, if needed. There is no standard emergency department screening for child abuse/neglect.[31,32,33,34]

✔**Take Home Message**: Abuse does escalate, therefore, it is imperative to make the diagnosis early (bleeding gums in our case) before the infant suffers from a more serious injury (subdural bleeding) or worse.

References

1. Committee on Fetus and Newborn. American Academy of Pediatrics, Policy Statement, Controversies concerning vitamin K and the newborn. Pediatrics. 2003;112(1):191–2.
2. Clemetson CAB. Capillary fragility as a cause of subdural hemorrhage in infants. Medical Hypotheses and Research. 2004;1(2/3):121–9.
3. Clemetson CAB. Caffey revisited: a commentary on the origin of "shaken baby syndrome." J Am Phys & Surg. 2006;11(1):20–1.
4. Morris AAM. Glutaric aciduria and suspected child abuse. Arch Dis Child. 1999;80:404–5.
5. Hedlund GL, et al. Glutatric acidemia type 1. Am J Med Genet C Semin Med Genet. 2006;142(2):86–94.
6. McIntosh N, et al. Epidemiology of oronasal hemorrhage in the first 2 years of life: implications for child protection. Pediatrics. 2007;120:1074–8.
7. Ewing-Cobbs L, et al. Neuroimaging, physical, and developmental finding after inflicted and noninflicted traumatic brain injury in young children. Pediatrics. 1998;102:300–7.
8. Griscom NT. John Caffey and his contributions to radiology. Radiology. 1995; 194(2):513–8.
9. Caffey J. The classic: multiple fracture in the long bones of infants suffering from chronic subdural hematoma. Radiology. 1946;194:163–73.
10. Caffey J. On the theory and practice of shaking infants: its potential residual effects of permanent brain damage and mental retardation. Amer J Dis Child. 1972;124(2):161–9.

11. Caffey J. The whiplash shaken infant syndrome: manual shaking by the extremities with whiplash-induced intracranial and intraocular bleedings, linked with residual permanent brain damage and mental retardation. Pediatrics. 1974;54(4):396–403.
12. Duhaime AC, et al. The shaken baby syndrome: a clinical, pathological, and biomechanical study. J Neurosurg. 2012;66:409–15.
13. Donohoe M. Evidence-based medicine and shaken baby syndrome, Part 1: literature review, 1966–1998. Am J Forensic Med Pathol. 2003;24(3):239–42.
14. Piteau SJ, et al. Clinical and radiographic characteristics associated with abusive and nonabusive head trauma: a systemic review. Pediatrics. 2012;130:315–23.
15. Findley KA, et al. Shaken baby syndrome, abusive head trauma, and actual innocence: getting it right. Houston J Health Law & Policy. 2012;209–312.
16. Walter AJ. Misdiagnosis of abuse. CMAJ. 2003;169(7):651–2.
17. Kemp AM. Investigating subdural haemorrhage in infants. Arch Dis Child. 2002;86:98–102.
18. Blumenthal I. Shaken baby syndrome. Postgrad Med J. 2002;78:732–5.
19. Keenan HT, et al. A population-based comparison of clinical and outcome characteristics of young children with serious inflicted and noninflicted traumatic brain injury. Pediatrics. 2004;114(3):633–9.
20. Vichon M, et al. Confessed abuse versus witnessed accidents in infants: comparison of clinical, radiological, and ophthalmological data in corroborated cases. Childs Nerv Syst. 2010; 26(5):367–45.
21. Kellogg ND. Evaluation of suspected child physical abuse. Pediatrics. 2007;119:1232–41.
22. Kemp AM, et al. Patterns of skeletal fracture in child abuse: systematic review. BMJ. 2008;337.
23. Jussey JM, et al. Child maltreatment in the United States: prevalence, risk factors, and adolescent health consequences. Pediatrics. 2006; 118:33–42.
24. Child Abuse Prevention and Treatment Act. Public Law 93-247. 1974.
25. Sedlak AJ, et al. Fourth national incidence study of child abuse and neglect (NIS-4): Report to Congress, Executive Summary. Washington, DC: U.S. Department of Health and Human Services, Administration for Children and Families. 2010.
26. World Health Organization and International Society for Prevention of Child Abuse and Neglect. Preventing child maltreatment: a guide to taking action and generating evidence. 2006.
27. Mandatory reporters of child abuse and neglect. Child Welfare and Information Gateway. 2014.
28. Immunity for reporters of child abuse and neglect. Child Welfare and Information Gateway. 2012.
29. Penalties for failure to report and false reporting of child abuse and neglect. Child Welfare and Information Gateway. 2014.
30. Making and screening reports of child abuse and neglect. Child Welfare and Information Gateway. 2013.
31. Benger J, et al. Simple intervention to improve detection of child abuse in emergency departments. BMJ 2002;324:780–2.

32. Louwers ECF, et al. Screening for child abuse at emergency departments: a systematic review. Arch Dis Child. 2010; 95:214–8.
33. Guenther E, et al. Randomized prospective study to evaluate child abuse documentation in the emergency department. Acad Emerg Med. 2009; 6(3)249–57.
34. Eveline CFM, et al. Effects of systematic screening and detection of child abuse in emergency departments. Pediatrics. 2012;130(3):457–64.
35. Isaacs H Jr. Fetal and neonatal leukemia. J Pediatr Hematol Oncol. 2003;(5):348–61.
36. Kellogg ND. Evaluation of suspected child physical abuse. Pediatrics. 2007;119(6):1232–41.

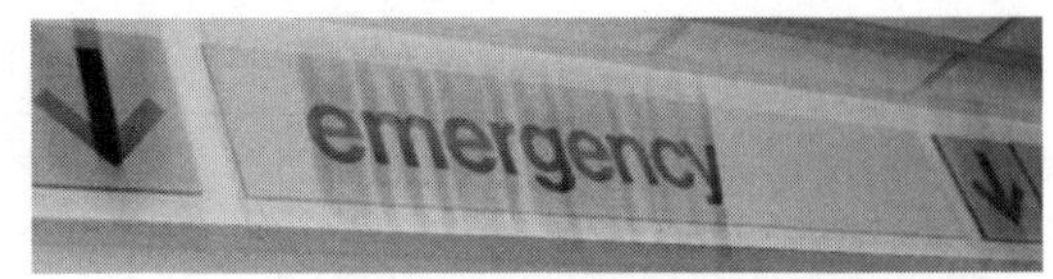

CASE 6

16-YEAR-OLD GIRL WITH EAR PAIN

Brittany L. Murray, MD
Emergency Medicine Specialist & Paediatric Emergency Medicine Specialist
Educational Programs Manager, Emergency Medicine Department
Muhimbili National Hospital, Dar es Salaam, Tanzania

Catherine Perron, MD
Assistant Professor of Pediatrics
Director Physician Quality Assurance and Compliance
Division of Emergency Medicine
Boston Children's Hospital/Harvard Medical School

Lise E. Nigrovic, MD, MPH
Assistant Professor of Pediatrics
Division of Emergency Medicine
Boston Children's Hospital/Harvard Medical School

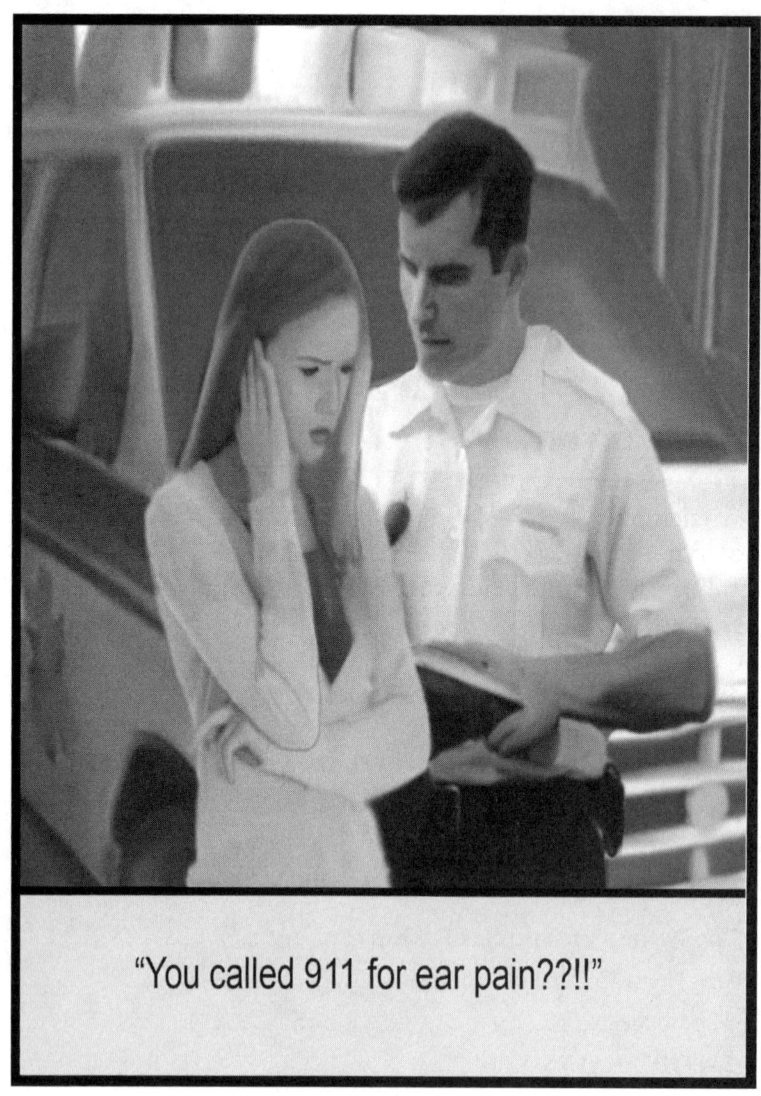

"You called 911 for ear pain??!!"

CASE 6

16-YEAR-OLD GIRL WITH EAR PAIN

PART 1—MEDICAL

I. The Patient's Story

Anna is a 16-year-old high school student who lives with her mother and her 19-year-old sister, Maria. Anna's mother works two jobs to support the family, and this often leaves Anna and her sister to attend medical appointments without her. Anna's family speaks Spanish at home, but English at work and school.

Anna has seen the same pediatrician since she was a toddler. She has never been seriously ill, been to the Emergency Department, or hospitalized. In late November, just days before Thanksgiving, she makes an appointment for 3 days of left ear pain, nasal congestion, and a sore throat. This is her first absence from school all year. She is diagnosed with left otitis media and given prescriptions for 10 days of amoxicillin and ibuprofen.

Despite taking the antibiotic and ibuprofen, Anna's ear pain worsens and over the next 24 hours, she develops a headache. Her mother calls the pediatrician's office at 9AM on Thanksgiving Day and is later called back by the nurse. By that time a pink fluid has started to drain from Anna's left ear and the pain has improved. The nurse asks the mother to continue the antibiotic and go to the ER if she has more pain or fever.

Over the next week, Anna improves, but the ear pain never fully resolves; she continues to have headaches and when the antibiotic course is finished, Anna's pain increases. Her left ear, the left side of her neck, and her whole head began to hurt more intensely, and she is nauseous and dizzy. She returns to the pediatrician, 16 days after her initial visit, and is diagnosed with cervical neck strain and headaches with a resolving otitis media.

The following day, Anna's mother calls the clinic and leaves a message that the ear pain and headaches are getting worse, and that Anna is unable to sleep or go to school. The clinic attempts to call Anna's mother back, but gets no answer. Anna's mother calls the clinic three additional times and leaves messages, but the clinic was unable to reach her when they return the calls.

Three days after Anna's second appointment (19 days after the initial visit), Anna's mother returns from work at 7pm and found Anna with severe ear pain and acting "out of it." She calls 911 and requests an ambulance to bring Anna to the Emergency Department affiliated with her pediatrician's office.

The paramedics arrived at Anna's house at 7:15PM. The prehospital run sheet reports:

"16 year old female found at home with complaint of left ear pain. Patient has been treated for one month without relief from pain. Patient completed antibiotics that ended more than 7 days ago. Patient took ibuprofen today at 4pm with no relief. Patient denies fever. She was transported to the Emergency Department without incident. On physical, the patient was a well-appearing adolescent with Glasgow Coma Score (GCS) of 15 with normal cardiovascular and pulmonary examinations."

The patient arrives at the Emergency Department at 7:19PM.

II. The Doctor's Version (the following is the actual documentation of the provider)

TRIAGE EVALUATION (RN)

19:30. Reporting ear pain for 1 month. Today left ear worse. Per family/EMS patient completed a course of antibiotics in the first week of illness. Triage examination: CV: normal, Resp: Normal, Abdominal: Normal, GCS: 15, Psych: Flat affect. Triage level 4. Placed in waiting room.

BASIC INFORMATION

Time seen by physician: 20:30
History source: Mother, Patient
Language: English

HISTORY OF PRESENT ILLNESS (MD): 16 year-old female who presents with left ear pain. Treated for left otitis media a month ago and completed antibiotics (amoxicillin?) as directed for 10 days per mom. Patient has been better, but now worse again. Mom states that patient has been seen by pediatrician a few times but no definite infection. Told to use compress to ear and ibuprofen for pain per mom. Patient not acting like herself, but otherwise well with no fevers, no vomiting/diarrhea, no cold symptoms, no rashes. Drinking.

REVIEW OF SYSTEMS

Constitutional symptoms: denies fever, denies chills.
Skin symptoms: denies rash, denies bruising.
Eye symptoms: denies discharge, denies redness.
ENMT symptoms: Ear pain: Left, denies nasal congestion.
Respiratory symptoms: denies cough, denies wheezing.
Gastrointestinal symptoms: no vomiting, no diarrhea.

HEALTH STATUS

Allergies: No known allergies
Medications: See HPI.

PAST MEDICAL/ FAMILY/ SOCIAL HISTORY

Medical history: Otitis media
Surgical history: Negative
Family history: Not significant
Social history: Lives with mother and sister. Spanish primary language in home.

VITAL SIGNS

Time	Temp(C)	Pulse	Resp	Syst	Diast	Weight(kg)
19:30	37.3	84	16	132	69	60

PHYSICAL EXAMINATION

General: Appropriate for age. Well hydrated.
Skin: No rash
Head: Normocephalic
Neck: Supple. No lymphadenopathy.
Eye: Pupils are equal, round and reactive to light. Normal conjunctiva. No discharge.
Ears, nose, mouth and throat: no oral lesions. no rhinorrhea. right tympanic membrane normal and left tympanic membrane red/fluid.
Cardiovascular: Regular rate and rhythm. No murmur.
Respiratory: Lungs are clear to auscultation
Gastrointestinal: Soft. Nontender. Non-distended. Normal bowel sounds. No organomegaly.
Musculoskeletal: Moves all extremities

MEDICAL DECISION MAKING: 16 year-old female who presents with left otitis media. Will give prescription for Augmentin given recent course of amoxicillin. Ibuprofen for pain control. Follow-up with PMD within the week to be sure patient is improving, sooner if concerns.

IMPRESSION AND PLAN (20:41):

Diagnosis: Otitis media
Condition: Stable.
Patient was given the following educational materials: Otitis Media.
Counseled: Family regarding treatment plan. Discharged to home

III. Greg Henry Comments

"There is not even a basic neurological examination on the chart"

What do you do with a 16-year-old with ear pain? Although otitis media is an extremely common diagnosis in emergency medicine, it is not necessarily common in a 16-year-old. Careful examination is required. Pushing on the pinna and pushing on the tragus produce intense pain in patients with otitis externa. Otitis media has very little discomfort on palpation, but should have an abnormality on pneumatic otoscopy.

There is no question in this case that a 16-year-old, awake and alert patient with ear pain and a red ear drum would be discharged on antibiotics in the hope that this would take care of the problem. I have no complaints with this initial approach.

It is stated in the history that the family speaks Spanish at home but English at work and school. The job of the healthcare professional is to determine whether adequate communication is taking place. In the vast majority of Spanish speaking patients, who also work in the broader community, their English will be found adequate to communicate. This is not true with other languages. The phone systems, which claim to have "170 different languages" forget to tell you they may not have the specific dialect that the patient speaks. Most of the legislation in this area was short sighted.

I would like to reproduce a phrase from the chart, "Patient not acting like herself, but otherwise well." This is an odd juxtaposition of words; who is she acting like and do we care if *that* person is well?? This short statement may be our diamond in the rough. At the least, it requires better differentiation. A flat affect could go along with someone simply not feeling well, but a true encephalopathy based on an infectious process is a completely different matter. More defined history and a directed physical examination is necessary to distinguish a neurological as opposed to a physiological cause. It is interesting to note that there is not even a basic neurological examination on the chart.

IV. The Bounceback

Anna goes home after her ED evaluation and starts the Augmentin that evening. The next day she stays home, as she is feeling too unwell to go to school. When her sister arrives home at 8pm, she notes that Anna was not acting like herself and is having difficulty speaking. Anna's sister calls a friend to bring Anna back to the hospital. The three girls arrive at the Emergency Department just after 10PM.

EMERGENCY DEPARTMENT CHART: Visit #2—25 hours after initial ED visit

- **Triage Evaluation (RN)** 22:15. Patient here. Sibling brought patient in to ED again tonight because she reports "she can't talk" since 8pm tonight. Patient awake, alert and follows commands, but tearful and not speaking to staff or sibling. Will not talk at triage. Triage level 3. Placed in waiting room.

- **Resident evaluation**
  History of Present Illness (Resident at 22:45): Her sister states that she came home from work around 8 pm tonight, and Anna was unable to talk or say anything. Anna was able to nod "yes" or "no" to her sister's questions. Anna has also been having "blank expressions" over this past week and has needed some things repeated more than usual. When patient's sister is out of the room, patient responds "I can't talk", but will not say anything else. She reports that her hands felt funny this morning but is unable to elaborate further.
  PMH: Medications: Augmentin, Ortho Tri-Cyclen Lo, vitamin D, ibuprofen
  PE: Temp 36.8, pulse 68, respire 18, BP 121/78, sat 99% (RA)
  - **General:** Alert. Cooperative. Smiling.
  - **Neck:** Supple. Trachea midline. No tenderness. No lymphadenopathy.
  - **Eye:** Pupils are equal, round and reactive to light. EOMI. Normal conjunctiva.
  - **Cardiovascular:** RRR. No murmur. No gallop. Normal perfusion.
  - **Respiratory:** Lungs are clear to auscultation.
  - **Neurological:** Alert. Normal coordination observed. Normal gait and coordination, Romberg negative, no pronator drift. Speech slow.

- o **Psychiatric:** Cooperative. Non-suicidal. Oriented x3, odd affect.

MDM: Given her recent behavioral changes, and missing school, a psych diagnosis is likely. Plan to send urine pregnancy and drug screen. May consider Neurology evaluation for other source of symptoms.

- **Attending note - shortened (23:30) -** This evening, when her sister arrived home from work, she noted patient would not speak to her. She asked her to write down what was wrong and the patient only wrote scribbles. My examination revealed the patient to be alert, intermittently flat affect vs. smiling, no acute distress. HEENT with cloudy left tympanic membrane (TM) with a small inferior defect. No mastoid tenderness, neck was supple. Neuro exam showed shows PERRL, EOMI, face symmetric, uvula and tongue midline, hearing grossly intact, motor 5/5 throughout, moves all extremities symmetrically. Her affect was initially flat, but then she began smiling. Her speech was slow speech and she does not seem to understand all directions and occasionally responds inappropriately. Concern for complication of otitis media. Neurology consulted and MRI, labs ordered.
- **02:42 ED MD called by Radiologist.** MRI/MRV Brain showed:
  - o Left mastoid and middle cavity fluid consistent with mastoiditis.
  - o Associated thrombus in the left lateral transverse sinus extending into the sigmoid sinus, jugular bulb, and the proximal jugular vein.
  - o FLAIR signal abnormality in the left temporal and occipital lobe compatible with meningitis.
  - o Diffuse cortical diffusion changes in the left temporal, bi-frontal lobes, left thalamus, and left hippocampus that may be related to infection or ischemia.
  - o A T2 hyperintense collection between the left mastoid and the thrombosed sinus consistent with an epidural abscess collection.
- Pt. admitted to ICU. An EEG is performed on admission to the ICU due to persistent altered mental status. It shows active epilepsy with a focal mechanism of seizure onset in the left mid temporal region.

FINAL DIAGNOSIS: Mastoiditis with associated sinus venous thrombosis, intracranial abscess, meningitis, and seizures.

SUMMARY OF HOSPITAL COURSE:

- Anna was hospitalized for 10 days. The first 7 days of her stay were in the ICU.
- Broad-spectrum antibiotics, anticoagulation, and antiepileptic medications were started.
- On the morning after admission, she was taken to the operating room and bilateral myringotomy tubes were placed with purulent drainage from the left ear and a needle aspiration was performed of the left postauricular region.
- Two days later her symptoms and seizures had not improved and she was taken to the operating room for drainage of the epidural abscess and for mastoidectomy.
- Anna improved and was able to be transitioned to the neurology floor and then home.
- **Discharge**: She was discharged on antibiotics, antiepileptic medications, and anticoagulation. Upon discharge, she still had marked aphasia, was able to read very slowly, and could write only basic words.

PART 2—ANALYSIS

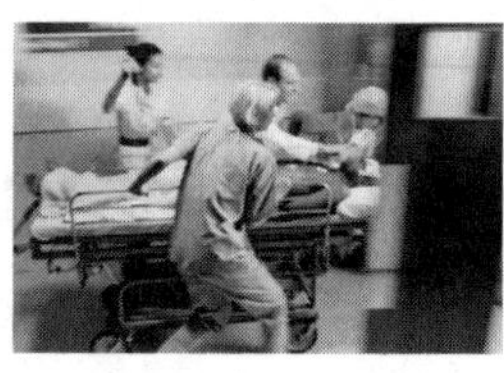

THE EVALUATION OF EAR PAIN, COMPLICATIONS OF OTITIS MEDIA, SINUS VENOUS THROMBOSIS

Brittany L. Murray, MD

Emergency Medicine Specialist & Paediatric Emergency Medicine Specialist
Educational Programs Manager, Emergency Medicine Department
Muhimbili National Hospital, Dar es Salaam, Tanzania

Catherine Perron, MD

Assistant Professor of Pediatrics
Director Physician Quality Assurance and Compliance
Division of Emergency Medicine
Boston Children's Hospital/Harvard Medical School

Lise E. Nigrovic MD, MPH

Assistant Professor of Pediatrics
Division of Emergency Medicine
Boston Children's Hospital/Harvard Medical School

"Acute pain of the ear with continuous high fever is dangerous, for the patient is likely to become delirious and die. " ~Hippocrates[1]

Introduction

Anna's chief complaint, "Ear Pain," is one that brings patients of all ages to the emergency department. Otitis media alone accounts for approximately 1.5 million ED visits in the US each year and is the second most common discharge diagnosis of pediatric patients, following only acute upper respiratory infections.[2] Although otitis media is a common cause of ear pain, the differential diagnosis is broad and includes otitis media, otitis externa, trauma, foreign bodies, complications of otitis media, and referred pain from other sources.

As demonstrated by Anna's case, an emergency provider must be vigilant and consider life-threatening processes in patients with otalgia. Although serious etiologies are rare, due to the sheer number of patients with otalgia that an emergency provider will see during their career, it is likely we will all see serious complications of otalgia. Luckily, in most cases of ear pain, a thorough history and physical examination are adequate to distinguish benign from serious causes.

ED evaluation of pediatric ear pain

Otalgia can be broadly divided into three categories:

- Pain related to the external ear
- Pain related to the middle ear
- Pain referred from other sources such as dental carries/abscess, or tonsillitis.

In some cases, the ED evaluation will not be able to pinpoint the exact cause of the pain, but it should be able to rule out serious etiologies of ear pain.

History

Anna's initial evaluation was her first visit to an Emergency Department, and she presented per EMS. This is an unusual presentation for simple otitis media.

The history for a patient with ear pain should include a careful description of the duration and evolution of symptoms. Outer ear pathology may start with skin changes and progress into the ear canal. Inner ear pathology may be associated with dizziness, a sense of a "blocked ear," hearing loss or deep ear pain. Pain referred to the ear from another source may be associated with other symptoms, such as tooth pain in the case of pain referred from a temporal or mandibular source. The history should elicit the exact location of the pain, progression of pain, radiation, aggravating factors, and associated symptoms. Specifically, inquire about recent antibiotic use, trauma and neurological symptoms.

Physical exam

The physical exam should begin with an evaluation of general appearance and vital signs. In young children who are unable to provide a reliable history, a complete examination should be performed even when a focal complaint exists. The examination in general should begin with examining areas that are not painful such as the head and neck and then proceeding to the areas of complaint. Additionally, examine the throat, dentition, face, neck, skin of the ear and surrounding area, mastoid area and lymph nodes of the head and neck. The cranial nerves should be tested, including a test of hearing in the involved ear.

The ear examination should begin with inspection and palpation of the outer ear. Both ears should be evaluated to look for any asymmetry in positioning or shape. The pinna should be inspected and palpated to assess for signs of trauma or infection. Pain with palpation or movement of the auricle or tragus can indicate pathology of the external ear. After examination of the external ear, otoscopy should be performed.

Otoscopy relies on good visualization of the ear canal and tympanic membrane. A prospective study that evaluated 221 otoscopes in Emergency Departments showed that more than half were not in proper working condition.[3] Ensure that the light is bright, then select the largest speculum that will fit comfortably into the ear canal and position the patient in an optimal way to inspect the ear. In older children and adults this may be as simple as asking them to remain still, but in younger children, immobilization for accurate visualization is often needed.

While inserting the speculum into the ear, initially examine the ear canal looking for evidence of infection or trauma. A normal TM should be in neutral position, translucent, pinkish gray, and move with insufflation. A middle ear effusion, inflammation, bulging, and immobility are typical findings in otitis media. The presence of otorrhea suggests a perforation of the TM even if it cannot be fully visualized. Tympanic membrane mobility by pneumatic otoscopy is strongly recommended if available.[4]

You look into the patient's ear and see an opaque, red, and bulging TM. It's time to diagnose otitis media, right?

Diagnosing Otitis Media? Don't miss these RED FLAGS

Historical Elements

- Patient age
- Aggravating factors
  - o Worsening pain with mastication or facial movements may indicate a primary etiology outside of the ear.
- Associated Neurological Symptoms
  - o May indicate a deeper space infection

Exam Findings

- Indication of a process outside of the ear is suggested by a normal ear exam
- Indication of deep space infection
  - o Mastoid tenderness/erythema
  - o Neurological abnormalities-—specifically cranial neuropathies, altered mental status, or stroke-like findings
  - o Signs of elevated intracranial pressure

Complications of otitis media

Complications of otitis media can have high morbidity and mortality. Prior to widespread antibiotic availability, complications such as meningitis, mastoiditis, and venous thromboembolism were common, occurring in more than 20% of pediatric patients with otitis media.[5] In the modern era, these complications are relatively rare. However, like Anna, many children presenting with these complications will have been treated and may not present with classic symptoms.

Mastoiditis classically presents in the setting of recent or concurrent otitis media, fever, deep pain localized behind the ear and systemic symptoms of illness including lethargy, malaise, irritability or poor feeding. On exam, these children often have a red, bulging TM and tenderness over the mastoid bone. In addition, the best way to appreciate the fullness in the mastoid area is to look for the ear being pushed forward (best seen from the back of the patient's head). However, in a recent case series of children with mastoiditis confirmed by radiology, more than 30% of children may present without localized pain and approximately 25% without documented fever.[6]

Furthermore, venous sinus thrombosis as a complication of otitis media is classically described as having an association with high fevers and unrelenting ear pain. However, in two recent retrospective case series at tertiary Children's hospitals, many of the patients diagnosed with lateral sinus thrombosis related to an otomastoid infection denied recent high fevers or ear pain. They were more likely to present with neurological symptoms such as cranial neuropathies, diplopia, headaches, vomiting and signs of raised intracranial pressure.

So, how do we avoid missing these rare complications?

Knowledge of the anatomy of the inner ear and mastoid can help a provider understand the complications of otitis media and to identify them. These complications are generally a result of direct extension of infection from the middle ear cavity into the surrounding structures. The mastoid sits immediately behind the middle ear and is separated from the middle ear by a mucous membrane. The posterior boundary of the mastoid forms the lateral sinus. The roof of the mastoid forms a portion of the brain cavity, and the temporal lobe of the brain sits on the mastoid. The facial nerve runs through the mastoid vertically, and the semi-circular canals are housed within the mastoid.

With this anatomical refresher, it is easy to imagine how otitis media can cause extracranial and intracranial complications.

Extra-cranial complications include:

- Mastoiditis (and sub-periosteal abscess)
- Petrositis (osteomyelitis of the petrous bone)
- Facial nerve paralysis
- Labryrinthitis
- Chronic suppurative otomastoiditis

Intracranial complications include:

- Temporal or cerebellum brain abscesses
- Epidural abscess
- Meningitis
- Sinus thrombosis
- Subdural abscess

What if you are worried about a complication of otitis media? It is time to image.

CT scans evaluate bones well and will show the mastoid air cells, the facial canal, the bone of the tegmen, the otic capsule, the posterior fossa and pathology of those structures in detail. A contrasted CT scan can also show abscesses and suggest sinus venous thrombosis. However, MRI/MRV is the ideal way to look for intracranial complications of otitis media. MRI is superior to CT in evaluating for sinus venous thrombosis, meningeal inflammation, intracranial abscesses, and intra-parenchymal edema. [5,6]

Treatment of sinus venous thrombosis

Emergency Department treatment of sinus venous thrombosis in the setting of otomastoid infection includes a combination of antibiotics and surgery in conjunction with ENT and neurosurgery to stop the extension of the infection and the thrombus to more distal sinuses. Anticoagulant usage in patients with isolated lateral sinus involvement is controversial, and initiation should involve shared decision making with the admitting and specialty teams. [7,8,9]

When thrombus is isolated to the lateral sinus, systemic anticoagulation is generally not needed, and may increase the risk of releasing septic emboli from clot breakdown as well as increasing the chances of serious hemorrhage. However, if the clot extends into the sagittal or sigmoid sinuses or there is evidence of increased intracranial pressure, systemic anticoagulation may be necessary.[7]

Summary of the case

Anna's infection likely started as otitis media, but despite treatment, progressed over weeks into her mastoid bone and extended into the surrounding structures resulting in an epidural abscess, meningitis, left lateral and sigmoid sinus venous thrombosis extending into her jugular veins, and temporal lobe involvement causing seizures and altered mental status. Interestingly, she was taking oral contraceptives but this information was not obtained until the second visit. By itself, it would not have been enough to make the diagnosis, but does emphasize the importance of asking detailed questions when there is an atypical presentation of otitis media.

✔Teaching points:

- Complications of otitis media can occur despite treatment with antibiotics.
- Fever and otomastoid symptoms may suggest complications of otitis media, but the absence of these symptoms does not rule out the diagnosis.
- Neurological symptoms in the setting of otitis media must raise concern for deep space infections and complications.
- You can gain valuable information by asking patients why they came by ambulance.

➢**Author's note (MW):** One final point of consideration, remember the resident's note upon admission, "Given her recent behavioral changes, and missing school, a psych diagnosis is likely." Well, turns out they were wrong, but kudos for thinking outside the box, and kudos for the rest of their note about involving neurology to ensure another diagnosis was not occurring. Caution in diagnosing a psychiatric etiology in patients without a psychiatric history, with isolated symptoms (confusion), following a recently treated illness (otitis media), or prior to cerebral imaging.

References

1. Hippocrates, Volume II: Prognostic, Loeb Classical Library Volume 148, translated by W. H. S. Jones, Cambridge, Mass.: Harvard University Press, 1923, p. 145.
2. Pitts S, Niska R, Xu J, Burt C. National Hospital Ambulatory Medical Care Survey: 2006 emergency department summary. National health statistics reports; no 7. Hyattsville, MD: National Center for Health Statistics, 2008.
3. Barriga F, Schwartz R, Hayden G. Adequate illumination for otoscopy. Variations due to power source, bulb, and head and speculum design. Am J Dis Child. 1986;140(12): 1237–40.
4. Lieberthal A, Carroll A, Chonmaitree T, et al. Clinical Practice Guideline: the diagnosis and management of acute otitis media, Pediatrics 2013. 131(3):e964–e994.
5. Van den Aardweg M, Rovers M, de Ru J, Albers F, Schilder A. A systematic review of diagnostic criteria for acute mastoiditis in children. Otol Neurotol. 2008;29(6):751–7.
6. Vazquez E, Castellote A, Piqueras J, et al. Imaging of complications of acute mastoiditis in children. Radiographics. 2003;23(2):359–72.

7. Bradley D, Hashisaki G, Mason J. Otogenic sigmoid sinus thrombosis: what is the role of anticoagulation? Laryngoscope. 2002;112 (10):1726–9.
8. Manolidis S, Kutz J,. Diagnosis and management of lateral sinus thrombosis. Otol Neurotol. 2005;26(5):1045–51.
9. Levine S, DeSouza S, Shinners M. Intracranial complications of otitis media. In: Gulya C, Minor L, Poe D. Glasscock-Shambaug's Surgery of the Ear. 6th. Ontario, British Columbia:Deckers; 2010:451–64.

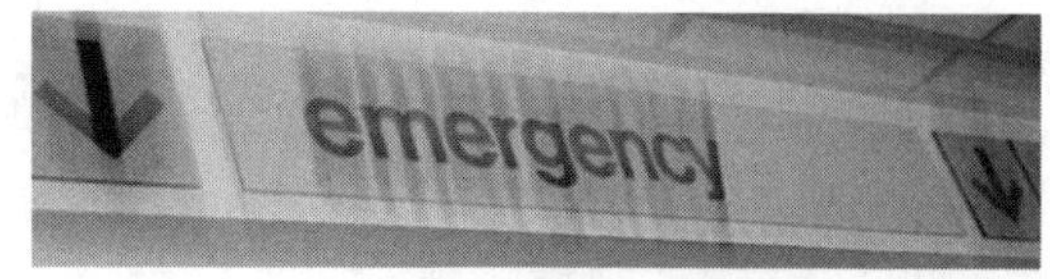

CASE 7

12-YEAR-OLD GIRL WITH PERSISTENT BACK PAIN

Cassie Zhuang, MD
Emergency Medicine Resident PGY-2
University of Texas Health Science Center at San Antonio

Gillian Schmitz, MD, FACEP
Associate Program Director
Department of Emergency Medicine
University of Texas Health Science Center at San Antonio

Paul Charlton, MD
Emergency Medicine Resident PGY-1
Division of Emergency Medicine, University of Washington
Master's degree, Conflict Resolution, Georgetown University

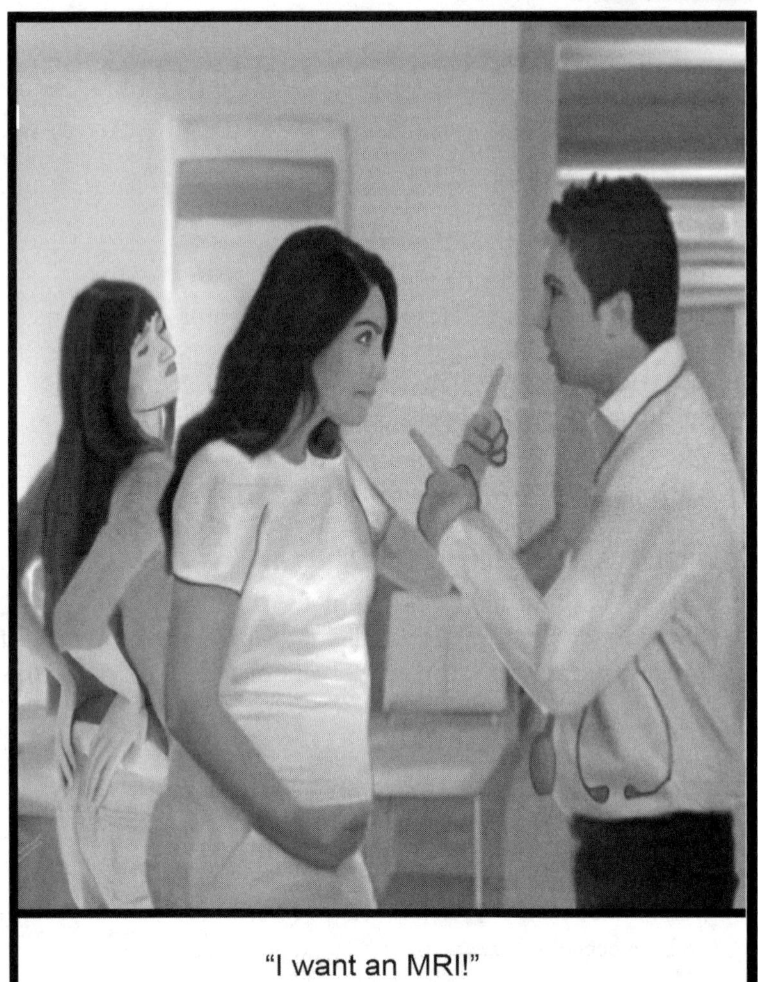
"I want an MRI!"
"It is not emergently indicated!"

CASE 7

12-YEAR-OLD GIRL WITH PERSISTENT BACK PAIN

PART 1—MEDICAL

I. The Mother's Story

"I initially brought my 12-year-old girl to the emergency department because she had back pain. She doesn't normally complain of pain, so I was worried. She is a gymnast so I thought it was reasonable when the first physician told me she had musculoskeletal pain and sent us home with Motrin."

"When she did not get better after a week, I brought her back to the same ED. This time, they checked a urine sample and told me she might have had a UTI and sent us home on antibiotics. She never had any fever or burning with urination though, which I thought was weird. The antibiotics didn't help."

"I brought her back a third time, and by this point, I was angry. I felt like no one was taking her seriously, and I wanted an MRI. The doctors kept telling me that an MRI was not indicated because she was able to walk okay and did not have any weakness or numbness. But why did my daughter's back hurt so much? I insisted on a MRI and was upset when we were sent home a third time after another negative urine sample and x-ray of her back. They told me to follow up with her primary doctor, but I couldn't get an appointment for a couple of weeks."

II. The Doctor's Version (the following is the actual documentation for ED Visit #3)

Date: September 18, 2007 11:23 AM
Chief complaint: Back pain
Nurse note: Pt. c/o low back pain 5/10. Patient seen in ED previously without improvement

HISTORY OF PRESENT ILLNESS – (Per Dr. Peterson): Patient complains of bilateral lower back pain. She rates it 5/10, non-radiating. Moving around or sitting up seems to maybe make pain worse. No fevers. No numbness or tingling. No weakness. No urinary symptoms. She was given Tylenol after the 1st visit, which has helped to some degree, but pain returns. She was treated with Cipro for UTI after 2nd visit, but this did not help either. On review of prior record, UA was contaminated on the previous visit with many epithelial cells and no culture was sent. Patient is a gymnast. She does not recall any specific trauma.

REVIEW OF SYSTEMS: Unless otherwise stated in this report, all other symptoms and systems were negative. Specifically, no abdominal pain. No fevers or chills.

PAST MEDICAL HISTORY:

Allergies: NKDA
Medications: None
PMH: None
Social history: Nonsmoker , lives at home with parents
Family history: non-contributory

VITAL SIGNS						
Time	Temp(F) Rt	Pulse	Resp	Syst BP	Diast BP	Pulse Ox
15:00	97.8	75	12	110	70	99% RA

Constitutional: Alert and well developed, No acute distress
Mental Status/Psychiatric: Affect appropriate for age
Head: Without temporal or scalp tenderness, masses, or lesions.
Eyes: PERRL, EOMI
Neck: Supple. No tenderness. No lymphadenopathy.
Lungs: Clear to auscultation and breath sounds equal.
Heart: RRR, nl heart sounds, without pathological murmurs, gallops, or rubs.
Abd: soft NT ND + bs
Back: no flank tenderness to palpation, no midline tenderness, + paraspinal tenderness to lumbar region, no bruises or evidence of trauma.
Neurological: Motor functions intact. 5/5 hip flexion bilaterally, 5/5 toe dorsiflexion, normal 2 point discrimination to upper and lower extremities. Normal gait but appears to have pain with movement. Negative straight leg test.

ED COURSE:

11:50 – Ibuprofen 400 mg PO given.
UA – neg for leukocytes, nitrites. WBC 3. No bacteria seen
Urine culture sent
X-rays LS spine: No fractures or acute abnormalities

Progress Notes (12:15): Results of x-ray and UA discussed with patient and family. Mother of patient is upset, requesting an MRI. I explained that an MRI could be obtained as an outpatient with her pediatrician, but was not clinically indicated at this time emergently. Her exam remained unchanged with no specific neurologic complaints or deficits. I explained return precautions with the patient and family.

DIAGNOSIS: Back pain

DISPOSITION (12:15 PM): Patient was discharged home by the ED physician with follow up with her pediatrician next week. Patient ambulated independently. Return precautions given. (Mother noted to be extremely upset that MRI was not performed.)

Lacey Peterson, MD

RESIDENT RECOLLECTION OF VISIT #3:

"I remember a healthy 12 year old girl who I evaluated on her 3rd ED visit. I reviewed her prior 2 visits and saw she had a contaminated urine specimen the week prior. Her vital signs had been normal on both prior visits and her exam was normal on both visits. On the 3rd presentation, I had a hard time talking to the patient because the mother was upset and continued to interrupt the history. The patient was sitting on the gurney and was not in acute distress. She had normal vital signs and an unremarkable examination except for bilateral paraspinal pain R > L. She had a normal gait, reproducible pain with movement or bending, normal strength in her lower and upper extremities and normal sensation. We asked the mother to step out of the room and inquired about illicit drug use, abuse or other things going on at home. The patient was quiet, but stated there was nothing else in the history. She denied sexual activity, any recent trauma and IV drug abuse. She stopped gymnastics because her back was sore, and she thought it was making it worse. No abdominal pain, pelvic pain, nausea, vomiting or diarrhea. When her mother came in the room, she demanded an MRI. We tried to explain that an MRI was not indicated emergently, as she had a normal neurologic exam. I ordered an x-ray of her LS spine, mostly to try and appease the mother, and we sent another urine sample and added on a culture. Her work up was negative; we sent her home with return precautions and follow up with her pediatrician. I thought this likely was a back strain."

MANAGING PARENTAL EXPECTATIONS AND DEMANDS: HOW TO NEGOTIATE AROUND INTERESTS, NOT POSITIONS

Paul Charlton, MD

Emergency Medicine Resident PGY-1
Division of Emergency Medicine, University of Washington
Master's degree, Conflict Resolution, Georgetown University

The EP in this case faces two tasks: addressing the patient's medical care and the mother's concerns. The mother's anger and demands require skillful negotiation. Such conflicts can be productive if harnessed in a positive way; destructive if not.[1] Three overarching principles should be used to defuse and reassure the patient/family:

1. **Identify and address the emotional components of the conflict.**[2]
    a. The mother's emotions are high, and the EP can utilize body language to help shift the tone: sit down, lean forward, and uncross your arms.
    b. Address your feelings and the mother's: "This seems like it has been frustrating for you ... You seem dissatisfied with how things have gone on your previous visits." Be willing to acknowledge our role in the conflict.
    c. If you feel your own emotions getting harder to control, consider stepping out of the room to recompose.
2. When a difficult conversation isn't going how we'd like, **listening is typically more powerful (and more time efficient) than talking.**[3] Listen for a purpose: to understand their "story" (how they perceive this conflict, and the reasons for their actions); and to identify their interests (goals, needs).

a. "Help me understand … what are you most worried about today?"
b. "What concerns you about this plan for your daughter's care?"
c. "What is most important for you in this visit?"

3. **Negotiate around interests, not positions.**[4] Positions are what people ask for. Interests are the needs, goals, or concerns that underlie those positions. Common interests include the need to feel respected, to feel listened to, and to feel like we are fulfilling our obligations (as a parent, or as a health care professional).
    - Mother's *position:* "I want an MRI for my daughter"
    - Mother's *interests:* "I want to be a good parent … I want to know that she doesn't have a serious illness … I want to know that there is a plan for treating this in the future … I want to know that my physicians are listening to me and understand how bad I feel."

The next step—get on the same page

Use interests to identify common, shared goals. "We both want to make sure that your daughter is safe … We both want your daughter to receive all of the medical care that she needs and none of the extra tests or procedures that could hurt her."

The management plan

Craft the management plan around meeting each side's interests. "Tell me if I have understood you correctly: It seems that your goals for this visit today are to (make sure that nothing serious is wrong with your daughter), (ensure that we have a management plan for getting your daughter feeling better), and (to feel comfortable when you leave here that we've done everything that is medically indicated for her). Is this accurate?"

1. *Explicitly spell out the plan and document it in the medical record* when the risk for a bounceback or unsatisfactory outcome is likely. "We've talked about a plan today where we will do X, and Y, and Z, does this seem like a reasonable approach? Are there other concerns that we need to address?"
2. *Close the loop* by calling the primary care provider/pediatrician (or offering definitive time to return to the ED if they don't have a PCP) to ensure they understand coordination and agreement with plan of care and availability of follow up.

In our case, such a discussion might have allowed the mother to feel heard and addressed her difficulty accessing timely pediatric follow up. While it is not uncommon for a patientto be told about a 2 week follow up, a call from the ED to the pediatrician/PCP may ensure much more rapid follow up.

1. Azouley E, et al. Prevalence and factors in intensive care unit conflicts: the conflicus study. Am J Respir Crit Care Med. 2009;80(9):853–60.
2. Stone D, Patton B, Heen S. Difficult conversations. New York NY: Penguin Books, 2010.
3. Shell GR. Bargaining for advantage. 2nd ed. New York NY: Penguin Books 2006.
4. Fisher R, Ury W, Patton B. Getting to yes. 3rd ed. New York NY: Penguin Books 2011.

III. The Bounceback (2 weeks later)

- **Hisory:** Patient presents to a different emergency department because of worsening back pain and urinary retention.
- **Examination:** Vital signs normal. Examination reveals severe bilateral paraspinal back pain.
- **Testing:** MRI is ordered, but not yet performed.
- RN attempts to place a foley catheter and realizes "something is wrong" and goes to get the doctor.
- **Re-exam:** On external GU examination, patient noted to have intact bulging blue hymen
- GYN is consulted and diagnoses hematocolpos (accumulation of menstrual blood in the vaginal usually due to imperforate hymen).
- Patient admitted for hymenotomy.
- Mother was upset that a pelvic exam had not been performed on prior visits and diagnosis was not made until several weeks later.

FINAL DIAGNOSIS: Hematocolpos secondary to imperforate hymen

IV. Greg Henry Comments

"The examination of the pediatric patient changes markedly when they become an adolescent"

I've long held the belief that a third visit requires intervention by *somebody*. The patient was not in extremis; the debate now begins as to what further work up should be done. An MRI is relatively benign, but was not the diagnostic test of choice; *physical examination* was! Age 12 is a pivotal moment. Some young women at 12 will look 20, some will look 5. The comment in the physical exam under constitutional is alert and well developed—what does that mean? The examination of the pediatric patient changes markedly when they become an adolescent.

In this case there was no inquiry as to her menstrual history. We now enter a difficult realm; a discussion needs to be held as to why a pelvic examination might be required. Discussions of everything from intercourse, menses, drug usage, and a whole host of other subjects become more difficult in the presence of the parents. To think that a 2-year-old and a 12-year-old should both be considered to have similar pediatric examinations is not to understand the maturation of the species.

PART 2—THE ANALYSIS

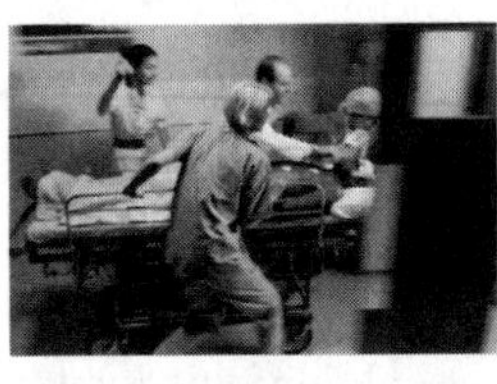

EVALUATION OF BACK PAIN, WHEN TO DO A GU EXAM IN AN ADOLESCENT, HEMATOCOLPOS

Cassie Zhuang, MD
Emergency Medicine Resident PGY-2
University of Texas Health Science Center at San Antonio

Gillian Schmitz, MD, FACEP
Associate Program Director
Department of Emergency Medicine
University of Texas Health Science Center at San Antonio

Evaluation of the Adolescent with Back Pain: The differential diagnosis

Adults presenting with back pain trigger consideration of a number of life threatening pathologies including AAA, epidural compression syndrome (cauda equina), and pancreatitis, to name a few. In contrast, *children and adolescents* are less likely to have these diagnoses. Benign musculoskeletal disease and trauma account for most cases of back pain in children and adolescents, however other causes, including congenital conditions, infection, inflammatory disease, and neoplasm, also must be considered.

In most large published series, including those from referral centers, the majority of children with back pain receive no definitive diagnosis.[16-19]

More common pathologies include:

- Urinary tract infections (pyelonephritis)
- Musculoskeletal injuries
- Spondylolysis and spondylolisthesis
- Scoliosis

Less common pathologies, particularly in a patient who has bounced back several times, include:

- Malignancy such as osteoid osteoma
- Physical or sexual abuse
- Sickle cell crisis
- Infections including discitis (vertebral osteomyelitis) and spinal epidural abscess
- Non vertebral infections such as pyomyositis, pneumonia and PID (in adolescent females)
- Fracture
- Primary renal disorders

Factors that warrant additional evaluation include patient age younger than 4 years, persistent symptoms, self-imposed activity limitations, systemic symptoms, increasing discomfort, persistent nighttime pain, and neurologic symptoms.[5]

History and Physical exam

Interviewing the adolescent patient can be difficult when trying to elicit information that can change the direction of a workup. It is critical to allow an opportunity to interview the patient alone and ask questions regarding sexual behavior, sexual orientation, gynecologic symptoms and drug and alcohol use. It is crucial to gain the adolescent's trust by stating that the information they share with the physician will be kept confidential unless there is a risk for the safety of the adolescent.

In addition, it is important to assure the parents that information regarding the safety of their child will be communicated. However, if state statute qualifies the patient as an emancipated minor, parental/guardian consent is not required and confidentiality with the patient must be maintained, only discuss their protected health information with the parent/guardian if the disclosure is authorized by the patient.

Asking about the last menstrual cycle (to rule out possible pregnancy) would have informed the physician that the patient did not have her first period, The history should also include questions regarding low grade fever, night sweats and weight loss to rule out leukemia and other malignancies presenting with bone pain.

A thorough physical exam to include a neurologic exam, along with a urinalysis and urine pregnancy test (regardless of whether the patient admits to sexual activity) should make up the core data. For most cases, that's as far as you will need to go. It is important to remember that in treating the adolescent, or any pediatric patient, you are not only treating the child, but the parent(s) as well!

Testing

Consideration may be given to ordering CBC, CRP or ESR or blood cultures with suspicion of infection, osteomyelitis, or abscess, but the results are not 100% sensitive and even less specific. Hematogenous spread with seeding of the epidural space is the suspected source of infection in most children of spinal epidural abscess.

Reported sources of infection are numerous and include bacterial endocarditis, infected indwelling catheters, urinary tract infection, peritoneal and retroperitoneal infections. Direct extension of infection from vertebral osteomyelitis occurs in adults, but rarely does in children. Additional imaging may be required and will depend on the patient's examination, access to outpatient follow-up and reliability of both patient and family. Communicating with the family is crucial. In a patient with a benign examination on their initial visit, MRI is unlikely to be helpful and may be misleading, but explaining that to the parent is important.

When to do the GU exam?

If the patient admits to sexual activity or if the patient complains of pelvic pain, vaginal discharge, bleeding or discomfort, a gynecologic examination should be considered. Whether or not a speculum exam is necessary will depend on the specific presentation. The physician must balance the trauma of performing a speculum exam, particularly on an adolescent who is not yet sexually active, against what information one may gain from the exam, realizing the speculum and/or internal exam rarely change the course of treatment.[6] In some cases, a limited external exam may be warranted to evaluate for signs of infection, trauma or foreign body or abuse. A pelvic exam is generally not indicated on a patient who complains only of back pain, but an external exam might be considered if the patient continues to have symptoms remaining unexplained.

Hematocolpos

Hematocolpos, the accumulation of menstrual blood in the vagina, as the result of an imperforate hymen has a reported occurrence of 1 in 2,000 girls.[7] An imperforate hymen is an isolated abnormality that often goes undetected until the onset of menstruation. Only 50% of cases are detected during the neonatal period.[8] Retained blood accumulates and leads to hematocolpos, hematometra (retained blood in the uterus), and hematosalpinx (retained blood in the fallopian tube). The typical presentation is cyclical lower abdominal or pelvic pain in a premenarchal female.[9]

Hematocolpos in any presentation is rarely seen in the emergency department, with less than 20 case reports found. Current literature cites that the most common (40–60%) presentation of hematocolpos is urinary hesitancy or dysuria.[6] Six case reports of hematocolpos presenting with back pain were found. Many of the case reports, regardless of the primary presenting symptom, presented scenarios in which the patient was misdiagnosed/undiagnosed at the first several visits, with alternate diagnoses such as urinary tract infections (as in our patient), appendicitis, nephrolithiasis, and abdominal tumor.[8]

One case report presented a 14-year-old girl who had been experiencing lower back and abdominal pain for 6 months and was being seen by an orthopedic surgeon when she was found to have acute urinary retention (sound familiar?) When the patient was catheterized for urinary retention, a bulge was noted in the vulva.[11] Another paper presented four cases of lower back pain in adolescent females seen at an orthopedic office; all four of these patients presented with large pelvic masses.[12] A presentation of low back pain, positive straight leg raise test, and signs of L5 radiculopathy was found in a patient found to have hematometra due to congenital absence of the lower third of the vagina, although this would not have been diagnosed by simple visual inspection.[13] Constipation has also been documented as a possible presenting symptom of hematocolpos, although more rare in isolation and more often associated with abdominal pain.[14, 15]

Making the Diagnosis

Although the diagnosis of imperforate hymen associated with hematocolpos can usually be highly suspected by visual inspection, ultrasonography should be performed to confirm the diagnosis, determine the direct cause of hematocolpos (imperforate hymen, vaginal septum, etc.) and rule out any other urogenital anomalies. Renal anomalies have been suggested to be associated with concurrent genital anomalies.[10]

Despite variations worldwide and within the U.S. population, median age at menarche has remained relatively stable, between 12 and 13 years, across well-nourished populations in developed countries.[20] Of note, higher gain in body mass index (BMI) during childhood is related to an earlier onset of puberty.[21] Delay in the expected start of menstruation should trigger the questions regarding regular monthly abdominal pain/cramps to think of hematocolpos. In this case, the patient was still in the acceptable age range for the start of her period.

Treatment

Treatment for imperforate hymen involves creating and maintaining an opening in the hymen. Hymenotomy may be followed by various techniques to minimize vaginal scarring to include surgical procedures or conservative treatment with indwelling intra-vaginal catheters.[10]

Consequences of a missed diagnosis

A missed diagnosis of hematocolpos can lead to hematosalpinx, which may place patients at a higher risk for developing infertility. Increased pressure within the fallopian tubes can destroy ciliary action and clotted blood can produce adhesions and obstructions; both of these scenarios can lead to blockage or difficulty passing the ova from the ovaries to the uterus. Endometriosis may develop from the refluxing of menstrual blood through the fallopian tubes into the peritoneal cavity. [14]

Back to our case

Although our patient's mother asked specifically for an MRI, it seems that she was *really* asking for a plan to find the cause of her daughter's back pain. She felt like she was being blown off. Directly addressing her concerns and expectations was attempted, but rejected, likely because the EP started behind the 8-ball. This was already her third ED visit. Though this would not have made the diagnosis, engaging the mother and daughter and primary care doctor/ pediatrician in a pre-discharge plan may have helped demonstrate concern for the patient.

✔ Teaching Points

- Children/adolescents (unlike adults) do not usually have chronic or worsening back pain. Have a higher threshold to look for other pathology. Warning flags include pain in toddlers, night pain and neurologic or progressive symptoms such as urinary retention or constipation.
- Assume the adolescent patient is sexually active and/or pregnant until proven otherwise, obtain a pregnancy test and consider an external genital examination with persistent or unexplained symptoms.

➤**Author's note (MW):** This case demonstrates some important principles in pediatric emergency medicine; the importance of an age-focused differential diagnosis, management of patient *and* parental expectations, and the value of an expanded history and physical on the third visit. I think Madeline would agree, *children* are not small adults ... and neither are *adolescents!*

References

1. Azouley E, et al. Prevalence and factors in intensive care unit conflicts: the conflicus study. Am J Respir Crit Care Med. 2009;80(9):853–60.
2. Stone D, Patton B, and Heen S. Difficult conversations. New York NY: Penguin Books, 2010.
3. Shell GR. Bargaining for advantage. 2nd ed. New York NY: Penguin Books 2006.
4. Fisher R, Ury W, Patton B. Getting to yes. 3rd ed. New York NY: Penguin Books 2011.
5. Bernstein R, Cozen H. Evaluation of Back Pain in Children and Adolescents. Am Fam Physician. 2007;76(11):1669–76.
6. Brown J, et al. Does pelvic exam in the emergency department add useful information? West J Emerg Med. 2011;12(2):208–12.
7. Adali E, et al. An overlooked cause of acute urinary retention in an adolescent girl: a case report. Arch Gynecol Obstet. 2009;279(5):701–3.
8. Hingorani R, Swain A. An unusual cause of lower abdominal pain in pubertal girls. Emerg Med J. 2009;26(12):909–10.
9. Kumar K, Waseem M. An uncommon cause of abdominal pain in an adolescent. South Med J. 2008;101(10):1065–6.
10. Chircop R. A case of retention of urine and haematocolpometra. Eur J Emerg Med. 2003;10(3):244–5.
11. Buick RG, Chowdhary SK. Backache: a rare diagnosis and unusual complication. Pediatr Surg Int. 1999;15(8):586–7.
12. Letts M, Haasbeek J. Hematocolpos as a cause of back pain in premenarchal adolescents. J Pediatr Orthop. 1990;10(6):731–2.
13. Deathe AB. Hematometra as a cause of lumbar radiculopathy. A case report. Spine. 1993;18(13):1920–1.
14. Isenhour JL, Hanley ML, Marx JA. Hematocolpometra manifesting as constipation in the young female. Acad Emerg Med. 1999;6(7):752–3.
15. Dickson CA, Saad S, Tesar JD. Imperforate hymen with hematocolpos. Ann Emerg Med. 1985;14(5):467–9.
16. Selbst SM, Lavelle JM, Soyupak SK, Markowitz RI. Back pain in children who present to the emergency department. Clin Pediatr (Phila). 1999;38:401–6.
17. Combs JA, Caskey PM. Back pain in children and adolescents: a retrospective review of 648 patients. South Med J. 1997;90:789–92.
18. Feldman DS, Hedden DM, Wright JG. The use of bone scan to investigate back pain in children and adolescents. J Pediatr Orthop. 2000;20:790–5.
19. Bhatia NN, Chow G, Timon SJ, Watts HG. Diagnostic modalities for the evaluation of pediatric back pain: a prospective study. J Pediatr Orthop. 2008;28:230–3. Nonspecific musculoskeletal pain accounts for at least 50 percent of cases [Kim HJ, Green DW. Adolescent back pain. Curr Opin Pediatr. 2008;20:37–45].
20. Chumlea WE, Schubert CM, Roche AF, et al. Age at menarche and racial comparisons in US girls. Pediatrics. 2003;111:110–3.
21. Wang Y. Is obesity associated with early sexual maturation? A comparison of the association in American boys versus girls. Pediatr. 2002;110:903–10.

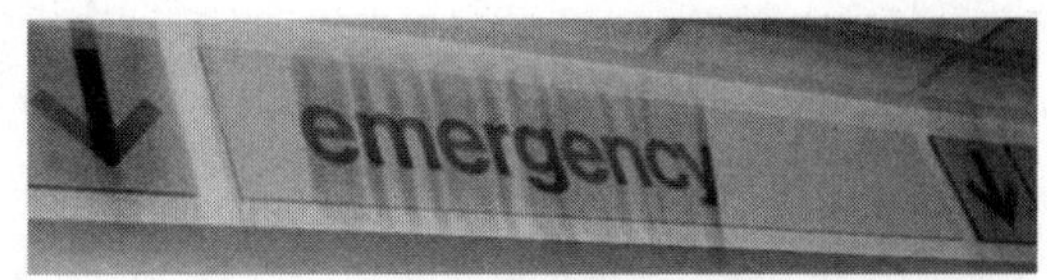

CASE 8

8-MONTH-OLD INFANT WITH POSSIBLE INGESTION

Ilene Claudius, MD
Associate Professor of Clinical Emergency Medicine
Keck School of Medicine of the University of Southern California

Michael Levine, MD
Assistant Professor of Clinical Emergency Medicine
Keck School of Medicine of the University of Southern California

PART 1—MEDICAL

PART 2—THE ANALYSIS

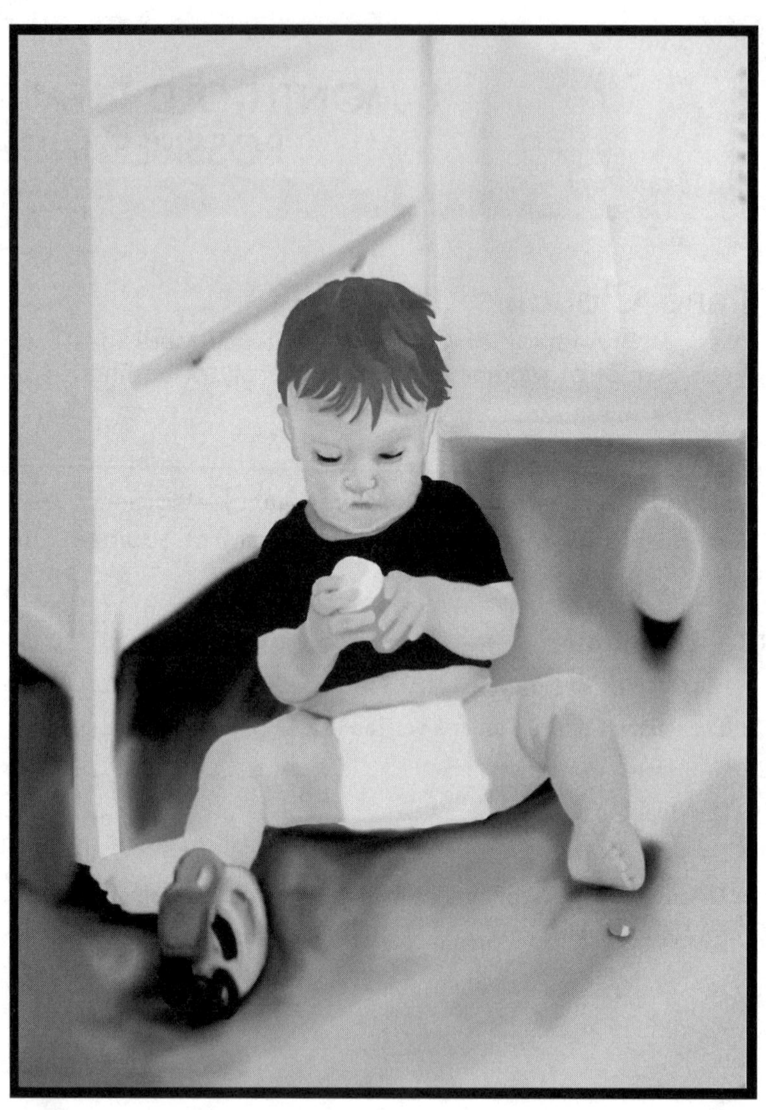

CASE 8

8-MONTH-OLD INFANT WITH POSSIBLE INGESTION

PART 1—MEDICAL

I. The Doctor's Version (the following is the actual documentation of the provider)

Date: 7/15/2009 at 11:20
Chief Complaint: Ate pill
Nurse note: Possible ingestion of an unknown pill 1 hour ago. Patient acting normal per mother.

History of Present Illness: Patient is an 8 month old infant presenting 1 hour after possible ingestion of an unknown pill. He was crawling in a department store dressing room when he ingested a pill he found on the floor. Per the mother, who witnessed the event, there was no emesis, and his behavior has been at baseline.

Review of Systems: All systems reviewed and are negative.
Past Medical History: None

VITAL SIGNS

Time	Temp(C)	Pulse	Resp	Sat
11:25	36.5	116	22	99%

PHYSICAL EXAM: Note: The chart's physical exam relied on check boxes. The following boxes were checked
General: Nontoxic
Lungs: Clear
CV: Regular Rate and Rhythm
Abdomen: Soft, nontender
Neuro: Awake and oriented x3

ED Course: Glucose was checked on admission and found to be 81 mg/dL. Urine toxicology was performed, and was negative. The patient was observed in the department for 4 hours and remained asymptomatic.

Progress Note (15:00): playful, interactive

Diagnosis: Unknown ingestion

Disposition: Home at 15:30 on 7/15/2009

II. The Poison Control Center's (PCC) Version

➢**Authors' note (MW):** When there is an adverse event, the primary source of information is the documentation of the provider. But don't rest on your chart being the only record.

Dr: I have an 8 month old here who was in a changing room at a department store. Mom thinks he ate a pill he found on the floor, but isn't 100% sure and has no idea what it was. She doesn't take any medicines and didn't have anything in her purse that might have fallen out.

PCC: In this situation, we recommend admission. It's possible it was a sulfonylurea, a long-acting calcium channel blocker, Lomotil, bupropion, or some other drug which requires a prolonged period of observation.

Dr: But even if the patient took one of these, the chance of a complication is small. That's a lot of "mights." To argue that the patient might have taken one of these pills and then might have a complication from it. It sounds overly conservative.

PCC: That is our recommendation. Would you like to talk to the toxicologist?

Dr: No. Thank you

Note: The PCC called back several hours later to check on the patient and was informed the child had been discharged home.

➢***Chapter Authors' comments:***

Sounding arrogant on medic, transfer, and PCC calls (which are routinely taped) is a bad idea, particularly if coupled with a refusal to follow the center's advice. Additionally, why ask a question when you don't want to know the answer? While I sometimes balk at bad advice from consultants, I wouldn't call the PCC if I was going to send the kid home in 4 hours regardless of what they told me. Not following a consultant's advice is often worse than deciding not to contact them in the first place.

➢**Author's note (MW):** Below is a slightly different take on this interaction from Greg Henry.

III. Greg Henry Comments

"If this child has a bad outcome, such as brain damage from prolonged hypoglycemia, the tape from the poison control center will be the smoking gun which turns this case into your worst medical legal nightmare."

When are we ever going to learn that you never ask a question you don't want to know the answer to? Why in the world was poison control called? We didn't have a specific medication to get information about. All this call did was place the EP in greater medical legal jeopardy.

Except for consideration of re-checking the blood glucose an hour before discharge, I think this child was handled appropriately. The child looked well at discharge; it's hard to beat normal. The chances that a child found a sulfonylurea, long-acting calcium channel blocker or other life-threatening medication on the floor of a dressing room, as mentioned by the PCC, has got to be amazingly small. If every child who looked normal was admitted, there would be no place to put them all. I commend the emergency physician for not doing something silly, like placing an NG tube, giving IV fluids or charcoal, or in any other way torturing the child.

Going back to the PCC call, If this child has a bad outcome, such as brain damage from prolonged hypoglycemia, the tape from the poison control center will be the smoking gun which turns this case into your worst medical legal nightmare.

IV. The Bounceback

Date: 7/15/2009 at 18:50 (3 hours 20 minutes after initial ED discharge)
CC: Altered Mental Status

History of Present Illness: Patient is an 8-month-old male seen previously today for ingestion of an unknown pill, which occurred while he was crawling around the floor of a dressing room. He was observed for 4 hours and discharged home. Approximately 3 hours after discharge, he was noted to be somnolent by his mother who called EMS. On their arrival, he was unresponsive except for the occasional weak cry. An accucheck was 18 mg/dL. He was given 0.5 mg glucagon IM by medics prior to transport.

ED Course:

18:50 Arrived in ED escorted by medics
18:53: Repeat glucose 45 mg/dL
19:01: IV established and 5 mL/kg of D10W administered
19:05: Repeat glucose 158 mg/dL
20:00 Repeat glucose 68 mg/dL
20:05: In response to the fall in glucose over one hour, 1mcg/kg of octreotide was administered subcutaneously and the patient transferred to the PICU for admission

Hospital Course:

In conjunction with a toxicology consult, the decision was made to treat the patient as a sulfonylurea ingestion. He was encouraged to maintain his normal feeding regimen and monitored overnight with glucose checks every 1–2 hours. He had one additional episode of hypoglycemia to 40 mg/dL three hours after admission to the PICU, which was treated with a 5 mL/kg bolus of D10W. Otherwise, his hospital course was uneventful, and he was discharged after 19 hours of monitoring without additional hypoglycemic episodes.

Final diagnosis: Altered consciousness secondary to hypoglycemia secondary to sulfonylurea ingestion

PART 2—THE ANALYSIS

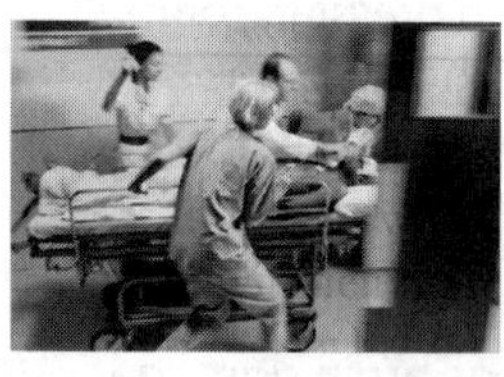

RECOGNITION, EVALUATION AND MANAGEMENT OF PEDIATRIC INGESTIONS

Ilene Claudius, MD

Assistant Professor of Clinical Emergency Medicine
Keck School of Medicine of the University of Southern California

Michael Levine, MD

Assistant Professor of Clinical Emergency Medicine
Keck School of Medicine of the University of Southern California

Our patient:

Certainly, this patient experienced an acceptable outcome. Would that have been the case if the ingestion had occurred in the evening, rather than the morning? Unlikely. The drop in serum glucose from sulfonylurea overdoses is delayed, but when it occurs, glucose plummets quickly. Were the child and family asleep at the time, chances are good that the diagnosis would have been ultimately made at autopsy.

Ingestions in pediatric population:

Ingestions are common in young children, but most are benign, commonly involving household cleaning and cosmetic products, analgesics, and topical preparations. Ingestions of medications, which can lead to significant morbidity, even in small quantities, are rare, and those with a delayed onset are even more rare. As reflected in the Poison Center call, the bad actors include:

1. Sulfonylureas
2. Sustained release calcium channel blockers
3. Sustained release bupropion (Wellbutrin)
4. Diphenoxylate/atropine (Lomotil)

These 4 meds will be the focus of our review. Cases involving these agents, or an unknown agent that may fall into these categories, are particularly challenging for the provider who must convince not only him or herself, but the family, the staff, the accepting physician and the insurer that admission or prolonged observation of the asymptomatic, well-appearing child is necessary.

Sulfonylurea ingestion:

Most of the "one pill can kill" medications aren't ubiquitous in the population, or are they occult when a child ingests them. People don't walk around with a purse full of quinine, and there is a contributory history when a child ingests gun bluing fluid (selenious acid).

However, with nearly 20 million diabetics in America alone,[1] sulfonylureas are common inhabitants of grandma's purse. In 2008, 4,308 sulfonylurea ingestions were reported to US Poison Control Centers.[2] They bind to the SUR1 receptor on the surface of the pancreatic â-cells, closing potassium channels, and releasing insulin.[3] This effectively lowers the blood glucose in diabetics, but also places non-diabetic patients at risk for hypoglycemia.

Depending on the specific sulfonylurea, peak plasma concentrations and subsequent rise in insulin levels occur between 1 and 8 hours after ingestion in adults taking therapeutic doses.[4] These drugs have a long duration of action. In a child under age 4 years, as little as a single tablet of chlorpropamide (250 mg), glipizide (5 mg), or glyburide (2.5 mg) can cause profound hypoglycemia.[5]

A Poison Center review of sulfonylurea ingestion in children 1–16 years of age found hypoglycemia to occur in 27% with an onset of 0.5–16 hours post ingestion (mean 4.3 hours).[5] A more recent review found hypoglycemia in 44% of ingestions, with an upper limit of 13 hours after ingestion.[6] Current recommendations vary, but observation for 16 hours, or up to 24 hours from time of ingestion, is most commonly considered safe.

When hypoglycemia occurs from a sulfonylurea ingestion, urgent treatment with IV dextrose is appropriate (D10W at 5 mL/kg for infants; D25W at 2 mL/kg for toddlers and older children and D50W for adolescents 1 mL/Kg). When IV access is not available, glucagon delivered IM will mobilize glycogen stores. Unfortunately, repeated administration of glucose or glucagon will further stimulate pancreatic release of insulin, exacerbating the underlying problem which results in recurrent hypo-glycemia.

Octreotide, a somatostatin analogue, inhibits release from pancreatic islet cells, and is ideal treatment for sulfonylurea-related hypoglycemia (1–1.5 mcg/kg subcutaneously or intravenously up to every 6 hours if hypoglycemic).[7] Glucose should be monitored every 1–2 hours, and the patient maintained on their home diet.

Other considerations in the hypoglycemic child following an unknown ingestion include:

1. Ethanol
2. β-blockers
3. Salicylates

Calcium channel blocker ingestion:

Long-acting calcium channel blockers are also a realistic concern, and sustained release versions of diltiazem, verapamil, nifedipine, felodipine, nisoldipine and nicardipine exist. Recommendations for young children with ingestion include observation for 6 hours if immediate release and 12–24 hours if sustained release.[1]

The risk of an adverse outcome for an infant or toddler ingesting one adult pill is far less clearly delineated. Deaths of this nature are certainly reported, but seem to be less common than adverse outcomes with sulfonylureas.[8] Unfortunately, there are no clear means of determining which child is likely to have an uncommon adverse outcome.

If a patient becomes symptomatic, hypotension can occur in the setting of either bradycardia or reflex tachycardia.[7] AV conduction disturbances, orthostasis, alteration of mental status, pulmonary edema and hyperglycemia can also occur. One case series noted the onset of symptoms to be up to 14 hours following ingestion of a sustained release preparation.[9]

Typical treatment includes IV fluid boluses, atropine, calcium, and norepinephrine. High dose insulin (positive inotrope)/glucose therapy has shown some promise in calcium channel blocker overdoses, and there may be a role for IV lipid emulsion specifically in diltiazem or verapamil at a dose of 1.5 mg/kg over 1 minute.

Diphenoxylate/atropine (Lomotil) ingestion:

Lomotil contains diphenoxylate and atropine, and is typically avoided as an anti-diarrheal in the pediatric population due to its potential for severe and delayed toxicity. Absorption of the drug is usually rapid, but the more potent metabolite, difenoxin, may take time to build up and has a long half-life, 12–14 hours.

"Classic" presentation of early onset anticholinergic symptoms, followed by delayed onset opioid toxicity is rare; most patients experience only the delayed phase. Additionally, the opioid-related symptoms of respiratory depression and coma can resolve then recur up to 2 hours later.[10] Toxicity has been reported after ingestion of half a pill.[11] Observation of 24 hours or more is recommended. Treatment is for symptomatic opioid toxicity.

Bupropion (Wellbutrin) ingestion:

Bupropion is an aminoketone class of antidepressant, which is often used for smoking cessation. Toxicity can result in tachycardia and delayed seizures. Because of the risk of delayed seizures, patients who ingest more than 450 mg (adults) or more than 8 mg/kg (pediatric) of extended release bupropion should be admitted to a monitored bed for 24 hours.

Chapter Summary

Although not an issue relevant to this case, another common medical legal pitfall in pediatric ingestions is clinician failure to consider intentional poisoning. In children outside the typical age range (those < 1 year or 5–11 years), children exposed to unusual or illicit substances or those with inconsistent or suspicious histories, consideration of child abuse may prevent future fatal abuse-related events.[12]

Unlike many bouncebacks, in this particular case, the presentation was not subtle. The history was handed to the clinician, and the recommendations clearly outlined. The diagnosis was initially missed in the same way sepsis is missed in normotensive children, the same way that abuse victims are sent home, and the same way patients with conditions like Pertussis or intussusception (who look completely fine between symptomatic episodes) are dismissed; we expect ill children to look ill. Even the most astute clinicians overlook the fact that children may appear well until only moments before they decompensate.

Finally, if you choose to ignore a consultant's recommendations, give a clear explanation of your thought process and medical reasoning, outlining the rationale for not following the recommendation(s) because If there is an adverse outcome, you can be sure someone will be looking at your chart.

References

1. Cowie CC, Rust KF, Byrd-Holt DD, et al. Prevalence of diabetes and impaired fasting glucose in adults in the U.S. population: National Health and Nutrition Examination Survey 1999–2002. Diabetes Care. 2006;29:1263–8.
2. Bronstein AC, Spyker DA, Cantilena LR, et al. 2008 Annual report of the American Association of Poison Control Centers' National Poison Data System: 26th annual report. Clin Tox. 2009;47:911–1084.
3. Fowler MJ. Diabetes treatment, Part 2: Oral agents for glycemic management. Clinical Diabetes. 2007;25(4):131–4.
4. Ferner RE, Chaplin S. The relationship between the pharmacokinetics and pharmacodynamics effects of oral hypoglycaemic drugs. Clin Pharmacokinet. 1987;12:379–401.
5. Quadrani DA, Spiller HA, Widder P. Five year retrospective evaluation of sulfonylurea ingestion in children. J Toxicol CLin Tox. 1996;34:267–70.
6. Levine M, Ruha AM, Lovecchio F, Riley BD, Pizon AF, Burns BD, et al. Hypoglycemia after accidental pediatric sulfonylurea ingestions. PEC. 2011;27(9):846–9.
7. Barrueto F, Gattu R, Mazer-Amirshahi M. Updates in the general approach to the pediatric poisoned patients. Ped Clin N Am. 2013;60:1203–20.
8. Ranniger C, Roche C. Are one or two dangerous? Calcium channel blocker exposure in toddlers. J EM. 2007;33(2):145–54.
9. Belson MG, Gorman SE, Sullivan K, Geller RJ. Calcium channel blocker ingestions in children. Am J EM. 2000;18:581–6.
10. Michael JB, Sztajnkrycer MD. Deadly pediatric poisons: nine common agents that kill at low doses. EM Clin N Am. 2004;22(4):1019–50.
11. Wasserman GS, Green VA, Wise GW. Lomotil ingestions in children. Am Fam Phys. 1975;11:93–7.
12. Calello DP, Henretig FM. Pediatric toxicology: specialized approach to the poisoned child. Emerg Clin N Am. 2014;32(1):29–52.

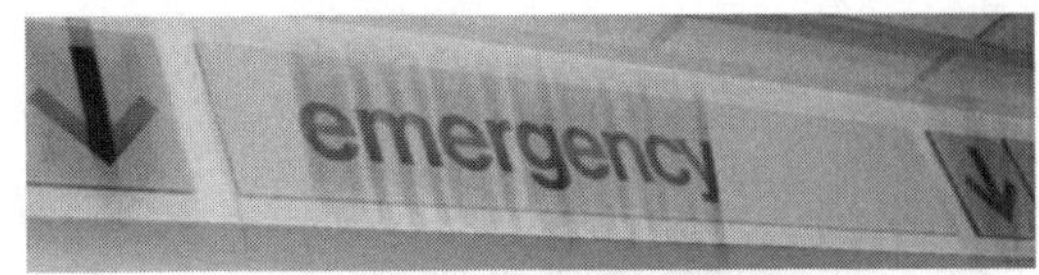

CASE 9

17-YEAR-OLD BOY WITH ABDOMINAL PAIN

Matt Dawson, MD, RDMS, RDCS
Director of Point of Care Ultrasound
Assistant EM Program Director
University of Kentucky

PART 1—MEDICAL

PART 2—THE ANALYSIS

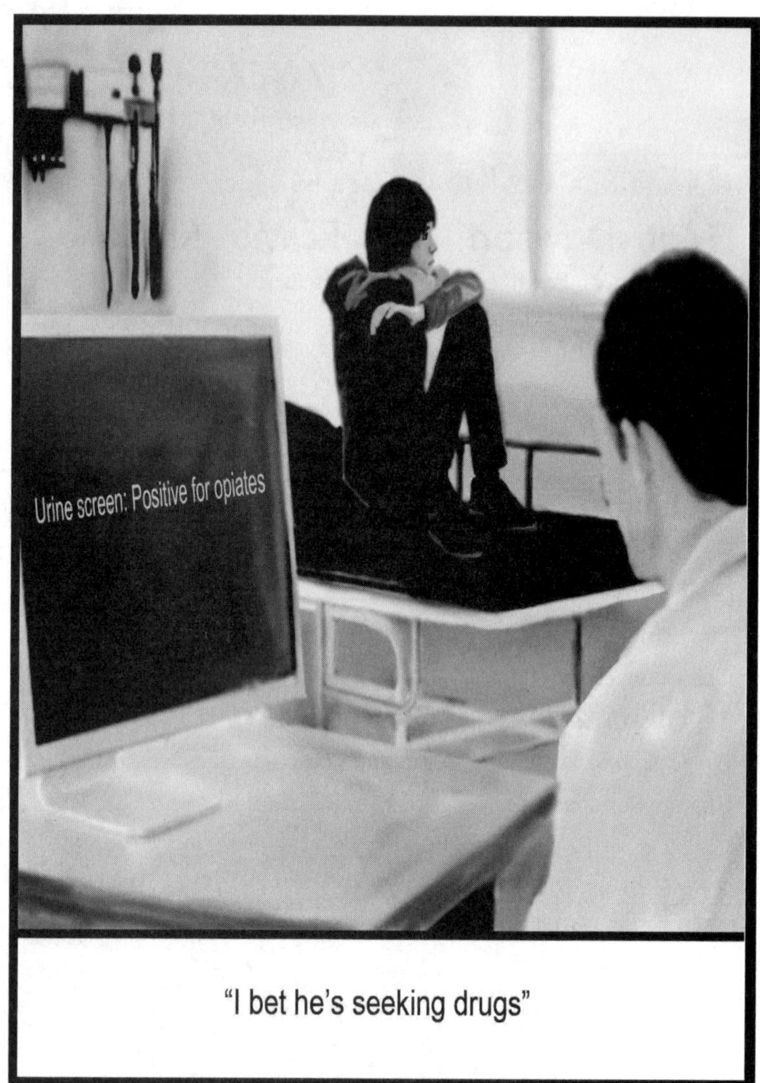

"I bet he's seeking drugs"

CASE 9

A 17-YEAR-OLD BOY WITH ABDOMINAL PAIN

PART 1—MEDICAL

I. The Doctor's Version (the following is the actual documentation of the provider)

Date: March 4th, 2010 at 23:57
Chief complaint: Abdominal pain
Nurse note: Pt complains of generalized abdominal pain for 4 hours. 10/10.

HISTORY OF PRESENT ILLNESS – Patient complains of abdominal pain since about 5pm. He appears comfortable, but states that he has intense abdominal pain since last eating. He has had nothing to eat since that time except a beer. Nausea, but no vomiting. No diarrhea or other complaints.

REVIEW OF SYSTEMS: Normal review of systems except noted in HPI.

PAST MEDICAL HISTORY:
Allergies: Ibuprofen
Medications: Lortab
PMH: Back injury
Social History: smoker. Denies drugs. Social EtOH.

EXAM:

VITAL SIGNS					
Time	Temp(F)	Pulse	Resp	Syst	Diast
00:15	99.9	94	16	115	62

General: NAD.
Skin: No lesions, but extensive tattoos
HEENT: No lesions or TTP, PERRL, EOMI, no lesions, TMs Normal, Normal mucosa, Pharynx without injection, exudate, or hypertrophy. Airway patent.
Neck: Supple. NTTP
Lungs: Clear to auscultation and breath sounds equal bilaterally
Heart: RRR, nl heart sounds, without pathological murmurs, ectopy, gallops, or rubs.
Abdominal: Diffuse TTP. No focal tenderness, rebound or guarding. Non-surgical abdomen.
Neurological: Cranial and cerebellar functions normal. Motor functions intact.
Psychiatric: Normal

ED COURSE:

0020: Labs ordered
0035: IV placed and 1 L NS, 4mg morphine, and 4mg Zofran given.
0112: CBC, UA, and BMP WNL. Drug screen positive for narcotics.

MDM: Pt complains of abdominal pain, but he appears comfortable when checked on. He is sleeping comfortable when re-examined and doesn't seem to be in distress. He asks for more pain medication, but he has no signs of abdominal pathology on testing and we are concerned he may be drug seeking with positive drug test for narcotics. He is discharged to home and instructed to follow up with his PCP.

DIAGNOSIS: Abdominal pain

Nursing discharge note:

VITAL SIGNS

Time	Temp(F)	HR	RR	Syst	Diast	Pain
01:30	100.1	97	16	107	74	8/10

DISPOSITION (0145): Pt discharged to home with a prescription for Zofran and instructed to follow up with PCP or return if worse. His mother arrives and takes him home.

William Savage, MD

II. Greg Henry Comments

"Males are relatively simple creatures; beside the appendix, everything else you want to check on is out in the open"

There are some interesting aspects to this case. Emergency physicians, like everyone else, can be derailed by elements of the history. It is unusual that a 17-year-old would be on a narcotic pain medication for back pain. We need a better history of why he is being treated in this fashion.

Secondly, a 17-year-old boy with lower abdominal pain is appendicitis till proven otherwise. Males are relatively simple creatures; beside the appendix, everything else you want to check on is out in the open.

I am not certain why the physical exam does not comment on the genitalia—intermittent testicular torsions can present like this. A word of clarification; there is no literature supporting a rectal exam to help diagnose lower abdominal pain. If patients have rectal complaints, that's different.

Considering the patient's temperature it gets into the "close but no cigar" game, which no one ever wins. It is or it isn't. There is very little data to suggest that the temperature is in anyway definitive in diagnosing appendicitis. It is about as accurate as the white blood count, which in teenage boys can be grossly inaccurate.

Abdominal pain in healthy young men can be followed as an outpatient. Pronounced vomiting, localizing of pain, or unresolved pain should result in a re-examination within the next 8–12 hours. The concept of re-examination has been lost in this country. The surgeon who waits until the temperature or WBC count goes up is going to have an increased rate of ruptured appendices.

The diagnostic modalities are never a 100%. In the old days when we made clinical decisions, we were probably 10% wrong, now with CT scans and/or ultrasound we are 5% wrong. Young males, with a good story and the right examination findings, need to have their abdomen explored. This is what I would do for a family member. Never let the skin stand in the way of a diagnosis.

III. The Errors—Risk Management/Patient Safety Issues

Risk management/patient safety issue #1:

Error: Blowing off an adolescent's complaint.

Discussion: Adolescents are a difficult to assess and treat. Of note, under the American Board of Pediatrics, Adolescent Medicine is a subspecialty that requires three additional years of training after pediatric residency! We are all guilty of attributing complaints in this age group to drama or malingering, but maybe this patient was in an MVC recently with back injury that required pain medication. No one asked him any questions to why he was on pain meds.

✔ **Teaching point:** Fight the temptation to quickly dismiss adolescent complaint.

Risk management/patient safety issue #2:

Error: Patient was discharged with significant pain.

Discussion: At discharge, the patient was still complaining of 8/10 abdominal pain. It is hard to say if the doctor was aware of this. If the complaint of pain was attributable to drug seeking, consideration of mental health evaluation could have been considered. If this was not a definitive diagnosis, then the exam would be cursory. Consideration of imaging or plan for imaging if the pain persisted, should have been explored. Of note, the initial examination of this patient did not include a detailed examination of the abdomen and genitalia.

✔ **Teaching point:** With a complaint of abdominal pain, ongoing exam and definitive d/c plan is necessary.

Risk management/patient safety issue #3:

Error: Too narrow differential.

Discussion: There are a myriad of possibilities in adolescents with abdominal pain including the obvious and the not so obvious; does the patient have sickle cell disease? Perhaps this is why he was taking narcotics?

✔ **Teaching point:** Simple pertinent questions in the past medical history could change the course of treatment significantly.

V. The Bounceback

March 5, 2010 (Morning after initial ED visit)

0720: Following morning patient returns with worsening abdominal pain, still diffuse. This is a small ED with single coverage and the patient is in the waiting room when the new physician comes on. At checkout the physician from the night before sees the patient in the waiting room and informs the new physician that the "17 y/o kid with the tattoos" was there the night before and is obviously drug seeking. He had a benign exam and normal labs other than a positive drug screen.

0730: The new physician sees the patient and informs him that he won't be getting any more narcotic medication but that we can repeat his vital signs and lab tests.

VITAL SIGNS

Time	Temp (F)	HR	RR	Syst	Diast	Pain
07:30	99.7	98	16	129	81	10/10

0800: Pt complains that pain is getting worse and wants to know why more isn't being done for him.

The new physician then brings in the bedside ultrasound machine to look at the patients kidneys, gallbladder, and appendix. The ultrasound shows no hydronephrosis, normal gallbladder, but an enlarged 1cm non-compressible appendix (see similar images below). The general surgeon is called.

0820: Surgery arrives to evaluate the patient. Repeat labs including WBC count are still within normal limits, but the exam has changed and the patient is now tender in the RLQ. The images are reviewed with the surgeon and the patient is taken to the OR where the diagnosis of acute appendicitis was confirmed.

FINAL DIAGNOSIS: Acute appendicitis

PART 2—THE ANALYSIS

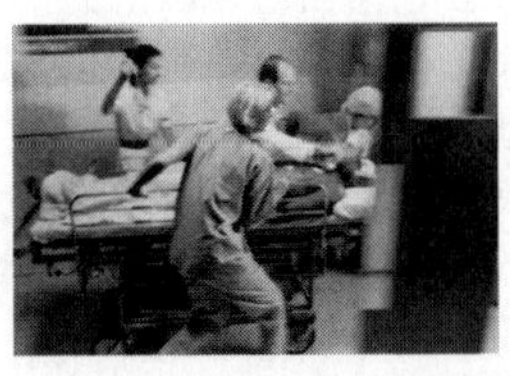

DIAGNOSIS OF APPENDICITIS AND THE ROLE OF ULTRASOUND

Matt Dawson, MD, RDMS, RDCS
Director of Point of Care Ultrasound
Assistant EM Program Director
University of Kentucky

Dr. Dawson is the co-author of Introduction to Bedside Ultrasound Volumes 1 and 2 digital textbooks and the co-creator of The Ultrasound Podcast, One Minute Ultrasound smartphone app, Sonocloud.org, and The Ultrasound Leadership Academy. He has recently received the CORD Innovations in Medical Education Award, ACEP Award for Contribution to EMUS, AEUS Ultrasound Education Award, UKEM Instructor of the Year Award, and UK Distinguished Young Alumnus Award.

Introduction

No harm, no foul, right? I remember this case very vividly because it was one of the first cases of acute appendicitis that I diagnosed with bedside ultrasound and I was very impressed with the surgeon's willingness to take the patient to the OR without any other studies. It was also a memorable case because it illustrated several important points about the diagnosis of appendicitis ... and the possibility of missing it.

Acute appendicitis and WBC counts

Appendicitis is a very common disease. Approximately 80,000 patients are diagnosed with appendicitis each year in the United States.[1] If the patient has a classic presentation, then great! Unfortunately, many patients, like this one, present atypically. He had a normal WBC count, diffuse pain, and simply didn't look like an appy on the initial presentation. He was also a frequent flyer, which colored the initial physician's evaluation.

Point one: WBC counts and appendicitis scores are not sensitive or specific.[2-4]

The normal WBC count and non-classic presentation may have been due to the patient presenting early in the course. This patient's exam did become more "classic" during the second visit with the pain moving to the RLQ. The normal WBC count gave the first provider false confidence that this was benign. He documented a benign abdomen, but the patient's pain was unchanged during the ED course.

Point two: Pain which is not improved needs reassessment and explanation in the chart. Stating "we are concerned he may be drug seeking with positive drug test for narcotics" is curious; there is really not great evidence for this from the chart. In fact, the patient had a reason for the positive drug screen as he freely stated he was taking Lortab (hydrocodone/acetaminophen). Yes, the physician states the patient was sleeping when he checked on him, which seems to be a statement also backing up the thought that this patient had nothing really bad going on. However, if someone has been in extreme pain for some time and they finally gets relief with medication, it would be expected that they fall asleep, especially in the middle of the night (sometime between 1 and 2AM); it certainly doesn't rule out any pathology. It seems that the patient's appearance and demeanor may have affected the physician's evaluation demonstrating:

Point three: As much as we'd like tattoos to be protective against appendicitis or other pathology, they don't seem to be. (I was unable to find a randomized, prospective trial to support this statement, so you'll just have to trust me on this one)!

Radiologic evaluation of appendicitis—CT v. US

The workup and radiologic evaluation of appendicitis is still evolving. The initial physician could have performed a CT scan, but with such a low pre-test probability, the harm may outweigh the benefit. Possibly a better approach to this patient at initial presentation would have been either observation, an ultrasound, or both.

Ultrasound doesn't have the risk of radiation and can be applied in conjunction with observation. Even if no imaging was indicated yet, more observation in the ED seems to have been warranted with a pain level that hadn't changed during the visit. If the patient was still to be discharged, a time and action-specific discharge plan would serve to inform the patient that appendicitis had not been definitively excluded.

Ultrasound has been used for the evaluation of appendicitis for 30 years now and has been reported to have sensitivities ranging from 76–100% and specificities of 88–100%.[5-12] Ultrasound is a user dependent modality, but in experienced hands the sensitivity and specificity for making the diagnosis of appendicitis is similar to CT scan. It may be slightly less sensitive, but can deliver a diagnosis without any harmful radiation.

At the time I saw this patient, I did not have a lot of experience with US and my personal sensitivity was probably quite low. I would not have used it to rule the disease *out*. However, bedside ultrasound is specific. If it's obviously there, as it was in this case, then that's very useful. A test doesn't have to be both sensitive and specific if you know its operating characteristics and use it appropriately. In this situation, I used it as a *rule-in* test to decrease radiation and speed time to diagnosis.

US studies—sensitivity and specificity

In one large prospective study conducted by Stanford University, [13] a protocol for the use of ultrasound and CT for diagnosing appendicitis was found to be very helpful. In moderate probability patients, ultrasound was performed first and if equivocal, then a CT scan was done to increase the sensitivity of finding the disease. This approach was found to have a sensitivity and specificity of 98.6% and 90.6%, respectively, for appendicitis. The negative appendectomy rate was only 8.1% with an impressive missed appendicitis rate of 0.5%.

Again, ultrasound was not used to completely rule out the disease with its sensitivity being probably in the 80's, but this protocol succeeded in its goal of decreasing the utilization of CT by 53%, significantly reducing radiation exposure. Of patients with an equivocal ultrasound, 34% were managed solely with observation with no missed appendicitis. Many of these patients got better and were discharged without a CT scan and others became more "classic" and went to the OR based on clinical assessment. Out of 207 of these equivocal ultrasound patients there were no missed cases of appendicitis and only one negative laparotomy.

Observation is probably not used enough in our EDs, and it may be that an equivocal US study gives the physician the benefit of "observation" and re-evaluation, which may be enough in many cases. So the choice is probably not one of ultrasound or CT, but a combination of the two in a well-defined protocol. In the future the use of MRI may play a bigger role, but for now, this seems to be the most reasonable algorithm.

US specifics—which transducer to use, normal and abnormal US appearance

The choice of which ultrasound transducer to use really depends on the body habitus of the patient. For larger body habitus patients and adults, one may need to use a lower frequency transducer such as the 3 MHz curvilinear transducer.[14] For thin body habitus patients or children, the higher frequency (5 to 7 MHz) linear transducer gives a better image and is sufficient.[15] The lower the frequency of the probe, the deeper it can penetrate, but you lose resolution. When you are evaluating a small structure, such as the appendix, this resolution is important, so one should use the higher frequency probe if the patient is small enough.[16] This patient was basically an adult, but he was thin, which meant that I was able to use the linear, high frequency probe.

Appendicitis is diagnosed as a tubular structure greater than 6 mm in the right lower quadrant that is non-compressible and lacks peristalsis.[17-19] It is frequently found lying just over the iliac artery and vein. It also is frequently found just lateral to this lying just over the psoas muscle. You can sandwich it between the psoas muscle and the probe in many cases.[20]

An inflamed appendix will be >7mm, non-compressible, and may have a "target" appearance due to edema of the mucosal walls. However, once an appendix perforates, then you will no longer see the target sign. Instead you will see a hypoechoic area and possibly free fluid. This patient had a beautiful target sign and a non-compressible appendix almost 1cm in size. It hurt directly over the appendix as I scanned it. (Figures 1 and 2 on next page)

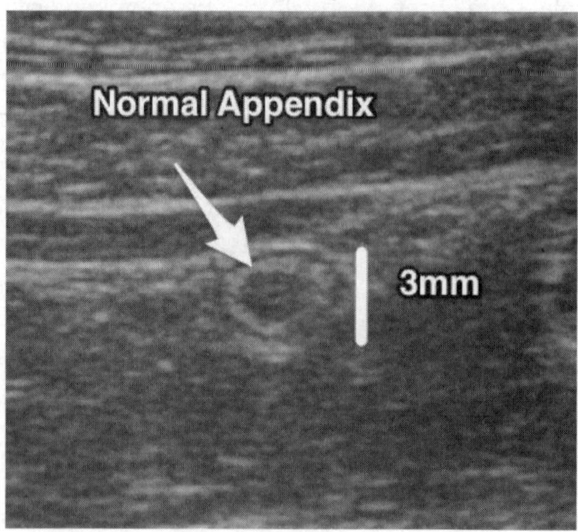

Figure 1: Normal cross section of appendix. <7mm, compressible, and rarely found when completely normal.

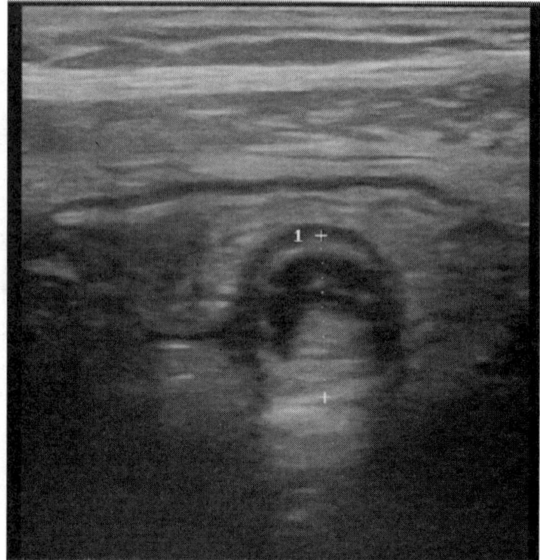

Figure 2: 9 mm noncompressible transverse view of appendix. This is appendicitis. You can see the hyperechoic area around the edges that represent edema of the walls. Just outside the appendix, especially superficial you can see hyperechoic fat stranding from inflammation.

Summary of ultrasound sensitivity, specificity, and user expertise

If you have a high pre-test probability of disease, the sensitivity of ultrasound may not be sufficient to rule out the disease.[5-12] Making this mistake would be very similar to "ruling out" appendicitis with a normal WBC count. It doesn't rule it out in high likelihood patients. Instead, these patients should be placed in an algorithm such as in the Stanford study. A positive ultrasound for appendicitis does have sufficient specificity to rule in the disease.[5-12]

As mentioned, it is also important to keep in mind that ultrasound for appendicitis is operator dependent. Experience and skill increase with each subsequent exam by the sonographer. The benefit of safely reducing radiation exposure and possibly improving operational savings and time continue to justify its use in diagnosing appendicitis.

Final thoughts: Consulting the surgeon

This patient benefited from the fact that the surgeon working had great experience with ultrasound for appendicitis from a previous job, so he "believed in it." The surgeon had worked extensively in a resource-limited setting where it was used out of necessity, not just for the radiation saving benefits. A different surgeon who didn't have this experience may have demanded a CT.

Lastly, in a patient with a very high likelihood of disease and a very classic presentation, it is completely reasonable to call surgery immediately. This patient's exam became more "classic" a little later during his second visit, just before surgery demonstrating the importance of a repeat exam with progression of disease. Most cases are not "classic," and the algorithm of ultrasound, then CT if US is equivocal seems to be the best current strategy for imaging of appendicitis.

Chapter Summary

1. Don't judge your patients based on appearance or behavior. Even if they were a drug seeker in the past, it doesn't mean they don't have real disease now.
2. A normal WBC count doesn't rule out appendicitis.
3. A "classic" presentation of appendicitis does not require radiologic testing, but it's rarely "classic."
4. Early appendicitis may not have the classic features. A trial of time in the ED may be useful, especially if the patient is complaining of unrelenting pain.
5. Start with an ultrasound for appendicitis. The sensitivity may not be high enough to rule out the disease, but the specificity is good enough to rule it in.

References

1. Lund DP, Folkman J. Appendicitis. In: Walker WA, Durie PR, Hamilton JR, et al, eds. Pediatric gastrointestinal disease: pathophysiology, diagnosis and management. 2nd ed. St. Louis: Mosby; 1996:907–15.
2. Bolton JP, Craven ER, Croft RJ, et al. An assessment of the value of the white cell count in the management of suspected acute appendicitis. Br J Surg. 1975;62(11):906–8.

3. Fee HJ, Jr. Jones PC, Kadell B, et al. Radiologic diagnosis of appendicitis. Arch Surg. 1977; 112(6):742–4.
4. Lewis FR, Holcroft JW, Boey J, et al. Appendicitis. A critical review of diagnosis and treatment in 1,000 cases. Arch Surg. 1975;110(5):677–84, 1975.
5. Puylaert JB. Acute appendicitis: US evaluation using graded compression. Radiology. 158(2):355–60, 1986.
6. Crady SK, Jones JS, Wyn T, et al. Clinical validity of ultrasound in children with suspected appendicitis. Ann Emerg Med. 1993;22(7):1125–9.
7. Hahn HB, Hoepner FU, Kalle T, et al. Sonography of acute appendicitis in children: 7 years experience. Pediatr Radiol. 1998; 28(3):147–51.
8. Karakas SP, Guelfguat M, Leonidas JC, et al. Acute appendicitis in children: comparison of clinical diagnosis with ultrasound and CT imaging. Pediatr Radiol. 2000;30(2):94–98.
9. Lessin MS, Chan M, Catallozzi M, et al. Selective use of ultrasonography for acute appendicitis in children. Am J Surg. 1999;177(3):193–6.
10. Rice HE, Arbesman M, Martin DJ, et al. Does early ultrasonography affect management of pediatric appendicitis? A prospective analysis. J Pediatr Surg. 1999; 34(5):754–8; discussion 758–9.
11. Roosevelt GE, Reynolds SL. Does the use of ultrasonography improve the outcome of children with appendicitis? Acad Emerg Med. 1998; 5(11):1071–5.
12. Lowe LH, Penney MW, Stein SM, et al. Unenhanced limited CT of the abdomen in the diagnosis of appendicitis in children: comparison with sonography. AJR Am J Roentgenol. 2001; 176(1):31–5.
13. Ramarajan N, Krishnamoorthi R, Barth R, et al. An interdisciplinary initiative to reduce radiation exposure: Evaluation of appendicitis in a pediatric emergency department with clinical assessment supported by a staged ultrasound and computed tomography pathway. Acad Emerg Med. 2009; 16(11):1258–65.
14. Caterino S, Cavallini M, Meli C, et al. Acute abdominal pain in emergency surgery. Clinical epidemiologic study of 450 patients. Ann Ital Chir. 1997; 68:807–17; Discussion 817–818.
15. Simmen HP, Decurtins M, Rotzer A, et al. Emergency room patients with abdominal pain unrelated to trauma: prospective analysis in a surgical university hospital. Hepatogastroenterology. 1991; 38:279–82.
16. Storm-Dickerson TL, Horattas MC. What have we learned over the past 20 years about appendicitis in the elderly? Am J Surg 2003; 185:198–201.
17. Siegel MJ, Carel C, Surratt S. Ultrasonography of acute abdominal pain in children. JAMA. 1991;266(14):1987–9.
18. Skaane P, Amland PF, Nordshus T, et al. Ultrasonography in patients with suspected acute appendicitis: a prospective study. Br J Radiol. 1900;63(754):787–93.
19. Worrell JA, Drolshagen LF, Kelly TC, et al. Graded compression ultrasound in the diagnosis of appendicitis: a comparison of diagnostic criteria. J Ultrasound Med. 1990;9(3):145–50.
20. Hahn H, Hoepner F, Kalle T, et al. Sonography of acute appendicitis in children: 7 years experience. Pediatr Radiol. 1998;28:147–51.

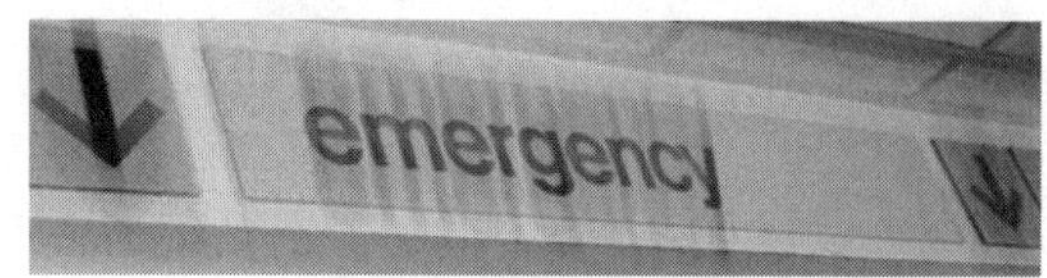

CASE 10

5-YEAR-OLD BOY WITH HEADACHE

David Andrew Talan, MD, FACEP, FIDSA
Professor of Medicine, UCLA School of Medicine
Chair, Department of Emergency Medicine, Olive View-UCLA Medical Center
Faculty, Division of Infectious Diseaes, Olive View-UCLA Medical Center

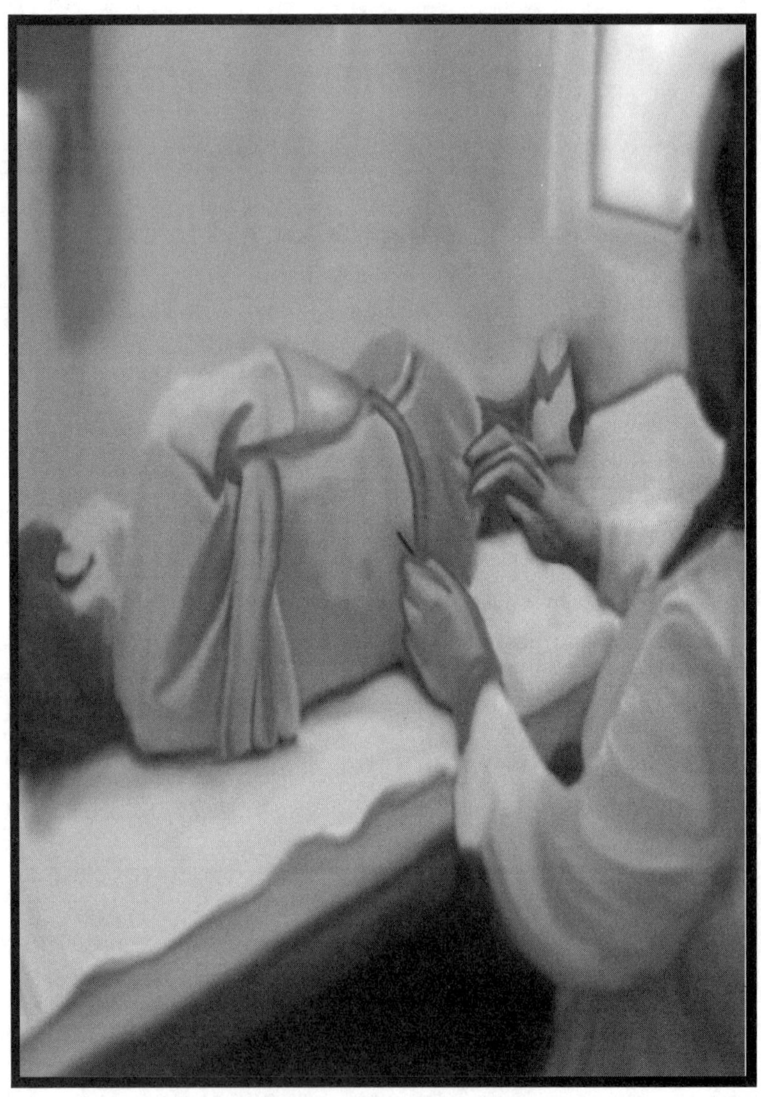

CASE 10

5-YEAR-OLD BOY WITH HEADACHE

PART 1—MEDICAL

I. The Doctor's Version (the following is the actual documentation of the provider)

CC (15:49): 2 days fever, vomiting

HPI (16:26): This five year old boy presents with both parents with history of abdominal pain, fever, vomiting for 2 days. Pain is described as colicky in character, sometimes localizing in right lower quadrant. No prior abdominal or surgical history. No testicular pain. Parents state has been taking clear liquids, no unusual or hematemesis character of emesis. No diarrhea. Last Tylenol at 0700.

PMH:

PMH/PSH: Negative for any medical or surgical history

FH: Sister with recent febrile illness, resolved

Pt has a fever since 6:30 this morning and complaints of right sided abdominal pain. Two days of vomiting

VITAL SIGNS

Time	Temp(F)	Pulse	Resp	Syst	Diast
15:57	101.7	110	22	72	

PHYSICAL EXAM:

Constitutional: A&O, NAD, WNWD

HEENT: Pharnyx unremarkable, neg for OM

Ears: TM's normal

Oral/Throat: Well hydrated, no erythema, exudate, edema

Eyes: Sclera white without injection or icterus

Neck: Supple

Lungs: CTA, neg for cough

Card: S1, S2 without murmur

Abd: careful deep palpation of abdomen with special attention right lower quadrant no significant localized tenderness, no rebound. No tenderness to testicular palpation.

Skin: Warm and dry. No rash

Neuro: Somewhat quieter than often seen in 5 yr. old male. Parents state this has happened before with fever and Tylenol. Does complain of headache. Neck supple.

MDM: This 5 yr old male appears well-hydrated. Abdomen shows no diagnosable evidence appendicitis at this time. Discussed fever management, alternation of Tylenol/ Ibuprofen with family. Return for any continuing or increasing right lower quadrant pain or for any/other new, worse problems of any kind.

DIAGNOSIS: Vomiting, Viral etiology.

Discharge Instructions: as above.

ADDENDUM (18:18): I did go back and check on the patient regarding mental status. Parents again state this is not unusual for patient with fever and Tylenol. Kernig's, Brudzhinski sign: equivocal. On re-evaluation he now appears to actually have some discomfort with flexing of the neck. I discussed with the mother that I do have a concern there could be meningitis and discussed the risks and benefits of an LP and she agrees to proceed. I will also order a CBC. IVF with .9NS, versed prior to LP

Procedure (1945): After some delay for IV start in busy ED . Patient required sedation with aliquots of Versed, Fentanyl. Pt on continuous pulse ox, monitor. Sat never lower than 92% on room air. With patient in left lateral decubitus position, after betadine preparation and sterile draping the L4-L5 interspace was entered with 22 gauge-1½ inch lumbar needle easily on first attempt. Patient tolerated well.

RESULTS:
CBC: WBC count 17.5, Hb 14.2, plt 323
CSF RESULTS (21:03):
CSF: Clear and colorless
RBC: 281 (0-5)
WBC 8 (0-5)
Glucose 65
Protein < 10
Gram stain: No organisms seen, rare WBC

MEDICAL DECISION MAKING: (21:17) In light of RBC count, this WBC count is strongly suggestive of viral meningitis, however we can never be 100%, but certainly is pretty strong evidence against a bacterial meningitis.

IMPRESSION: Viral syndrome

PLAN: Symptomatic therapy, return if symptoms worsen

RN Notes (2130): Pt. left ED ambulatory

Charles Chase, MD

II. Greg Henry Comments

"I applaud the emergency physician for the thoroughness of the evaluation, a second evaluation, and performance of the spinal tap"

This 5-year-old febrile child looks like most 5-year-old febrile children. The physical examination seems complete and well done. I applaud the emergency physician for the thoroughness of the evaluation, a second evaluation, and performance of the spinal tap.

It is hard to claim that 281 red blood cells represent anything other than mild traumatic tap; we are not considering a subarachnoid hemorrhage. A white blood count of eight is within the realm of statistical variability. With a gram stain being negative and only rare white blood cells and a protein of 10, this child appears to have labs consistent with a viral illness.

I see nothing on this initial workup which would require admission to the hospital or consideration of bacterial meningitis. I have seen this case hundreds of times.

III. The Bounceback

- Pt. is put to bed when he gets home, but around 5:30 parents are awoken to a loud noise. They go into patient's room to find that he has fallen out of bed and is unable to be aroused
- EMS is called and they rapidly arrive on scene to find the patient seizing, which is brief and spontaneously resolves
- They transport and arrive at the ED within 14 minutes
- Triage: "Pt to ER per squad with parents c/o unresponsiveness with onset after receiving Tylenol/mortin this AM at 0500. Pt had similar reaction to Tylenol in the past (per parents)"
- Initial vitals: Temp 100.0, pulse 105, R 30, BP 140/66
- HPI: Was seen in our ED last night. Two day hx of fever and some HA. Pt acting normal before going to bed. Received Motrin at 1:00 and Tylenol at 5:00. He was subsequently unable to be aroused – would shout "mommy" or "Daddy" and flail arms around. Per father left arm seemed limp.
- PE: Pt responsive to painful stimuli by moaning or flailing his upper extremities and rolling to his right side. Exam otherwise normal.
- Testing CBC and chem 7 done. Review of labs documented from last night including CSF differential of 94% PMNs and 6% monos. (Author's Note: This was not seen by the initial treating physician the night prior)
- Decision made to transfer to tertiary peds ED. Discussion with ED physician recommended starting ceftriaxone and vancomycin.
- Diagnosis: Altered mental status. Rule out encephalitis. Rule out meningitis.

IV. The Bounceback (per tertiary center)

- Brain CT is negative
- Pt is continues on IV ATB
- Pt. is admitted to the ICU
- Early the next morning the pt goes into full cardiopulmonary arrests and is resuscitated
- Within a few hours he arrests again but is unable to be resuscitated.
- CSF culture returns showing strep pneumo

FINAL DIAGNOSIS: Strep pneumo meningitis

PART 2—LEGAL

I. The Accusation/Cause of Action

The accusation here is that the results of the CSF were misinterpreted and there was subsequent failure to diagnose. There is a dispute in the testimony how the WBC count in the CSF is adjusted with the presence of RBC's or if it should even be adjusted. There is a contention that the patient should have been admitted initially and started on IV antibiotics. There is a dispute about how the clinical appearance is factored in when the child is non-toxic in appearance ... or was he? And where was the CSF differential?

II. What Would Greg Do (WWGD)? Part 2 of Greg Henry Comments

"The legal problem is that you are running the magic show of the court room against scientific concepts"

There is no question that this is a tragedy. The death of children is never good, but the emergency physician has an extremely strong position that what was done was defensible. It is also difficult for the plaintiff to prove that the physician's action or inaction caused harm. The plaintiff can always state that the child should have been admitted and given antibiotics, but you could say this about any child. If we admitted all these children we would kill more than we would save.

The legal problem is that you are running the magic show of the court room against scientific concepts. No juror understands sensitivity or specificity. Bad things happen to perfectly good people. Discussion with the parents prior to discharging the patient the first time would have been important and seems to have been done. To say that the emergency physician fell below the standard of care in interrupting the CSF and blood results is to me ridiculous. Would I settle this case, knowing what we know at this moment in time? I would not.

III. The Deposition

➢**Author's note (MW):** This is an incredibly tragic story, for the patient, the family, and the initial treating physician (more on this later—see anonymous interview below). But now we are way past the medical care, we have entered the legal arena where many doctors would prefer to be facing a lion than a plaintiff attorney—Let the games begin!

What follows next is a condensed summary of the deposition of the defendant physician, the ID expert for the plaintiff, the EM expert for the plaintiff and then a direct and cross of the EM expert. We have drastically shortened the testimony, but left a significant amount to show how attorneys' think and the questions they ask. This is the only chapter with legal testimony, so we wanted to include as much as possible since it is difficult to find this information unless you have received it from your own attorney! It is interesting to hear the testimony of these experts—they all have excellent credentials, there are no "hired guns"—it is easy to see how different physicians can look at the same data but come to different conclusions. As you read this passage, consider:

- How difficult it is to be objective after the final diagnosis and outcome are known
- Not only if *you* would have handled things in a similar or different fashion, but if the physician's actions seemed reasonable and meet the standard for other similarly-trained and concerned physicians
- If a call to arrange follow up would have blunted the impact of the plaintiff's arguments
- Whether the failure to initiate antibiotic therapy was a "proximate cause" in this patient's death (or if there was such a rapidly progressive inflammatory response, whether this would have made a difference)

Cast of characters (names changed):

Patient: Ty Thompson
Defendant physician: Dr. Charles Chase
Plaintiff's attorney: Karl Spachler
Plaintiff's ID expert witness: Dr James Spalding
Plaintiff's EM expert witness: Dr. Lanny Underwood
Defense attorney: Rodney Danninger
Defense EM expert witness: George Christopher

Table of contents:

E. Plaintiff's attorney (Karl Spachler) cross-examination of defense ER expert (Dr. George Christopher): page 154

A. Plaintiff attorney (Karl Spachler) direct of Plaintiff's expert infectious disease (ID) witness (Dr. James Spalding):

Q. Doctor, would you please state your name for the record.
A. Dr. James Spalding.
Q. Doctor, my name is Karl Spachler and I represent the family. I would like you to tell the jury about your background.
A. I graduated from medical school in 1962 and completed my pediatric training. I was assigned to the CDC and then completed an infectious diseases fellowship. I have a special interest in meningitis.

➤**Author's note (MW):** The plaintiff's attorney starts by establishing the credibility of the expert by asking him to give a brief summary of the history of meningitis. Whether we agree with his testimony or not, we have to admit, this guy has spent more than a few hours studying meningitis.

Plaintiff's attorney to Plaintiff's expert ID witness (continued):

Q. I wonder if you could hold off on this specific case and talk about meningitis in a global sense. Just give a brief summary of the history of meningitis and how it has changed [over the years].
A. Meningitis is one of the most severe ailments that can occur in individuals. It's essentially an inflammation of the brain, and may result in death or disability. So that is a feared complication of infectious diseases. Before antibiotics were available, almost all patients with bacterial meningitis died.

I should make a distinction between the organisms that cause meningitis. The bacterial organisms are very severe, and they have been Hemophilus organisms, meningococcus and pneumooccus. We are very fortunate that Hemophilus, which was the most comment cause of bacterial meningitis in infants and children, has now almost been eradicated by the use of an effective vaccine. So all children receive the HIB vaccine, and we rarely see a case of meningitis due to that organism. Then that left the two most common bacterial organisms causing meningitis. The meningococcus and the pneumococcus. In 2000, a vaccine similar to the HIB vaccine was introduced for pneumococcal disease, and we are beginning to see a decrease in the number of cases of pneumococcal meningitis as well. Every infant gets this new conjugate pneumococcal vaccine which has the trade name of Prevnar. Unfortunately, Ty's case occurred in the fall of 1999, just before the introduction of this new vaccine. So he did not have the availability of this effective preventive product.

In the fall of 1999, then, with the Hemophilus almost eradicated, the bacterial meningitides would have constituted about 10 to 25 percent of all of meningitis. The rest of the cases of meningitis fall into a category called aseptic meningitis, and aseptic simply means that it's not bacterial, and there are a lot of causes. Some of them are bacterial, like, but the vast majority [are]viruses. The viruses may be severe, such as herpes simplex, the cold sore virus, and that can lead to death or severe seizures and other forms of disability. But many of the viruses resolve when the patient does not have apparent severe complications from the viruses. Then almost every category of microorganism is represented in this area of nonbactcrial meningitis. So organisms like syphilis, fungi, mycoplasma, even parasites, may cause aseptic meningitis. But in the US, in a child in the fall of 1999, the vast majority would be viruses.

Q. On thc ordcr of what, 80 percent or so?

A. Yes. It would be dependent on the time of year, and in the fall there are still a lot of the summer viruses hanging around. But about 10 to 25 percent would be bacterial. The vast majority would be viral.

Q. Is it correct to say that bacterial meningitis would be the more deadly meningitis, whereas viral normally is not?

A. With the exception of herpes. Herpes is a very severe form of meningitis, and can be even worse than some of the bacteria. But the majority of viruses are, the summer viruses, enteroviruses, and they usually don't lead to long-lasting consequences.

Q. Whereas the bacterial?

A. Whereas the bacterial can lead to severe disabilities of the pneumococcal meningitis, and Ty had pneumococcal meningitis About a third of the surviving children do have hearing loss and another 10 to 20 percent have other forms of permanent disabilities.

Q. Let's talk about pneumococcal meningitis before antibiotics. First of all, when did antibiotics come into play?

A. The first antibiotics [were] introduced in the mid 1930s, and those are the sulfonamides, and then you have the penicillins. But before the introduction of antibiotics, 100 percent of patients who had pneumococcal meningitis died. If you survived, there was possibly a mistake in the diagnosis or it was miraculous. It was in that order of magnitude, but it was virtually a death sentence.

Q. What about after the antibiotics?

A. The antibiotics [brought about] a remarkable change. The mortality rate started coming down with the sulfonarnides to more than 50 percent survival, than with penicillin, to 80 to 90% survival, and now with the array of antibiotics that are available to us, survival occurs in virtually all children, and perhaps only about three to five percent die.

Q. Would that have been the case in 1999?

A. Yes

➢**Author's note (MW):** Is that true—100% of pneumoncoccal meningitis died? Fun fact: At the turn of the last century the life expectancy in America was 47 years of age. Maybe this was one of the reasons why ...

Q. Doctor, would it be acceptable to withhold antibiotics under these circumstances when you've got the presence of polymorphonuclear cells in the CSF?

DEFENSE: Objection!

A. No, and I think for the reasons we stated. If the child has a 10 to 25 percent chance of having bacterial meningitis, with the consequences that we know may occur as a result of bacterial meningitis, then that's a treatable disease.

Q. You mentioned the risk and benefit analysis that a doctor has to go through in a situation like this. Why don't you talk about that? Obviously the risk of bacterial meningitis is neurological injury or death. What is the risk of going ahead and treating a patient?
A. The risk of the antibiotics, the intravenous, the hospitalization, are small. They are not without consequence. But when you're balancing it against a life-threatening event, then admitting a child to a hospital, putting an intravenous line in place, and administering an antibiotic, is a very small risk. You could get irritation of the vein from the intravenous. You could get an allergic reaction from the antibiotic. You could get an infection in the hospital. All of these are relatively paltry adverse events in contrast to death or disability…

➢**Authors' note (MW):** Sure, good argument, minimal effect. But wouldn't this be the case with everything that occurs rarely? I should add that Dr. Spalding chaired a task force on Diagnosis and Management of Meningitis by the American Academy of Pediatrics. He has researched meningitis for around 40 years. He is a very accomplished physician, but has never practiced emergency medicine. Does this matter?

Q. Okay. Something just occurred to me as you're talking here. You are not an emergency physician?
A. I'm not.
Q. One could argue why should an emergency physician be held to the same standard as you who studied this disease for most of your career?
DEFENSE: Objection!
A. The emergency physician who orders a lab test should know how to interpret the results of the test, and WBC counts in the blood or the results in the lumbar are the responsibility of the physician. This is not rocket science. This is very basic information about interpretation of a lab test.

➢**Authors' note (MW):** This guy is moving past the question and has his dagger at the throat and decides to go for the kill. Not rocket science? Easy as pie? Sure … after you know the diagnosis!

➢**Author's note (MW):** So what has the plaintiff expert said? That most causes of meningitis are viral, but even if there is a chance that it is bacterial, it is worthwhile treating. If you are a juror, this would be pretty compelling testimony, especially after you have heard about a child who died. My guess is that most of the patients he sees on the floor during inpatient rounds have bacterial meningitis. Like the surgeon who retrospectively sees a case of missed appendicitis – "how could you have not done a CT scan?" Well… for every case of missed appendicitis, acute coronary syndrome, subarachnoid hemorrhage, we see many more that we are concerned about, but do *not* turn out to have the disease. Let's hit the "elephant in the room"; what was the thought process of the emergency physician? I call to the stand … Dr. Charles Chase!

B. Planitiff's attorney (Karl Spachler) examination of defendant emergency physician (Dr. Charles Chase):

Q. Would you please state your name for the record, sir?
A. Charles Chase

Q. Dr. Chase, my name is Karl Spachler. I represent the family. If I ever ask you a question you don't understand, please ask me to rephrase the question instead of answering it.
A. Yes.

➢Author's note (MW): Aaaahhh! This is tough stuff. Who wants to be sitting in this chair, particularly when there was significant concern for this child, a re-exam which prompted a change in management, and a lumbar puncture was done quickly and efficiently.

Q. Doctor, when is the first time you considered the diagnosis of meningitis for Ty?
A. As I was doing his initial dictation.
Q. Is it fair to assume that you were considering the diagnosis almost immediately?
A. I would not phrase it that way. I considered it to the point where I thought it was worthy of further investigation after my reassessment.
Q. Your addendum note says that on reevaluation of the patient, he now appears actually to have [some] discomfort and seems to wince a little bit upon flexing his neck. Whereas on your initial note, you note that the neck is supple. Isn't that a change? . . .
A. I would attribute the differences in the documentation to reflect [that] on reevaluation I approached him with a different mindset, therefore reexamined him very, very, carefully.
Q. Am I correct that he—so are you saying you think he had neck stiffness initially but you just didn't pick it up?
A. Often on reexamining a patient, depending on what one is thinking, one will be attentive to different sets of clues.
Q. You did actually examine his neck in your initial exam, because in your physical exam it does say neck is supple, so that would be an indication that you did examine his neck initially, correct?
A. That's correct.
Q. But you're saying this is not a change?
A I'm saying it's a reexamination.
Q. And you also did a Kernig sign on your reexamination. Can you tell us what that is?
A. Kernig sign is where one flexes the hip and then has the patient extend the knee.
Q. Did that cause neck pain?
A. A positive Kernig signs indicates neck pain, yes.

➢Author's note (MW): In the haze of a million snotty nosed kids with fever, this EP was vigilant and went back and re-examined the patient, detected a change in the presentation, and acted on it. A LP was done and the results were discussed in the progress note.

Q. Looking at the results of the CSF count then. First, the white count is elevated correct?
A. Referenced on this laboratory sheet, it does list it as high.
Q. Are you saying that this is normal for Joshua?
A. Yes.
Q. What is your basis for saying that?
A. Reference ranges for pediatric white blood cell counts range 0 to 7.
Q. He is an 8.
A One has to evaluate the 8 since there is presence of blood in the CSF

Q. Well, is the presence of blood going to affect the number of white cells?
A. Yes, it will.
Q. So you attribute the 8 to the presence of the RBCs then. Is that what you did?
A. I attributed up to 7 of the 8 to be within normal.

➤**Author's note (MW):** So there are several issues at play here:

1. Is there a "correction" in the WBC count when there is an elevated RBC count?
2. How concerning is a WBC so minimally above the normal range?
3. Was this the correct reference range for children (note: 0–5 WBC is listed on the chart), or is this the CSF reference range for adults and the range for children is 0–7, as alleged by Dr. Chase?

These issues will be the centerpiece of the continuing testimony. Predictably, the plaintiff's experts will say this was either an obvious case of meningitis or predictive enough to admit and treat. The defense experts will say that this physician was correct in his interpretation of the lab result and met the standard of care. What do you think? Would you like to use a "lifeline" and call a friend? How about calling Dave Talan, double boarded in Emergency Medicine and Infectious Diseases? He was not there for the legal action, but reviewed this case and testimony a few weeks ago for this chapter. Stay tuned, after the testimony is complete, we'll let Dr. Talan break the tie!

Q. So in other words, I think you said this, but you considered this a normal finding despite the fact that the lab said it was high?
A. The lab reference here for this paper that we're looking at, my understanding is an adult reference, and, in fact, on pediatrics reference ranges up to 7 white blood cells. Even without presence of blood is normal.
Q. Even in a five-year-old?
A. Yes.
Q. What about the polynuclear—polymorphonuclear. It says polynuclear here, but the PMN count is 94 percent. Do you also think that's normal?
A. With a very low white blood cell count, it is difficult to attach a lot of specificity to a PMN count.
Q. Can you explain that, please?
A. You have a very low sample size. And if one is considering, for example, the diagnosis of possibly viral meningitis, polynuclear counts can be elevated also.
Q. Is the reason that you did the lumbar puncture basically because you were thinking he might have meningitis and you were trying to distinguish whether it was viral or bacterial?
A. What is the question again?
Q. Is the reason that you did the lumbar puncture because you were thinking he might have meningitis and you were trying to determine whether this was a viral illness or a bacterial illness?
A. I began doing the lumbar puncture with the mindset that it would prove to within the limits that he did not have meningitis.
Q. You diagnosed him with meningitis after the lumbar puncture, correct?
A. My written diagnosis is not a diagnosis of meningitis.

Q. What was your diagnosis upon discharging Joshua?
A Viral syndrome slash possible viral meningitis.
Q. This predominance of PMNs in the CSF, isn't that more suggestive of a bacterial problem than a viral problem?
A. No.
Q. Do you have any literatures that you can point to that you can say otherwise?
A. I do not have it with me at the moment.
Q. Have you seen it?
A. Yes.
Q. Do you know where?
A. I would have to consult again to see exactly which volumes it's in to quote those to you.
Q. Dr. Chase, is it true that the CSF findings that we see here are consistent with very early bacterial meningitis?
A. They are consistent with possibly viral meningitis.
Q. But my question was, aren't they consistent with early bacterial meningitis?
A. No.
Q. Why is it inconsistent with that?
A. The white blood cell count is very low within range of normal.
Q. Well, I mean at some point in time the bacteria invades the CSF, but there's no inflammatory response yet, correct?
A. That is correct.
Q. Based upon the CSF findings here, you're saying that the CSF findings are normal for Joshua. Is that your testimony?
A. Normal or suggestive of viral meningitis.
Q. Can you rule out bacterial meningitis with these findings?
A. Yes.
Q. And did you, in fact, do that?
A. I believe so.

➢**Author's note (MW):** What do you think? This guy is holding up pretty well. What's the best way to answer questions during testimony? Let's take a quick break and ask Greg Henry, expert witness in over 2000 legal cases:

IV. Greg Henry Comments

"Insinuating the doctor's clairvoyance is an offense to the ears of God"

My thoughts are very clear. I am very pleased that the defendant physician held his ground in deposition. He did what most of us would have done, in fact, probably a little more. I'm not going to call the plaintiffs' experts lying whores and intellectual sluts, but I certainly could.

To think that the allegation of an existing literature base proving that eight white blood cells equals meningitis is just plain wrong. With no organisms, essentially normal chemistries, insinuating the doctor's clairvoyance is an offense to the ears of God. Reading this exchange does not make me a happy camper.

My advice to the physician is hang tough, go forward and hope that your defense experts can carry the day. This case has nothing to do with science; it is about a dead child.

V. The Deposition (continued)

Continued cross-examination of Dr. Chase:

Q. I would like to ask you about the bottom paragraph of your addendum. The sentence that reads: "In light of the fact that there is contamination with red cells also, this seeing of an eight may be suggestive of viral meningitis. However, we cannot be 100 percent." Does that mean that it's also consistent with bacterial?

A. What that meant was that I could not be 100 percent sure that it was, in fact, diagnostic of viral meningitis.

Q. Sorry?

A. What that meant was that I could not be 100 percent sure that it was diagnostic of viral meningitis.

Q. Okay. If it's not viral, then bacterial?

A. If it's not viral, then normal.

Q. Then normal. The last remark there says, "it is pretty strong evidence against a bacterial meningitis particularly in light of a child which has been sick for two days." Can you explain what you mean by that?

A. What I mean by that is in reference to a child who had been sick that long, that if there had been a bacterial meningitis, we would have expected that he would have progressed well beyond the stage you referred to in which this was early bacteria in the CSF, but not an inflammatory response yet.

Q. So in other words if— so because he was ill for two days then, you would have expected to see a very high white count?

A. In the thousands.

Q. Doctor, if you had—Doctor, what—if you would have had the impression that you could not be sure based upon the CSF findings whether he had bacterial or viral meningitis, what would you do?

A. If I could not be sure?

Q. Right.

A. If I could not be sure, the child would be treated with—be observed probably in the hospital and/or treated with antibiotics.

Q. In this case, you were sure, correct?

A. Yes.

➢**Author's note (MW):** Whether you agree or don't agree that sending the patient home with a very minimally elevated WBC count in the CSF was OK, we all agree that the sentence in the medical decision making (MDM) section at 21:17 was very important during the testimony. It was quoted multiple times during the proceedings. If it had not been present at all, it would be very difficult to see what the thought process of the provider was at the time, demonstrating the importance of the MDM.

C. Plaintiff's attorney (Karl Spachler) to plaintiff's emergency medicine expert witness (Dr. Lanny Underwood):

Q. This is Karl Spachler, I just have a few questions for you this morning and I'm going to let you get back to practicing medicine
A. That would be good. Thank you.
Q. I need your full name, please
A. Dr. Lanny Underwood
Q. Are you licensed?
A. Yes
Q. Do you actively practice?
A. Yes
Q. Are you a member of any professional organizations?
A. Yes. Two of them. Advanced ER Services. And Underwood consulting.

➤**Author's note (MW):** So this continues for several more pages. How much he is paid. Which type of cases he has testified in. Then the plaintiff's attorney cuts to the chase:

Q. Why don't you just tell me in global terms, doctor, what your opinions are regarding Dr. Chase's assessment, evaluation, and care of this patient?
A. Assessment, I have no problems with. Evaluation, I have no problems with. But I think the patient should have been given antibiotics pending a culture results, or the patient could have been admitted and be seen promptly, and I'll define promptly within an hour, maybe an hour and a half, who could then make their own judgment whether they wanted to start antibiotics. These two approaches would have met the standard of care. And that is because the patient was 5 years old, had enough question of his neck that the spinal tap was done, had an elevated white count and a fever, and the result of the spinal tap showed some white blood cells.
Q. Just in the interest of completeness, is there any further testing or evaluation which Dr. Chase should have done?
A. I think it would have been very reasonable to do a blood culture, but I have to tell you if that were the only thing left out, I would not be critical.
Q. Do you think Dr. Chase appropriately interpreted the results from the spinal fluid?
A. Well, that's a really interesting question. He certainly reviewed the results and made an impression this could be viral meningitis. I would agree that it could be viral meningitis. However, regardless of the results of the spinal fluid, he still had a patient with a fever, and elevated WBC count, and enough neck changes on exam to justify the spinal tap, and therefore I felt that antibiotics should have been used anyhow.
Q. Could he have been treated as an outpatient with an antibiotic?

➤**Author's note (MW):** So this is a curious question. Why would the plaintiff's attorney bring up outpatient treatment when his expert just said that the patient should have been admitted? Maybe to show how easy it would have been for Dr. Chase to give an injection of rocephin and treat with oral antibiotics as an outpatient … you simply check a box and the patient lives …

A. Okay. I would say that Dr. Chase could have met the standard of care by doing what he did plus giving the patient an injection of antibiotic, most likely Rocephin, and sending him home.

Q. And the antibiotic is an injection?

A. Correct

Q. And then send the child home with oral antibiotics? Under those circumstances, do you believe this child's course would have been any different?

A. I think he would have more than not—more likely than not have never developed the full blown meningitis because of the antibiotic.

Q. And on what do you base that opinion?

A. Nothing in the record. We just know from the literature and from practice that this particular bacteria is sensitive to [ceftriaxone] and it usually, not always, but usually kills it.

➢**Author's note (MW):** Do you get the feeling that this guy is answering a question that he has not been asked? Who speaks like this, "more likely than not"? Well ... to prove causation, to prove that the antibiotics would have made a difference, the plaintiff needs to prove that "more likely than not" they would have saved the boy's life. So in this context, this expert sounds like a *professional* expert. The kind that advertises for their services. Underwood consulting. Can someone just "Google" them?

Q. Okay, more likely than not, as you know, is a little more than 50% standard.

A. Right. I can go beyond that. I think it would be like probably 70%. But if you ask me the next question, which I'll ask for you: Can I base that on the literature? The answer is no.

➢**Authors' note (MW):** You think this guy is good? Turns out, he is not only an expert witness, but also asking the attorney's questions for him! Can you charge extra for that? You may see him in 20 years sitting in a park somewhere, feeding nuts to the squirrels, and playing chess against himself ... but dressed quite nicely!

Q. Well, actually, the next question would have been: Can you be more specific than more likely than not?

A. Yes, and the answer is I don't have a basis on which to—it's just that we know that when we do have these infections, a significant majority of patients get better. I'll say it is significantly over 50%, but that doesn't help you with a number. Is it 72% or 84%, I don't know.

Q. Earlier the 70% number came out. I just wondered if that is your opinion, whether you can cite literature or not, as to what his chance of survival was if treated as you suggested?

A. I would expect if I were seeing this patient myself that he would have a very significant chance of not getting worse. In other words, like 80–85%.

➢**Author's note (MW):** OK. So just to break the tie I did a literature search and found the exact number of people who get better with an injection of [ceftriaxone] in this exact situation is 63.24%. On Tuesdays. In January. If you change the situation and he is being treated on a Thursday in November, the exact number is 71.48% ... or so ... This guy is getting a bit out of control. Can the plaintiff's attorney ask for his money back?

Q. Let's assume hypothetically [that] he received an injection of [ceftriaxone] in the ED while Dr. Chase was caring for him. Is there a time delay between the injection and when the antibiotic begins to attack and kill the bacteria?
A. Sure.
Q. And what is that in your understanding?
A. Oh, it probably is an hour, hour and a half, that range, before it starts to do all the stuff you want it to do.
Q. Do you believe that had he gotten an injection the infection would have been under control?
A. I think it would have. The antibiotic would have commenced its work in killing the bacteria.

➢**Author's note (MW):** We better get Greg Henry in here. Greg, would you like to be the defense expert in this case. I can feel you squirming in your seat!

VI. Greg Henry Comments

"I would defend this physician and his approach vigorously"

My hands are fidgeting and my adrenalin is kicking in. I would love to be the defense expert on this case. I would defend this physician and his approach vigorously. There is a lack of literature to defend the fact that this child was pathognomonic for meningitis. On second visits, almost everyone can make the diagnosis. There is no evidence that a CSF/PCR would have been back in time to make any changes in therapy in this child and that there is considerable question as to whether antibiotics actually change the inflammatory response which goes along with such infections.

➢**Author's note (MW):** OK. Enough beating up the doctor. Now let's hear the defense response. We already heard from the EP defendant. Next is the emergency medicine expert from the defense counsel. This is not a "hired gun," but a well-respected emergency physician who has led a major department and emergency medicine residency program. The difficulty is always to look back and try to imagine how things would have been handled at the time of the initial encounter, before the diagnosis and outcome are known. If Mr. Lincoln could have known the end of the play, he would have seen a movie instead ....

VII. The Deposition (continued)

D. Defense attorney Rodney Danninger direct examination of defense emergency medicine expert witness, Dr. George Christopher:

Q. Okay. Do you have an opinion based upon the evaluation and examination, if you will, recorded in the medical records and the lab results what the reasonable diagnosis would have been of Ty's condition?
A. Well, the most reasonable diagnosis based on the setting here given the way the child appeared and given the results of the cerebrospinal fluid is that this is viral meningitis.
Q. How is viral meningitis treated?

A. Viral meningitis is treated symptomatically. By that I mean there's no antibiotics to take care of most viral meningitis. There's a few exceptions. If somebody has herpes meningitis, we would treat that, but that's not the case here. So for most viral meningitis what we do is we treat the symptoms. We give them Tylenol or Motrin for the fever [and pain] and they get better.

Q. Okay. Doctor, based upon your review of materials in this case including the medical records, the depositions that you've identified for us, based upon your background, training and experience as an emergency department physician, have you formed an opinion to a reasonable medical certainty as to whether Dr. Chase, my client, met or exceeded the standard of care for an emergency medicine physician in his evaluation and treatment of Ty Thompson?

A. Yes, I do.

Q. What's your opinion?

A. My opinion is that Dr. Chase met the standard of care in this instance.

Q. Would you explain for the court and the jury what you base that opinion on please?

A. Certainly. The child was seen and examined. Dr. Chase reexamined the child. On reexamination he had some indication to do a spinal tap, which he did in an appropriate manner. The question then comes to was his interpretation of the cerebrospinal fluid a reasonable thing? So we look at the cerebrospinal fluid and we have to make some judgment about whether this is viral meningitis or bacterial meningitis. The things that would make me think that it's bacterial meningitis are a very high number of white blood cells in the cerebrospinal fluid. Usually in bacterial meningitis that means over 1,000. In this case it was eight. The second thing is that we look to see if the glucose is low? In this case, it was not. The third thing we look at is: is the protein very high? In this case, the protein was low. The fourth thing we look at is the Gram stain. Are there bacteria seen on the Gram stain? In this case it was not.

The last thing that we sometimes take into consideration is what's the mix of white blood cells in the cerebrospinal fluid. But that's not a very useful measure for us because in viral meningitis you can have a lot of polys and in bacterial meningitis you can have initially a lot of lymphs. So the distinction early in meningitis doesn't really help us any. Both patterns, viral and bacterial meningitis, can look the same early.

So it's really the total number of white blood cells, the Gram stain, the glucose, and the protein. In this case all those things point to a viral meningitis. Given that it's a viral meningitis, you then make a decision about how sick does this child look; that is, is this child throwing up repeatedly in front of you so that you don't think they can keep down fluids. Sometimes you have to admit kids with viral meningitis just because you have to give them intravenous hydration. That doesn't seem to be the case here. So all you have to decide then is are these reliable parents, can they see their pediatrician the next day. If the answer to that is yes, then you send the child home. This is done every day in every emergency department across the country.

Q. Dr. Christopher, again based upon the medical records you reviewed, the depositions, the other materials you've referenced earlier in your deposition and your background, training and experience, do you have an opinion within a reasonable medical certainty as to whether Dr. Chase did or failed to do for Ty in the emergency caused his death?

A. Prospectively I think his actions were reasonable. I think it's the same actions that physicians would take across the country every day. They would look at this and say this looks like viral meningitis. I'm going to send this child home.

Q. Okay. If you make that judgment, the one you just indicated, it looks like viral meningitis, I'll send the child home, and you as an emergency department physician are wrong and it's a — and this is a strep bacterial meningitis that actually led to Ty's death as I understand; am I right?

A. That's correct.

Q. Let's assume hypothetically that you think it's viral, you send the child home, and he in fact has a strep meningitis. Do all of those children die?

A. Fortunately most of them do not. The course in most children [is that] the child gets slowly more ill, comes back to see their doctor or to the emergency department, the diagnosis is made, they're given antibiotics and most of those children do well. There are a few children and adults actually also who have what we call a fulminant meningitis; that is they have a rapid downhill course whether the diagnosis is initially not made or even if the diagnosis is made and treated, they progress very rapidly and unfortunately die. But under most circumstances if we think it's viral meningitis and then later on we find out it's bacterial, we usually make that diagnosis in the next 12 to 24 hours, start antibiotics, and the child does well.

➢**Author's note (MW):** Do you think they spoke about this first? Seems like the EM expert just threw the defense attorney a softball. Next he will ask questions about fulminant meningitis. They will attempt to distinguish between "run of the mill" meningitis which responds to antibiotics and a meningitis so extreme and so advanced already, that even if antibiotics would have been given, it would not have altered the outcome ... can anyone say, "Causation?"

Q. You mentioned fulminant meningitis. What does that mean to physicians?

A. Well, what that means to a physician is a child or an adult who comes in and is awake and not looking too ill, and then over the course of hours they go downhill. What causes this is when you have bacteria around the cerebrospinal—around the brain, sometimes you get—well, you almost always get some inflammation action, that is some irritation of the brain. The body reacts against the bacteria and you get brain swelling. And in some cases that brain swelling is dramatic and they die from that. Unfortunately it's not predictable who is going to get that, and unfortunately it's not treatable.

Q. Well, are antibiotics effective in either stopping or preventing fulminant meningitis?

A. Unfortunately not. The antibiotics are effective at killing the bacteria, but once the inflammation starts, it's going to run its course. It's sort of like if you're out in the mountains and you throw a rock at a pile of snow and you might get an avalanche. If you get that avalanche it's going to run its course—there's nothing you can do.

➢**Authors' note (MW):** So we have a well-respected defense EM expert saying that the EP met the standard of care (SOC), as they did an H&P, re-exam, LP and based on the cell count that was known, made a diagnosis which other EP's would have made; viral meningitis. Further, even if the diagnosis of bacterial meningitis would have been suspected, antibiotics would not have mattered because the inflammatory response was already too advanced. How did the plaintiff's attorney respond. Hint: Reading the next section, you can *feel* the tension and animosity of this interaction. Here is where the sparks start to fly!

E. Plaintiff's attorney (Karl Spachler) cross of defense ER exert (Dr. George Christopher):

Q. Okay. You tell me what you would think a kid looks like who shows up in an ER with a seven on the glasgow coma scale.

A. It would be a child that was responsive to painful stimulus.

Q. And otherwise, he would appear unconscious; right?

A. He would appear to be unresponsive, not necessarily unconscious.

Q. Okay. And for a kid to look like that, as a result of pneumococcal meningitis, that means that meningitis had to have begun to enter the fulminate stage; right?

Defense attorney: Objection! Go ahead, Doctor.

A. What it likely means is that he had increased intracranial pressure.

Q. And what would have caused the increased intracranial pressure, if you could describe that to a lay person given that the kid has pneumococcal meningitis?

A. What it means is that the brain tissues have reacted to the bacteria and reacted in a way that is causing inflammation. And that inflammation is causing more swelling. And that's the piece that's not predictable. Some people have a very minimal inflammatory reaction to meningitis and some people have a fulminate reaction. And that's the case with Ty.

Q. And you don't know whether the antibiotics would have prevented or staved off that inflammatory process; right?

A. The antibiotics would not have prevented the inflammatory process, no.

Q. You mean even if the antibiotics are effective in treating the bacteria and keeping the bacteria from spreading, it will have no effect on the very inflammatory process caused by the bacteria?

Defense attorney: Objection.

A. They're two separate processes. The inflammatory response and the infectious response are related, but they're separate. The antibiotic treats the infectious process, but not the inflammatory process.

Q. You would agree with me there's no inflammatory process without the infection to begin with; right?

A. Yes, that's correct.

Q. So there's some link between the infectious process and the inflammatory process; right?

A. Yes, you have an infection first and then you develop the inflammatory process.

Q. And when the infection is treated so early on that the white cell count in the bloodstream is 17,500, the white blood cells in the CSF tap are only eight, you're saying that had antibiotic treatment been started that early it still wouldn't have had any effect on the interrelated inflammatory process?

A. Yeah, that seems to indicate when people look at this in the past in terms of timing of antibiotics and what appears to be the case that in people they're going to have a fulminate course of meningitis whether you give them the antibiotics early or later, they still develop the inflammatory response.

Q. Name one study that suggests that children who are given antibiotics very early in the course, i.e., with the lab values that Ty had, name one study that suggests that antibiotic therapy at that early stage has no impact on preventing the catastrophic inflammation.
A. You're asking me for a study of only children that have the same lab values as Joshua?
Q. Yeah.
A. Is that what you're asking me?
Q. Yeah.

➤**Author's note (MW):** You wanna mess with me? You wanna mess with *me*? Bring it on! So now they are getting into it. The plaintiff's attorney can't know all of the literature, but has decided to go out on a limb and is guessing that Dr. Christopher does not have an answer. Let's see how *this* plays out ...

Continued plaintiff cross of defense EM expert Dr. George Christopher:
A. I don't recall seeing any studies of children with CSF counts of eight. But there are studies that have looked broadly at this issue of the timing of antibiotics with meningitis.
Q. And they all suggest that the earlier they're started the better; right?
A. No, that's not correct.
Q. Okay. But when you say that antibiotics instituted as early as Ty's presentation in the ER.... once these lab values are established, when you say that antibiotics administered that early would have no effect on the inflammation process, you're making that up out [of thin air] because you've seen no such patient given that therapy, that early, right?
Defense attorney: Objection! Karl, you're entitled to ask the witness his opinions and the basis for his opinions. You're not entitled to argue with him or make your final argument now. You don't have to answer that question, Doctor.
Plaintiff's attorney: Rod, you're *really* going to instruct him not to answer that question?
Defense attorney: Yeah, I'm instructing him not to answer the way you phrased it.
Q. Doctor, have you ever read a study that suggests that a child who is given antibiotic therapy with Ty's lab values, i.e., early in the course, have you read a study that suggests that given that antibiotic therapy at that point has no effect on the anti-inflammatory process—or on the inflammatory process?
A. Well, I understand what you're trying to get at. It's just hard for me to answer the question the way that you're asking it.
Q. Let me put it another way. If you have seen a study that suggests that children who are given antibiotic therapy real early in the course, and by "real early in the course" I mean with the hypothetical lab values I've already discussed with you, can you name me one such study that shows that the antibiotic therapy has no effect on the inflammatory process?
A. Well, there's two studies that get to the issue you're asking about, which is the effect of the timing of the antibiotics on the outcome of meningitis. And the two studies, one was in the journal called Pediatric Infectious Diseases, I think it was in 1992 by Radetsky.
Q. When did you last read that?
A. And the second study was in the American Journal of Emergency Medicine, and it was after that, maybe '95, '96, and the author was Bonao, B-O-N-A-O, although I'm not certain about that. Both of those studies came to the conclusion that the timing of antibiotics over the course of hours didn't make a difference in the outcome of meningitis.

Q. Is a 101 degree temperature in a five-year-old abnormal?
A. 101 would be considered a fever.
Q Would it be considered abnormal?
A. Yes.
Q. Would eight white cells in the cerebrospinal fluid of a five-year-old be considered abnormal?
A. It would depend on the red cell count.
Q. What do you mean by that?
A. Well, if you have a traumatic tap, then sometimes you see white cells in proportion to the red cells, in which case you would consider you had a traumatic tap. If you did not have a traumatic tap, it would be normal.
Q. And there's no reason to think that Ty's tap was traumatic; right?
A. That's not correct.
Q. You saw evidence of a traumatic tap in Ty?
A. He had red cells in his cerebrospinal fluid.
Q. Define "traumatic tap," please.
A. Blood in the cerebrospinal fluid that is not coming from an intracranial course.
Q. Can you please tell me where in the labs you saw evidence of red cells or blood in the CSF?
A. Yes, it's in the lab report.
Q. Would you agree that if there are red cells in the CSF fluid, for it to be considered a traumatic tap you need more than one thousand red cells? Doc, isn't 281 red cells in the CSF normal?
A. So the answer is there are 281 red cells per cubic millimeter in this CSF specimen, that is probably evidence of a traumatic tap. No, you do not have to have more than one thousand red cells to be abnormal.
Q. Okay. So you' re saying 281 red cells in a spinal tap is an abnormal finding?
A. Most likely indicative in this setting of a traumatic tap.

➤**Author's note (MW):** Next they are going to ask about the interpretation of the CSF results, the total WBC count, the differential. Spoiler alert; the guy stands his ground.

Q. Is there anything about the results of the CBC that would have enhanced your suspicion about the possibility of meningitis?
A. No.
Q. And then let's discuss the CSF count and differential. Doctor, you know, we all have these. Do you consider these results to be normal?
A. I wouldn't consider them to me normal, but their interpretation is not straightforward.
Q. How would you interpret them?
A. Well, I think like most doctors looking at the spinal fluid, your first thought is this is either something or nothing. Eight white blood cells is a normal number, but seven of the eight blood cells are polys, which is not usual in an absolutely normal person. So I would, in looking at it, I would say maybe this is really a normal person without anything of concern. But there are few too many poly for complete comfort. So the second possibility is that it's something, not nothing. But the something is a very long list of things, which includes meningitis of some sort, it could be due to adjacent infections, sinus disease can cause something like this occasionally, there are other infections within the skull that could potentially cause this. But like I said, it could be nothing at all. It could be a funny variation

in a child that has no serious illness whatsoever. So I would say in looking at it that it's not entirely normal, it is a little bit unusual, the number of polys. The most generous interpretation would be that it is some form of non bacterial meningitis with a faint possibility that it's bacterial meningitis, but I'd say faint, because nothing is impossible in medicine.

Q. I assume that bacterial meningitis would be the most—the biggest concern for the physician?

A. Well, there are other possibilities that are just as bad as bacterial meningitis; herpes meningitis, brain abscess, subdural empyema, infectious thrombosis of a vessel in the brain, osteomyelitis of the skull. I mean, there are some pretty awful things out there. That is only one of them.

➢**Author's note (MW):** The hypothetical question asked after the fact—what would Dr. Christopher do?

Q. Dr. Christopher, what would you have done if you would have gotten these results?

A. I think, Mr. Spachler, that depends entirely on how I appraised the child's condition at the time. And if like Dr. Chase, I felt that this was a child that was not ill, six hours after he arrived and was still not ill, and whose clinical condition did not worry me in any way, I would have done what Dr. Chase did.

Q. Well, given what you know, Doctor, would you have gone ahead and hospitalized this child?

A. Given what I know now sir, sure. We all would.

Q. Certainly, in retrospect. But let's look at it prospectively, Doctor. Wouldn't you have given these CSF results, hospitalized the boy and started him on antibiotics?

A. As I said when I tried to answer your question last time, Mr. Spachler, it depends entirely on the clinical appraisal. Here is a child who if I were in Dr. Chase's shoes, I would have been observing for six straight hours and I would have a pretty good feel for the child's illness and whether the illness is progressive or not. So the answer is no, if I was content with the child's condition at the end of those six hours that he did not have a serious illness. I think a reasonable option was what was chosen. It's not the option everybody would choose. There are a number of other things that other people might choose, but they are all acceptable reasonable options that meet the standard of care.

Q. In your opinion, did Ty Thompson have bacterial meningitis on the 31st when he was in the emergency department?

A. Yes.

Q. And what's your own explanation as to the relatively small white count in these circumstances?

A. The explanation is that different people react with different patterns of white cell response in bacterial meningitis.

Q. Doctor, do you agree with the recommendations that I've found in several publications that if the emergency physician suspects that a child has the possibility of having bacterial meningitis that it is prudent for the doctor to go ahead and give the antibiotics and then wait for the cultures to come back?

A. I believe everything resides on the meaning of the word "suspects." I would say that it would be beneath the standard of care for an emergency room doctor not to think of bacterial meningitis when the circumstances are correct. But if in thinking about it he finds no real support for it or he feels the diagnosis is unlikely, then there are other management options that are available.

➢**Author's note (MW):** So there you have it. If you were on the jury, how would you vote? If you were the initial treating physician, how would you *feel*?

Stick around for the end—how was this resolved? We'll ask Greg Henry how the depositions went and how it likely ended. Then we'll interview the Emergency Physician and find out the "story behind the story."

Well, big surprise—the defense and plaintiff disagree. So we are finally ready … Dr. Talan, please break the tie!

VIII. DISCUSSION OF DIAGNOSIS OF INFECTIOUS HEADACHE, INTERPRETATION OF CSF RESULTS, AND ACUTE MANAGEMENT OF MENINGITIS

Guest author:

David Andrew Talan, MD, FACEP, FIDSA

Professor of Medicine, UCLA School of Medicine
Chair, Department of Emergency Medicine, Olive View-UCLA Medical Center
Faculty, Division of Infectious Diseaes, Olive View-UCLA Medical Center

Dr. Talan serves on the editorial boards of the Annals of Emergency Medicine, Emergency Medicine News, and Pediatric Emergency Care and is a reviewer for Clinical Infectious Diseases, JAMA, and The Medical Letter. Dr. Talan has written and researched extensively on infectious diseases. He is triple boarded in emergency medicine, infectious diseases, and internal medicine.

We asked Dave Talan to break the tie … who is "right" in their testimony, and who is taking liberties. He will also address meningitis in general as well as in the context of this case. Specifically:

- Is there an adjustment in the WBC count when there are RBC's present?
- When there is documentation that the CSF was easily obtained on the first attempt, are the RBC's related to an infectious process or a traumatic tap? (as alleged by the EM defense expert Dr. Christopher)
- What is the role of inflammation in meningitis?
- Then some "rubber meets the road" questions:
    - o Would initiation of antibiotics at the first visit made any difference (causation)?
    - o Did the experts testify truthfully or did they take some liberties or state things inaccurately?
    - o Would you take this case as an expert for the defense or plaintiff?

Bacterial meningitis—suspicion and diagnosis

Bacterial meningitis is an infectious disease emergency. Before antibiotics, nearly every patient with bacterial meningitis died. The current overall survival is about 85%. Among etiologies of bacterial meningitis, the most common, pneumococcal, has the worst prognosis; the mortality rate is 15–20% and 50% of survivors have some neurological impairment.

As such, if you work under a big red "Emergency" sign, you have an extra burden of diligence to diagnose these cases, and diagnose them as early as possible. In legal terms, however, that means diagnose as is *reasonably* possible. Negligence is decided by juries who determine the reasonableness of a provider's decision-making.

Clinical diagnoses are based on weighting various factors that affect the odds of a disease being present adjusted for the risk of missing an opportunity to effectively treat a life-threatening illness. Before we discuss the factors which we use to assess a patient's risk of having bacterial meningitis, one first has to suspect meningitis. This is not at issue in this case. I'd give the physician credit for his extra concern about a "quiet kid" despite his parent's dismissal of his countenance of his "typical response" to a febrile illness.

Some respected emergency medicine authorities have opined that one can safely diagnose viral meningitis, and "rule out" bacterial meningitis, based on clinical evaluation alone without LP and CSF analysis. My colleague at UCLA, Dr. Larry Baraff (who is also trained in pediatric ID) and I debated this in the *Annals of Emergency Medicine*.[1,2]

I think a lumbar puncture is necessary, but one could contend that a reasonable approach would have been to send this well-appearing child home straight away. Now, if you consider the CSF WBC abnormalities in this case to be important, then this highlights the extra value of CSF analysis beyond the clinical evaluation. Regardless, had an LP not been done, the child would have returned and been diagnosed with meningitis later, and the defendant emergency physician would still have been sued for not doing the LP. The CSF would have been presumed to have been even more abnormal than it actually was.

Interpreting a lumbar puncture

In this case, a spinal tap was done and the plaintiff's and defense's experts diverge as to the importance of a solitary CSF value, the white blood cell result. The plaintiff's expert argues that 8 WBCs almost all polys is so abnormal that it makes bacterial meningitis sufficiently likely that parenteral antibiotics were required to meet the standard of care, i.e., not giving antibiotics was unreasonable.

Alternatively, the defense's expert opines that this one value is not so abnormal such that the likelihood of bacterial meningitis could not be modified by the absence of many other risk factors that in sum made discharge home without antibiotic treatment reasonable.

The predictive value of a test is affected by the prevalence of disease. Here we have good data from the PECARN study by Nigrovic et al. of children presenting with meningitis who had LP conducted between 2001 and 2004.[3] Note that this is just after Prevnar was introduced so it would have little effect on a 5-year-old and did not yet have the full penetrance to provide generally protective herd immunity.

Of 3,295 children with meningitis, only 3.7% were found to have bacterial meningitis.*1 The prevalence might have been a little but not a lot higher in 1999. So the plaintiff's expert's claim of 10–25% is just plain wrong (see scoreboard in boxes). Of note, in this study CSF pleocytosis was defined as WBCs $\geq$ 10, supporting the defense's contention that 8 WBCs is "normal."*2

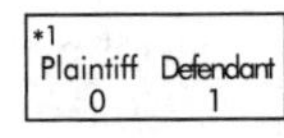

*2

Plaintiff	Defendant
0	2

So we start out with a low risk based on disease prevalence, and then this is modified by various epidemiologic, clinical, and laboratory risk factors. Nigrovic et al. suggested applying 5 low-risk criteria to minimize the risk of bacterial meningitis called the Bacterial Meningitis Score, which included absence of positive CSF Gram stain, CSF absolute neutrophil count of $\geq$ 1000, CSF protein of $\geq$ 80, peripheral blood ANC $\geq$ 10,000, and a history of seizure before or at the time of presentation. Note that the CSF differential, or % polys, did not fall out as an independent predictor of bacterial etiology.

Any of these criteria being present caught 98.3% of bacterial meningitis patients. In this case, the total peripheral WBC count was high 17,500 and the differential is not given but probably the ANC was > 10,000.*[3] While this could be used by plaintiff to justify their side of the argument, defense can also argue that the risk of bacterial meningitis overall was still small with the low prevalence of disease and 4 of 5 risk factors absent. While we all recognize the lack of specificity of peripheral WBC counts and differentials, these results do influence most doctor's decision-making in everyday practice, perhaps more than they should. It is also true that the more abnormal the result, the more specific the result is, in this case supporting the existence of bacterial infection. I was surprised that this was not raised as a point by the plaintiff's side to support the requirement of hospital admission and empirical antibiotics.

*3	
Plaintiff	Defendant
1	3

Several studies have reported on the predominance of CSF neutrophils in children with aseptic meningitis and the changes in CSF neutrophil proportions with illness duration among these patients, some suggesting that neutrophil predominance is more common early on.[4, 5]

The conclusion of the Negrini, et al.[5] paper says it all, "The majority of children with aseptic meningitis have a PMN predominance in the CSF. The PMN predominance is not limited to the first 24 hours of illness. Because the majority of children with a PMN predominance during enteroviral season will have aseptic disease, a PMN predominance as a sole criterion does not discriminate between aseptic and bacterial meningitis."*4

*4	
Plaintiff	Defendant
1	4

In trials, however, sometimes perception is more important than reality. If the jury perceives that the emergency doctor was careless in ordering and then not waiting to evaluate the CSF differential result, they may conclude he was negligent despite the fact that the differential count is not an important predictor of etiology.

Viral and bacterial meningitis

We are not given the time of year that this case was seen. However, note that the Nigrovic et al. study found enteroviral meningitis by CSF PCR testing in about two-thirds of cases across all seasons, not just the summer months when enterviral disease is supposed to be most prevalent.[6] *5

*5	
Plaintiff	Defendant
1	5

In a well-appearing child presenting with some GI symptoms, with a sib who recently recovered from a febrile illness, and who is found to have relatively normal CSF, it would be reasonable to suspect aseptic meningitis due to enteroviral infection. Hopefully, in the near future, more labs will provide rapid enteroviral CSF PCR testing to make these decisions more secure. In the meantime, for practitioners who are risk-adverse, there is always default hospitalization or one dose of ceftriaxone and good discharge instructions with next day follow-up. However, if, as mentioned above, some advocate a clinical diagnosis of viral aseptic meningitis without LP and discharge home, then these measures would not logically be required to meet the standard of care in most cases.

The issue of the red blood cells in the CSF is really irrelevant. With a traumatic tap, one could assume a similar proportion of WBCs to RBCs in the CSF as seen in the peripheral blood, or about a ratio of 1:250 in this case. So at most 1 CSF WBC was the result of the blood being introduced.

The legal equation

In my experience, the jury's conclusion regarding negligence trumps causation arguments. If a jury decides that an avoidable and unreasonable mistake was made, they typically accept the plaintiff's version of causation no matter how unreasonable. Causation is to a great extent best-guesswork since one could not conduct a trial randomizing presumed bacterial meningitis patients to immediate or delayed antibiotics. Since most died before antibiotics, and most live now, we can conclude that an infinite antibiotic delay is important. What we don't know is how important in relation to outcome a delay on the order of hours is in any individual.

Note that even the use of the term, "delay," is pejorative, suggesting the doctor was going to give antibiotics but decided he or she was hungry and instead went to lunch. Often there is time in considering the diagnosis among others, observing and re-evaluating as occurred in this case, testing, and in discussing with the patient and their family that leads to longer times to treatment. However, to a bored jury sitting on a hard wooden seat all day, even a 1–2 hour "delay" could seem like an unreasonably long amount of time.

Here the defense expert limits his opinion about the care needed to antibiotics, but one could also contend that steroids could have been additionally beneficial. The defense expert may not have thought this was standard of care in 1999. I have yet to see a successful malpractice case of meningitis be decided on the basis of steroid administration (and to be effective, they must be given before or concurrently with the first dose of antibiotics).

Observational studies based on duration of symptoms have not found a consistent relationship between time to antibiotics and outcomes, and others based on time to treatment once presenting for care suggest that antibiotics within 6 hours or before neurological deterioration may lead to better outcomes than when given later. Of course, observational studies have great potential for confounding, and it is circular logic to presume a patient who had neurological deterioration before antibiotics did worse only because he or she did not receive them, not instead due to having bad and advanced disease.

The defense expert's testimony on hyper-acute fulminant meningitis

The defense expert attempts to make the argument that there's two types of meningitis, the type that moves slowly with a good outcome for which sooner antibiotics make no difference, and the hyper-acute fulminant type for which sooner antibiotics make no difference. Hmmm? While it can be argued that there must be something different about this patient such that he deteriorated so quickly, it is illogical that antibiotic delays aren't important in the majority of patients. I doubt a jury would buy this, but good try.

In this case, the time between points A and B, i.e., from when earlier treatment was contended to have been necessary to meet the standard of care until it was given later, is about 8 hours. Besides time, other factors in causation are how neurologically intact or devastated the patient was at point A, their ability to respond to infection and comorbidities, and the treatability of the infection. As mentioned above, pneumococcal meningitis has bad outcomes but the bug itself is not generally resistant to our standard empirical treatments. Negligence and causation often have a ying and yang relationship. The same facts that support the lack of negligence, the well-appearance and good health of the boy, also support the case for causation.

On the other hand, 8 hours is a short amount time to turn things around. We've all had strep throat. After you take your first dose on penicillin, the pain and inflammation in your throat does not start to go away for at least a day. Why would we expect antibiotics to affect a much more serious bacterial infection and inflammatory process so much faster?

And then what is your experience with septic patients and, of those who survive, the rapidity with which they turn around? To me, with a pneumococcal infection and the rapid progression, 8 hours seems too short to argue that the boy would have survived to the legal, "more likely than not" standard.*[6] If you are interested in meningitis and encephalitis, I, along with my co-authors, have reviewed the topic and also discuss bacterial meningitis causation issues.[7]

*6	
Plaintiff	Defendant
1	6

IX. Greg Henry Comments

➢Author's note (MW): Greg, you read the deposition. Would you recommend this case goes to trial or that it be settled?

I am glad to see that the eminent Dr. Talon brings some rationality to the discussion of the science in this case.

I was not physically there. I do not know how good the doctor and the various experts look in person. Again, this is a case for emotion, not science. On a science basis, I would try this case in a heartbeat. On an emotion basis, all bets are off. One of the great skills of defense attorneys is knowing how much battering their client will take. Will their sense of guilt overwhelm them in the court room? Will the Stockholm syndrome take over? All of these questions need to be answered to consider settlement.

Hospitals also become involved in settlements. Do they really want this case being discussed in the local newspapers? Do they want the publicity that goes with it? Are they willing to pick up any overage and protect the physician's financial interest? Remember the longer a case goes on, the more destructive it is to the psyche of any physician. Also it is important to remember that settlement is not an admission of guilt. It is an open statement that parties refuse to discuss the matter anymore. Realignment of the thought process of what a settlement really means can often go a long way to helping a physician be more comfortable with the idea of the settlement process.

➢**Author's note (MW):** How did it end? We'll let the actual physician who managed this case tell the rest of the story:

X. INTERVIEW OF THE EMERGENCY PROVIDER WHO CARED FOR THE PATIENT ON THE INITIAL VISIT

Do you remember this child and your thought process at the time of initial evaluation?

I saw Ty, 5 years old, with both parents on a busy Sunday late afternoon. I had been called in early as my partner physician was not known to handle high volume well.

Ty was in bed 18 for fever and abdominal pain. After completing the H&P and exam, while doing the dictation a "caution-reset light" came on in my medical decision making. I teach students now to do their documentation real-time as I've often had these "caution-reset" intuitions during the documentation process. These "caution-reset" intuitions are to be heeded, always.

Ty's mental status had seemed a little subdued for a 5-year-old boy. His parents stated this had occurred before when Ty had had acetaminophen. With some discussion they consented to LP. This required IV sedation with midazolam and fentanyl.

CSF came back 262 RBC, 8 WBC. I reasoned this was so low that bacterial meningitis had been ruled out. Ty recovered nicely from sedation and walked out of the department with Mom and Dad. I had no more "caution-reset" thoughts, what with minimal suspicion for bacterial meningitis in the first place, I was confident this CSF result had excluded it from the differential diagnosis. I went on to help move more patients.

Do you remember getting the "letter in the mail"?

The certified letter, and my wife can tell you I still get nervous every time the mail truck comes up our driveway, came a year later. The letter was a smaller aftershock.

I learned Ty had died while I was working day shift on Tuesday. By now the CSF culture was back: *Strep Pneumo.* On the drive home it hit. "This boy died, he died, this is real, he died, he died!" On arrival home Ty's death was on the local television news. Grief counselors were being made available to Ty's kindergarten classmates. His Mom and Dad, both nice small-town folks, spoke little to the TV cameras.

So much pain, for so many, and it was my doing. I cried as I never had ever, with my wife crying and hugging me. Thus began years of years of the hardest and scariest experience I've ever had. Ty's family, his sister, twin brother and Mom and Dad beginning a similar, and I am sure worse, journey. The letter in the mail, a year later, was a smaller bump in the road.

How did this affect you and your family?

It hurt so long and so hard I feared for my mental health and ability to work and take care of my wife and children. I considered suicide. Listening to "Risk Management Monthly" I learned some Docs have done so. I remember reasoning that if I had already caused so much pain, then my suicide would just cause more. It was like falling down an elevator shaft that never ends. To resort to popular culture references it was like the scene in "Top Gun" when the engines have flamed out, they are in a flat spin, the warning buzzer is sounding and Goose is saying his last words "altitude 7,000, 6,000 this is not good, this is not good." I remember being in an evening church dinner a year after Ty's death, children were singing on stage. It was a December rain outside. I had to step out, overcome by thoughts of these children, including my own, singing, while cold rain pelted Ty's grave. It is better now—I write if it may help any reader who has been or may be in similar straits.

I sought help after my wife, finally exhausted after two years of this, said "You are stuck on that dead child—you have children of your own to take care of!" My wife later said it was like I was emotionally absent for years. I sought a counselor known for working with stressed police and fire-fighters. She said I had PTSD. Cognitive therapy and EMDR (Eye Movement Desensitization Response) helped. Fifteen years have helped.

How did the decision to settle get made? What did the attorneys recommend? What did you want to do?

I wanted to settle. I had consulted several pediatric EM texts, they all included those tables we are familiar with, that is viral meningitis WBC range here to there, bacterial meningitis WBC range much higher to much higher. BUT all these references included a sentence in the text noting that bacterial meningitis can occur with lower counts. The plaintiff's attorney (who looked like my residency director—and I told him so in the elevator) had the same and similar references. In contrast, I note the 2007 PECARN study Dr. Talan refers to showing up to 10 CSF WBC's to be acceptably low risk.

It was April 2002, seated in the courtroom awaiting jury selection. The above noted PECARN study was not out then. Even if it had been, I may have done the same. I told my attorneys I could not, would not give any lawyerly answers on the stand in front of Ty's Mom and Dad. If asked I would say I had made a mistake. My attorneys, given the fact that the CSF differential had been almost all neutrophils, were not sure we would win anyway. I agreed, noting that if we had won, I would feel morally and ethically compromised. I asked them to settle. We did for $1.1 million. Ty's parent came over hugging and crying and we finally got to talk. We have talked a lot since.

In closing, I told Mike Weinstock I was interested in possibly being of help to any readers who may have had or will have similar experiences. I hope so. The world is a painful place, we are blessed to have a job that alleviates some of that pain for all comers. As they say at the end of the EM-RAP CDs, what we do is important and it matters. I pray for you and for all of our patients.

XI. Greg Henry Comments

Closing Comments

Having spent much of my professional career counseling physicians involved in legal actions, all I can say is that the devastation to the confidence, personality, and family situation of the physician can be overwhelming. Nobody likes to have his or her name associated with the death of a child. Most people would like it forgotten. There is no question that during the time that a legal action is going forward the physician is unhappier, has more fights with his or her spouse, and moving on to some resemblance of normalcy is extremely difficult.

This case was low risk and if the child has a problem secondary to antibiotic therapy, there would be serious questions as to why such was given. There is no good news here for anyone, and I hope the plaintiff's attorney understands he did no one any good by bringing this case. There was no financial dependence on this child, and certainly the parents cannot be consoled with a few dollars as opposed to having their child back. This case is the ultimate reason why the current system used in the United States should be thrown out and a system fairer to the science, and less dependent on the cynicism and emotion, adopted.

References

1. Talan DA. Bacterial cause of suspected meningitis cannot be safely excluded without cerebrospinal fluid analysis. *Ann Emerg Med.* 2012;59:227–8.
2. Ciovacco WA, Baraff LJ. Lumbar puncture is not needed for all patients suspected to have viral meningitis. *Ann Emerg Med.* 2012;59:228–9.
3. Nigrovic LE, Kuppermann N, Macias CG, et al. Clinical prediction rule for identifying children with cerebrospinal fluid pleocytosis at very low risk of bacterial meningitis. JAMA. 2007;297:52–60.
4. Straussberg R, Harel L, Nussinovitch M, Amir J. Absolute neutrophil count in aseptic and bacterial meningitis related to time of lumbar puncture. Pediatr Neurol. 2003;28:365–9.
5. Negrini B, Kelleher KJ, Wald ER. Cerebrospinal fluid findings in aseptic versus bacterial meningitis. Pediatrics. 2000;105:316–9.
6. Nigrovic LE, Malley R, Agrawal D, Kuppermann N. Pediatric Emergency Medicine Collaborative Research Committee of the American Academy of Pediatrics. Low risk of bacterial meningitis in children with a positive enteroviral polymerase chain reaction test result. Clin Infect Dis. 2010;51:1221–2.
7. Fitch MT, Abrahamian FM, Moran GJ, Talan DA. Emergency department management of meningitis and encephalitis. Infect Dis Clin North Am. 2008;22:33–52.

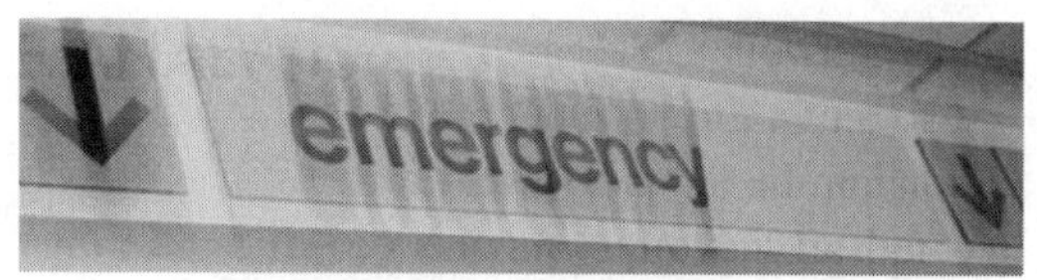

CASE 11

18-YEAR-OLD FEMALE WITH ARM PAIN

J. Matthew Blickendorf, MD
Chief Resident, Department of Emergency Medicine
Wexner Medical Center at The Ohio State University

Colin G. Kaide, MD, FACEP, FAAEM, UHM
Associate Professor of Emergency Medicine
Board-Certified Specialist in Hyperbaric Medicine
Department of Emergency Medicine
Wexner Medical Center at The Ohio State University

Frank Orth, DO, FACEP
Attending Emergency Physician, Immediate Health Associates
Emergency Department facilitator
Mt. Carmel St. Ann's Hospital, Columbus, OH

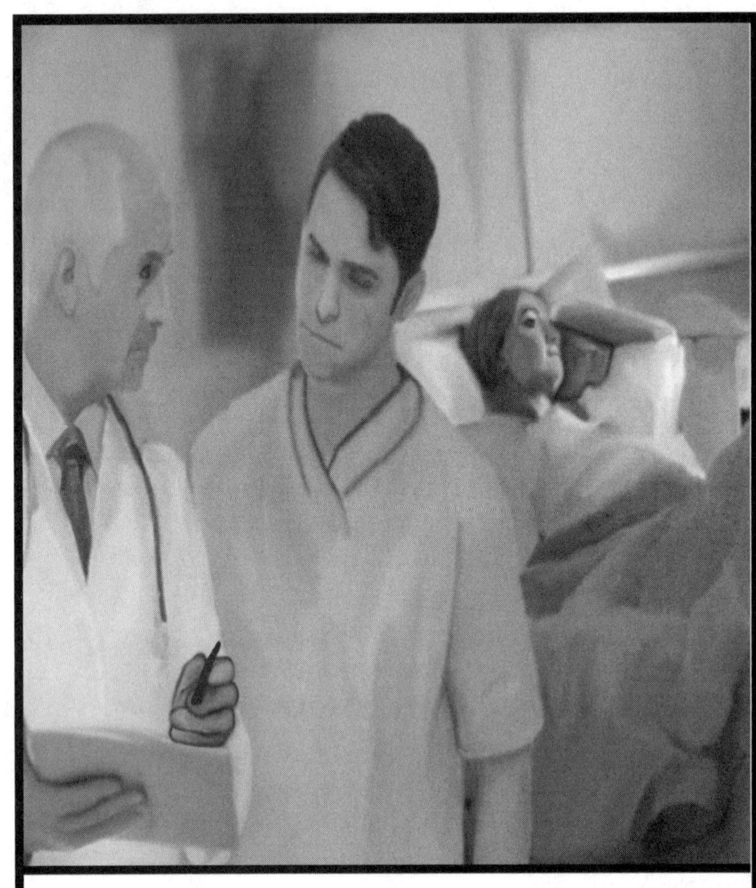

"She's having a panic attack."

CASE 11

18-YEAR-OLD FEMALE WITH ARM PAIN

PART 1—MEDICAL

The Patient's Story

Jessica is a college freshman with a little more than a month under her belt. She has a roommate and though they were only "Facebook friends" over the summer, over the last 4 weeks have become confidants. As the early fall leaves begin to change, Jessica develops chills and nausea, initially attributing her symptoms to the stress of a new environment, but the next day, Tuesday, she feels worse. Her symptoms do not resolve. Just before midnight, she presents to the local Emergency Department.

The Doctor's Version (the following is the actual documentation of the provider)

VISIT #1
Date 10/02/2008 @ 23:30
Chief complaint: body aches, fever 2 days

VITAL SIGNS

Time	Temp(F)	Pulse	Resp	Sat
23:36	100.0	94	18	99%

Disposition: After waiting over 3 hours, she approaches the triage desk and states she is feeling better. Signs paperwork for leaving before being examined (LBBE) and returns to her dorm room.

The Patient's Story (continued)

The next morning, Jessica still feels ill with fever, chills, and now has a new symptom of left arm pain. The pain in the arm is so severe she again seeks medical care.

The Doctor's Version (continued)

VISIT #2 (that same morning)
Date: 10/03/2008 @ 08:00
Chief Complaint: left arm pain, chills, HA

VITAL SIGNS

Time	Temp(F)	Pulse	Resp	Syst	Diast	Sat
08:06	98.1	not taken		97	63	

HPI: Patient is an 18 year old female who complains of fever and body aches for two days. Also has had a sore throat. This morning she developed pain in the left arm. No history of trauma to the left arm. Used Tylenol this AM 1 hour ago. No hx of mono or exposure to students with mono or strep

PMH:
NKDA
Meds: None
SH: No smoking

EXAM:
Constitutional: A&O, NAD
HEENT: Mild erythema posterior pharynx, no exudate, uvula midline. No drooling or stridor
Neck: Supple; some anterior cervical adenopathy
Lungs: CTAB
CV: RRR without m/r/g
Abd: Soft, NT without r/r/g
Ext: Pain with palpation left biceps tendon and also pain with flexion at elbow. Otherwise normal

DIAGNOSIS (09:23): Pharyngitis, muscle strain

DISPOSITION (09:25): Symptomatic treatment

PLAN: Symptomatic therapy to include acetaminophen, ibuprofen, gargles, vitamin pills. Return if worse

Chapter Author Commentary

FRANK ORTH, DO, FACEP

This sounds like a fairly routine visit for any type of viral infection—except for the pain in the arm, mentioned in the history, but with only minimal documentation on exam. There is a long differential diagnosis for a traumatic pain in an extremity and almost all are benign with one caveat; they are benign only *after* an *exam* of the arm. Checking neurovascular status including pulses, bony pain, skin changes, and signs of swelling would be helpful to rule out cellulitis, osteomyelitis, or septic joint. In fact, there was no documentation of a mechanism of an arm strain, yet that was in the diagnosis.

Making an accurate diagnosis is tough enough, but making one without adequate data on which to base it, makes it even tougher. An opportunity to gather some of this data was missed as the patient did present the prior evening, but there was no mention of this LBBE visit, made more important since the two visits were so close in time frame. Note the differences in chief complaint:

Visit #1:Chief complaint: body aches, fever 2 days
Visit #2: Chief complaint: left arm pain, chills, HA

What changed overnight? The patient now has not only infections symptoms ("fever" at the first visit and complaint of "chills" on the return visit) but on the second visit a *chief* complaint of left arm pain and also a HA. The arm pain is minimally explored, but the headache is not even mentioned in the history and there is no neurologic exam.

Finally, the disposition does not specifically mention either of its most essential elements; the importance of being 1) action and 2) time specific. There is a lack of instructions for follow up with increasing arm pain or concerning headache symptoms.

The Patient's Story (continued)

Jessica again goes back to her dorm room, but her arm pain continues to worsen and she becomes short of breath. She calls her father who tells her to go back to the ER and he will meet her there, but will not arrive for several hours (due to the drive time).

The Doctor's Version (continued)

VISIT #3 The patient returns several hours later. She is re-registered as a new patient and a repeat assessment is done by a different physician:

Date 10/03/2008 12:00
Chief complaint: arm pain is much worse, chest pain and shortness of breath
Triage (nurse): Feels like she may pass out. She is tearful. States this is the first time she has been away from home

VITAL SIGNS

Time	Temp(F)	Pulse	Resp	Syst	Diast	Sat
11:56	not done	108		102	60	99%

HPI: Was seen this morning and now has developed chest pain and left arm pain. Feels like she is going to pass out. Has SOB. No treatment initiated from first visit. No change in history except above.

EXAM:

Constitutional: A&O, NAD, anxious
HEENT: Mild erythema posterior pharynx, no exudate, uvula midline. No drooling or stridor
Neck: Supple; no adenopathy
Lungs: CTAB
CV: RRR without m/r/g

Abd: Soft, NT without r/r/g

Ext: Exam: arm still tender at area above the elbow. Subjectively could not move arm but was able to do so objectively. Neuro circ intact distally. No skin changes

MDM: Patient vomited twice. Feels like she may pass out so EKG will be done. She is given crackers. States cannot use left arm but is using it to drink water with her crackers. Per nurse she has a cool wash-cloth on her forehead.

EKG: Normal except slight tachycardia

MDM: Continued feeling of dizziness. She is now hyperventilating. Vomited. Given paper bag to breathe into. Waiting for father to arrive to take her home.

DIAGNOSIS: Hyperventilation/panic attack

Additional Chapter Author Commentary

There is a primary tenet in emergency medicine that a second visit should raise serious red flags with a stellar H&P and an expanded DDx. Jessica's symptoms were more severe in the arm. She had two episodes of vomiting. She had an elevated heart rate. Though she was short of breath, she did not have a respiratory rate measured. Something is going on—but what? Could increasing progressive severe pain with hyperventilation be from a panic attack? There are more than several elements arguing against this; the consistently localized unilateral arm pain, objective vomiting, lack of history of panic/hyperventilation, and no history of emotional disorders, to name a few. It is easy to be led astray upon hearing the nurse tell the patient to "stop breathing so fast." This patient is in trouble; it seems like this patient is being written off.

The Patient's Story (continued)

As the patient waits for her father to arrive, she continues to worsen, occasionally screaming out in pain. Upon the parent's arrival to the ED, the treating physician tells them "they can take their daughter home as she is having a panic attack." Upon entering the room, the parents see a different picture. Their daughter is diaphoretic, pale, and holding her left arm at her side, not moving it at all. The father makes a quick decision to take his daughter to a larger ED in the adjacent city, approximately 20 minutes away. On the drive she engages in minimal conversation, holding her arm, and complaining of severe pain.

The Doctor's Version (continued)

VISIT #4

Chief complaint (16:15): left arm pain. No injury. Pain scale 10/10

VITAL SIGNS						
Time	Temp(F)	Pulse	Resp	Syst	Diast	Sat
16:15	99.1	115	28	124	68	

Exam: Patient screaming in pain during examination of the arm. Ecchymoses noted on skin of upper arm with a 'bluish' discoloration 20 cm in diameter

- Testing:
  - o Plain film of arm shows subcutaneous air consistent with possible infection in tissues.
  - o Labs:
    - WBC 4.4 with 15% bands
    - Sodium 132, potassium 2.8, CO_2 19, glucose 138, creatinine 0.8
    - Sed rate 34
    - Pregnancy- negative
- Antibiotics are started immediately and she is given IV pain meds and IV fluids
- Air transport is arranged and she is flown to a tertiary care center
- Upon arrival, patient is taken directly to the operating room, where the left arm is amputated at the level of the chest wall musculature
- Secondary closure ensues
- Culture positive for clostridia species

FINAL DIAGNOSIS: Necrotizing fasciitis left arm

PART 2—THE ANALYSIS

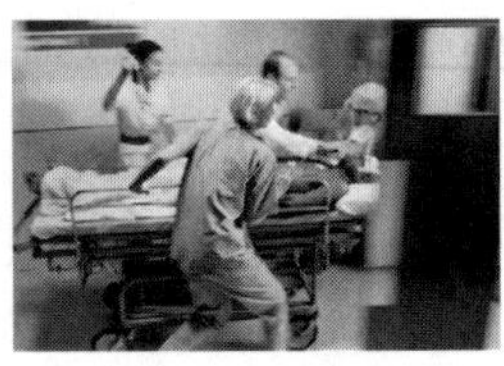

NECROTIZING SOFT TISSUE INFECTIONS (NSTIs)

J. Matthew Blickendorf, MD
Chief Resident, Department of Emergency Medicine
Wexner Medical Center at The Ohio State University

Colin G. Kaide, MD, FACEP, FAAEM, UHM
Associate Professor of Emergency Medicine
Board-Certified Specialist in Hyperbaric Medicine
Department of Emergency Medicine
Wexner Medical Center at The Ohio State University

This case is extremely humbling for emergency physicians—the diagnosis of necrotizing fasciitis (NF) requiring emergent amputation of a young girl's arm is made at her *fourth* ED visit in 24 hours. Documentation of the previous 3 visits provides a unique understanding of how this disease can progress rapidly from benign signs and symptoms to acute severe illness. Affecting 500–1500 patients annually in the US.[1, 2] NF produces a life-threatening infection with a mortality rate of 25–35%, despite maximal therapy.[3]

The Pathology

NF is an infection of soft tissue that quickly progresses to necrosis of subcutaneous tissues and muscle fascia. Endotoxins, exotoxins, protease enzymes, and activation of the clotting cascade produce local endothelial damage, tissue edema, and impaired micro-vascular blood flow blocking the delivery of antibiotics and decreasing the effectiveness of PMNs.[4-5] Expanding local tissue injury stimulates the inflammatory response cascade causing severe systemic toxicity and even cardiovascular collapse.[4] The infection can spread at the rate of one inch per hour without manifesting overlying skin changes until the infection is in an advanced state. Jessica's arm didn't demonstrate skin changes until she presented with a dusky ecchymotic area requiring emergent amputation. Patients who survive the initial infection often have significant ongoing morbidity after multiple surgeries for debridement and surgical reconstruction.

NF occurs in in two different but occasionally overlapping patterns. The majority of cases are Type I NF, a poly-microbial infection that tends to develop in older and sicker patients who have a history of chronic systemic disease such as peripheral vascular disease, immune compromise, or diabetes. While many patients have an inciting factor like a decubitus ulcer, postoperative wound, animal/inset bite, or insulin injection site, often there is no obvious source of injury.

The involvement of both aerobic and anaerobic bacteria distinguishes Type I from Type II NF. In Type I NF, wound cultures frequently grow *S. aureus*, *S. pyogenes*, *E. coli*, *B. fragilis*, and various species of *Enterococci*, *Peptostreptococcus*, *Prevotella*, and *Porphyromonas*. *Clostridium perfringens* is reported in Type I NF but has recently become less common.[5, 7] Fournier's gangrene, a form of NF that attacks the perineum and abdominal wall, is also poly-microbial but enteric organisms predominate.

Type II NF accounts for only 15–20% of cases.[8-10] It is the mono-microbial form previously caused almost exclusively by Group A Streptococcus (*S. pyogenes*). However, community-associated methicillin-resistant staph aureus (MRSA) has been increasingly reported as the sole organism.[11-12] Though type II NF can develop spontaneously in otherwise healthy people who have no known inciting factor or portal of entry,[13] most patients will have a history of minor skin trauma or blunt injury. IV drug use has emerged as another significant risk factor for Type II NF.[14]

Although not universally accepted, experts use the designation of a Type III to describe a rare, very virulent form of NF caused by *Vibrio vulnificus*. This is seen in coastal communities and is associated with exposure of an open wound to warm sea water.[15-16]

Clinical Presentation

Diagnosing NF clinically can be strikingly easy or extremely difficult depending on how advanced the infection is on presentation. The diagnosis hinges upon how quickly one recognizes that this "particular cellulitis" doesn't look like the other 1000 cases seen during the year! Jessica's case drives this point home; her first ED visit included nonspecific symptoms of fever, chills, nausea, and myalgias, but NF was at the top of the differential by her fourth visit when she presented screaming in intractable pain with a blue ecchymotic arm without history of injury.

Rapidly progressing pain, diaphoresis, and anxiety together with a history of skin trauma or injury only occurs in 10–40% of patients.[19-20] The initial presentation of NF most commonly appears like cellulitis: skin erythema, swelling, and pain. The striking feature that often distinguishes this infection is tenderness beyond the margins of the apparently infected area. The pain is frequently "out of proportion" to a garden-variety cellulitis. This may be the only clue that there is serious badness brewing just below the surface!

In addition to color change and crepitus, later skin findings include blistering and bullae formation. Various studies have reported crepitus in only 13% —31% of patients.[9] However, the probability of NF is very high if crepitus is found on exam. In the final stages, bullae convert to hemorrhagic bullae, and skin anesthesia and necrosis can quickly follow. Most patients seek evaluation for their severe pain before progressing to the end-stage presentation of fever, shock, altered mental status and impending cardiovascular collapse. If NF is strongly considered clinically, the goal is early evaluation by a surgeon for possible debridement or amputation, the only definitive therapy.

Lab & Imaging Workup

Commonly abnormal lab values in NF include an elevated white count (>15,000) and low sodium (<135). Other inflammatory markers are often elevated. A scoring system was devised to help risk stratify patients in whom NF is considered. A total of less than 6 points was reported to have a 96% negative predictive value for NF whereas a score of 6 or greater confers a positive predictive value of 92%. Subsequent, though less well-done, studies have failed to validate the predictive value of the system.[21-24]

Laboratory Risk Indicator for Necrotizing Fasciitis	
Variable	Score
C-reactive protein (mg/dL)	
< 15	0
≥ 15	4
Total white blood cell count (1000s per mm³)	
< 15	0
15–25	1
> 25	2
Hemoglobin (g/dL)	
> 13.5	0
11–13.5	1
< 11	2
Sodium (mmol/L)	
≥ 135	0
< 135	2
Creatinine (mg/dL)	
≤ 1.59	0
> 1.59	2
Glucose (mg/dL)	
≤ 180	0
> 180	1
A score < 6 suggests a 96% negative predictive value for NF, and a score of 6 or greater suggests a 92% positive predictive value	

Source: Su YC, Chen HW, Hong YC, et al. Laboratory risk indicator for necrotizing fasciitis score and the outcomes. ANZ J Surg. 2008;78(11):968–72. Table 1 at 969. © 2008 John Wiley & Sons. Used with permission.

Imaging can be helpful when NF is suspected but not clear enough to convince a surgeon to operate. Subcutaneous air on x-ray is highly specific but not sensitive for NF; it is a big mistake to assume that the absence of gas rules out NF. CT is more sensitive than plain films and allows for the identification of gas, fluid collections, and inflammatory changes in deeper tissue planes. Its sensitivity is traditionally quoted at 80% (Wysoki)[25] but up to 100% in a recent study (Zacharias).[33]

MRI remains the most definitive imaging modality with sensitivities of 90–100%. However, specificities are only reported at 50–85%.[26,27] MRI can be problematic in a patient who is developing systemic symptoms of disease since it is a time-consuming test which removes the patient from the critical care aspects of the ED. Regardless of imaging modality, gas is identified in only 25% of NF. Overall, imaging studies are generally only indicated in cases in which the diagnosis is questionable. Obvious cases of NF suffer when tests get between them and surgical steel!

Direct Exploration as Diagnostic Tool

A very effective but seldom performed way to diagnose NF clinically is to do a 2 cm bedside incision over the affected area, continued down to the muscle fascia. The ability to slide a finger easily along the disrupted fascia, along with the finding of gray-brown purulent fluid and necrotic tissue clinches the diagnosis![27, 28]

Treatment

Definitive treatment for NF is surgical debridement. The mortality of NF is directly proportional to the delay to operative management. Delays of 24 hours confer a nine fold increase in mortality.[29] A recent Australian study described a clear correlation with survival and early surgical debridement.[30]

Antibiotic therapy is not definitive because antibiotics do not penetrate into the areas of active infection. However it is very important in the treatment of sepsis and in controlling the spread of the disease. Empiric therapy should include coverage for MRSA and MSSA along with gram negative and anaerobic bacteria. Piperacillin/tazobactam, vancomycin, and clindamycin are a typical regimen.

Hyperbaric Oxygen Therapy (HBO) can be used as an adjunct therapy, but it should never delay definitive surgical therapy. Inhaled 100% oxygen at pressures of 2.5–3 atmospheres absolute generates a partial pressure of oxygen up to 2200 mmHg. The hyperoxic environment results in physiologic and biochemical changes that can have significant antibacterial effects and improve the effectiveness of antibiotics.[31] HBO is best used after debridement. Studies to date have shown a decrease in mortality, amputations, and surgical re-debridement when HBO is added to aggressive surgery.[31-32]

Closing Thoughts on Jessica's Case

Jessica's case was not classic for either form of NF since she was previously healthy without an inciting factor but had cultures grow primarily *Clostridium* species. It's interesting to note that her illness course began first with *systemic* signs and symptoms before localized arm pain. Though not evaluated by a physician at the initial visit, diagnosing a viral syndrome would have been consistent with her symptoms.

The MDM began to unravel at the back-to-back second and third visits. After presenting with chief complaints of arm pain, chills, and headache during her second visit, she is discharged with two distinct diagnoses of pharyngitis and arm strain. As stated above, an incomplete exam is recorded, and furthermore there are no documented historical elements to support the diagnosis of muscle strain. It would be a stretch to attribute her localized arm pain to a viral syndrome. Myalgias from a viral illness do not typically localize and progress in severity, as was the case with Jessica. Unfortunately for the physician taking care of her at the third visit, Jessica didn't have skin changes. However, she did have "pain out of proportion to exam" without history of trauma, injury, or overuse.

The fact that the patient—a young previously healthy college student without psychiatric or maladaptive behavioral history—does not leave because of uncontrolled pain and dissatisfaction with the diagnoses should be a red flag in and of itself. Panic and anxiety attacks are diagnoses of exclusion. Writing these in the chart should reflexively cause the discharging physician to pause and reflect as to whether there is any alternative explanation.

Of course patients can present with multiple distinct illnesses or injuries, but keep your guard up with these patients. Attempting to ascertain a single diagnosis that concomitantly explains all symptoms should be pursued before assigning multiple diagnoses to explain isolated symptoms—especially when tempted to include a diagnosis not supported by the H&P. This is the principle of Occam's razor: among competing hypotheses, the one with the fewest assumptions should be selected.

As physicians in a tertiary referral center, specifically one that provides hyperbaric oxygen, we see a good number of "de novo" and "referred for (possible) necrotizing fasciitis" patients. This diagnosis can be a "no man's land." It can fall into the domain of many specialties including general surgery, orthopedics, urology, and OB/Gyn. It is important for the emergency physician to take ownership of these patients, so their care is not delayed.

When the diagnosis is obvious—a patient with diabetes who presents with a rapidly progressive cellulitis, including blebs and blisters, abnormal vitals signs, and elevated inflammatory markers—things may still progress at an average pace if the consultants aren't made acutely aware of the degree of your concern. When the situation is less obvious and a person comes into the ED with a cellulitis that looks "different" than most of the cellulitis you have seen, the problem may stagnate to the point of disaster! No one wants to believe the patient has NF, especially over the phone in the middle of the night. In suspicious cases, it's imperative that the physician suspecting NF be decisive and confident when explaining why the surgeon must evaluate the patient immediately.

✔ Teaching points

- All documented chief complaints should be fully explored and documented
- Reported extremity pain warrants documentation of neurovascular status, soft tissue or bony pain with palpation, and the presence or absence of skin changes or swelling
- Bounceback visits should prompt an expanded H&P, differential diagnosis, and MDM documentation
- Be cautious when assigning diagnoses not supported by the H&P or your documentation
- Panic and anxiety attacks are always diagnoses of exclusion—*you* should hyperventilate and feel panicky a little when writing these diagnoses in the chart!
- Extremity pain "out of proportion to exam" should raise a red flag and broaden the differential to include diagnoses like compartment syndrome and necrotizing fasciitis
- Necrotizing fasciitis requires early surgical consultation and intervention—time is flesh!

References

1. Jallali WS, Butler PE. Hyperbaric oxygen as adjuvant therapy in the management of necrotizing fasciitis. Am J Surg. 2005; 189(4):462–6.
2. Levine EG, Manders SM. Life-threatening necrotizing fasciitis. Clin Dermatol. 2005; 23(2):144–7.
3. Shiroff AM, Herlitz GN, Gracias VH. Necrotizing soft tissue infections. J Int Care Med. 2014; 29(3):138–44.
4. Salcido RS. Necrotizing fasciitis: reviewing the causes and treatment strategies. Adv Skin Wound Care. 2007; 20:288–93.
5. Cainzos M, Gonzalez-Rodriguez FJ. Necrotizing soft tissue infections. Curr Opin Crit Care. 2007; 13:433–39.
6. Mandell GL, et al. Mandell, Douglas, and Bennett's principles and practice of infectious diseases. New York: Churchill-Livingston; 2005.
7. Brook I, Frazier E. Clinical and microbiological features of necrotizing fasciitis. J Clin Microbiol. 1995; 33(9):2382–7.
8. Hasham S, et al. Necrotising fasciitis. BMJ. 2005; 330(7495):830–3.
9. Sarani B, Strong M, Pascual J, Schwab CW. Necrotizing fasciitis: current concepts and review of the literature. J Am Coll Surg. 2009; 208(2):279–88.
10. VanUnnik A. Inhibition of toxin production in Clostridium perfringens in vitro by hyperbaric oxygen. Antonie Leeuwenhoek Microbiology. 1965; 31:181–6.
11. Jonsson K, Hunt TK. Oxygen as an isolated variable influences resistance to infection. Ann Surg. 1988; 208(6):783–7.
12. Wong CH, Chang HC, Pasupathy S, et al. Necrotizing fasciitis: clinical presentation, microbiology, and determinants of mortality. J Bone Joint Surg Am. 2003; 85(8):1454–60.
13. Miller LG, et al. Necrotizing fasciitis caused by community-associated methicillin-resistant Staphylococcus aureus in Los Angeles. N Engl J Med. 2005; 352(14):1445–53.
14. Lee TC, Carrick MM, Scott BG, et al. Incidence and clinical characteristics of methicillin-resistant Staphylococcus aureus necrotizing fasciitis in a large urban hospital. Am J Surg. 2007;194(6):809–12.
15. Childers BJ, et al. Necrotizing fasciitis: a fourteen-year retrospective study of 163 consecutive patients. Am Surg. 2002; 68(2):109–16.
16. Chen JL, Fullerton KE, Flynn NM. Necrotizing fasciitis associated with injection drug use. Clin Infect Dis. 2001; 33(1):6–15.
17. Kuo Chou TN, Chao WN, Yang C, et al. Predictors of mortality in skin and soft-tissue infections caused by Vibrio vulnificus. World J Surg. 2010; 34:1669–75.
18. Chen SC, Chan KS, Chao WN, et al. Clinical outcomes and prognostic factors for patients with Vibrio vulnificus infections requiring intensive care: a 10-yr retrospective study. Crit Care Med. 2010; 38:1984–90.
19. McHenry CR, Piotrowski JJ, Petrinic D, et al. Determinants of mortality for necrotizing soft-tissue infections. Ann Surg. 1995; 221:558–65.
20. Wong CH, Haw-Chong C, Shanker P, et al. Necrotizing fasciitis: clinical presentation, microbiology, and determinants of mortality. J Bone Joint Surg Am. 2003; 85:1454–1460.

21. Wall DB, Kleain SR, Black S, et al. A simple model to help distinguish necrotizing from non-necrotizing soft tissue infection. J Am Coll Surg. 2000; 191(3):227–31.
22. Wall DB, de Virgilio C, Black S, et al. Objective criteria may assist in distinguishing necrotizing fasciitis from non-necrotizing soft tissue infection. Am J Surg. 2000; 179(1):17–21.
23. Wong CH, Khin LW, Heng KS, et al. The LRINEC (Laboratory Risk Indicator for Necrotising Fasciitis) score: a tool for distinguishing necrotizing fasciitis from other soft tissue infections. Crit Care Med. 2004; 32(7):1535–41.
24. Holland MJ. Application of the Laboratory Risk Indicator in Necrotising Fasciitis (LRINEC) score to patients in a tropical tertiary referral centre. Anaesth Intesive Care. 2009; 37(4):588–92.
25. Wysoki MG, SantoraTA, Shah RM, Friedman AC. Necrotizing fasciitis: CT characteristics. Radiology. 1997; 203:859–63.
26. Seok JH, Jee WH, Chun KA, et al. Necrotizing fasciitis versus pyomyositis: discrimination with using MR imaging. Korean J Radiol. 2009; 10(2):121–8.
27. Kim KT, Kim YJ, Won Lee J, et al. Can necrotizing infectious fasciitis be differentiated from nonnecrotizing infectious fasciitis with MR imaging? Radiology. 2011; 259(3):816–24.
28. Andreasen TJ, Green SD, Childers BJ. Massive soft-tissue injury: diagnosis and management of necrotizing fasciitis and purpura fulminans. Plast Reconstr Surg. 2001; 107(4):1025–35.
29. Wong CH, Haw-Chong C, Shanker P, et al. Necrotizing fasciitis: clinical presentation, microbiology, and determinants of mortality. J Bone Joint Surg Am. 2003; 85:1454–60.
30. Kelly Bucca K, Spencer R, Orford N, et al. Early diagnosis and treatment of necrotizing fasciitis can improve survival: an observational intensive care unit cohort study. ANZ J Surg. 2013; 83:365–70.
31. Kaide CG, Khandelwal S. Hyperbaric Oxygen—Application in Infectious Disease. In: Martin, D, et al. Infectious Diseases—Emergency Medicine Clinics of North America. 2007.
32. Shaw JJ, Psoinos C, Emhoff TA, et al. Not just full of hot air: hyperbaric oxygen therapy increases survival in cases of necrotizing soft tissue infections. Surg Infect. 2014; 15(3):328–35.
33. Zacharias N, et al. Diagnosis of necrotizing soft tissue infections by computed tomography. Arch Surg. 2010;145(5):452–5.

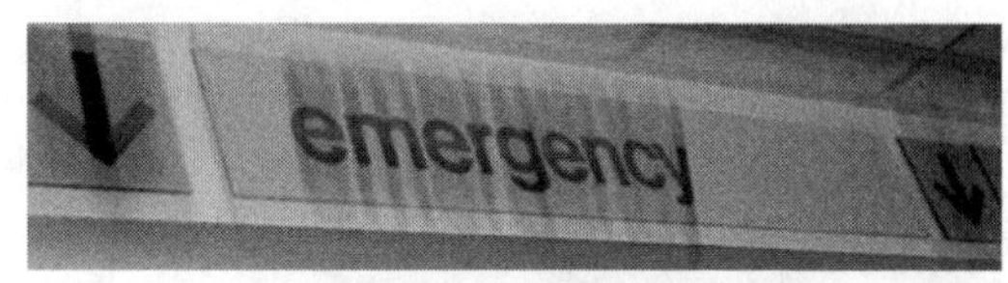

CASE 12

2-YEAR-OLD BOY WITH CONSTIPATION

Solomon Behar, MD, FACEP, FAAP
Assistant Professor of Emergency Medicine and Pediatrics
Los Angeles County Medical Center and Children's Hospital Los Angeles
Keck School of Medicine at the University of Southern California

PART 1—MEDICAL

PART 2—THE ANALYSIS

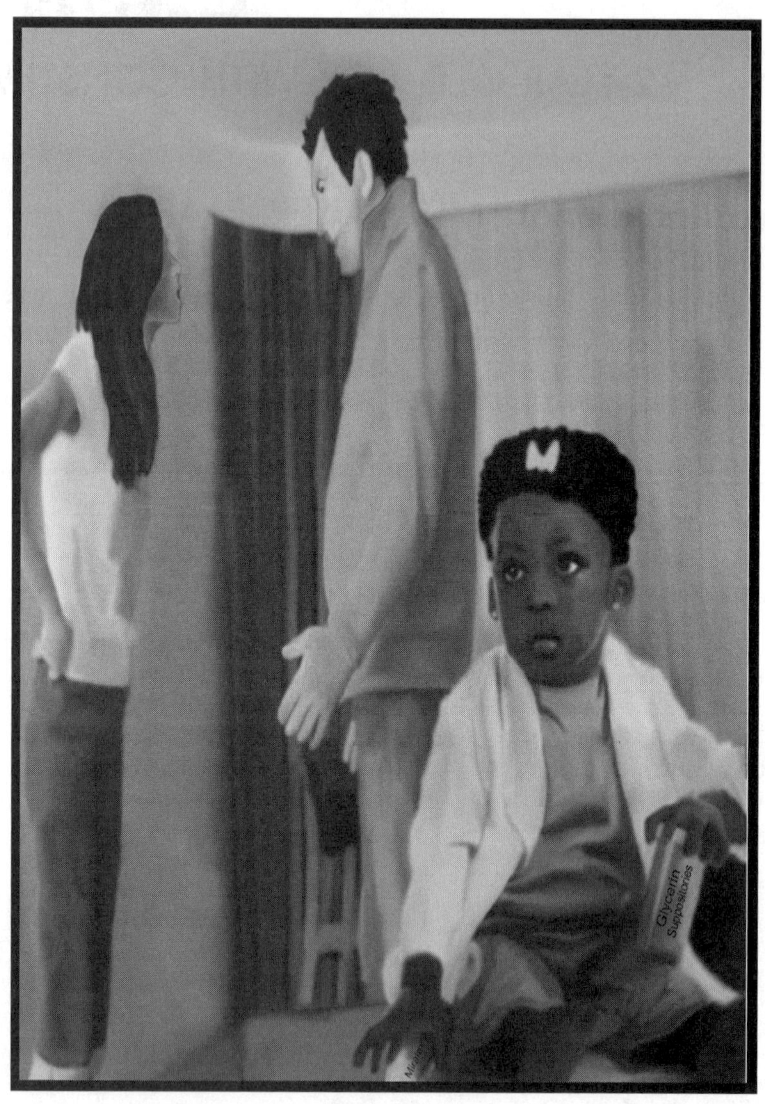
Glycerin
Suppositories

CASE 12

2-YEAR-OLD BOY WITH CONSTIPATION

PART 1—MEDICAL

I. The Doctor's Version (the following is the actual documentation of the provider)

Initial Visit (1405):

Chief Complaint: constipation, no BM x1.5 wks

VITAL SIGNS

Time	Temp(C)	Pulse	Resp	Syst	Diast	Sat	Weight	Pain
14:05	37.6	153	28	97	69	100%(RA)	11.9kg	4/10

RN Triage assessment: comfortable, a/a/o for age, pink, warm, well perfused, irritable but consolable, firm, distended abdomen, lungs with good aeration, normal color and temperature, delayed capillary refill time, regular rhythm, normal skin turgor, absent edema, no rash

HPI: (1440- resident) 2yo M brought in by parents. Constipation x1 yr, belly is hard, not tender to touch. No fever. Rhinorrhea x3 days. Cough this AM. Vomit x1, about 4wks ago. Drink only juice, milk, and no solid food. Little diarrhea today. Normal UOP. No food intake x3days. Glycerin suppositories last use 2 days, tried every week. MiraLAX yesterday

Review of Systems: Negative for derm, throat, GU, MSK, psych, neuro, exposures.

PAST MEDICAL HISTORY:
Medications: glycerine suppository, miralax
Allergies: NKDA
Birth hx: full term, c-section
PMHx/Hospitalizations: none
Immunizations: Up to date, no flu shot
PSH: none

PHYSICAL EXAM: (resident) - Check boxes marked:
Triage sheet reviewed
Alert, no distress,
Eyes PERRLA, Ears well formed
Normal external ears
Moist mucous membranes
Neck normal

No heart murmur
Clear breath sounds
Abdomen: No guarding, no rebound, Bowel sounds present
Extremities warm, well perfused
Neuro no abnormality
Psych no abnormality

Hand written notes: (resident) - Sleeping. Mass felt in all Q's. Normocephalic, PERRLA, well formed ears

Attending PE: (1450) - Comfortable, no resp distress, MMM(+), lungs clear, abd distended, soft, (+)TTP, palpable stool. Rectal w/decreased tone (+) palpable stool in vault, No mass palpable

Orders: (1500)
Pediatric fleet enema PR x1
Magnesium citrate 48mL PO x1

RN progress notes:
(1530) assumed care for this 2 yo who is FOS, Mixed Mag citrate w cherry syrup. Toddler will not drink
(1545)Peds enema x1 (+) sm amt stool
(1645) Repeat enema, child fights enema
(1735) Pt care assumed for d/c. Rx given. Pt awake and playful. Mom and Dad educated about constipation

MD PROGRESS NOTES: (resident- untimed): enema peds given, no change, adult enema

Attending
(1630): (+)stool with enema
(1720): abd soft, (+) more stool

DISCHARGE VITAL SIGNS

VITAL SIGNS					
Temp(C)	Pulse	Resp	Syst	Diast	Pain Scale
37.6	148	36	108	67	0/10

DIAGNOSIS: Constipation

Disposition (1750): d/c home, use miralax as directed. Constipation handout given. Increase H2O, high fiber diet. Return for unable to tolerate PO, or any other concerning symptoms. Follow-up with PMD in 2-3 days.

II. Greg Henry Comments

"Children do not need to have a daily bowel movement to obtain admission to Harvard."

Children present to the emergency department more commonly when they are first born as opposed to fifth born; I don't think there is a more common case than constipation. Parents need to figure these things out—despite all their beliefs, I have never seen a child's abdomen actually explode. Children less than 1 month of age may have organic process such as Hirschsprung's disease, but this is not a moment to moment type emergency.

The great danger of the diagnosis of constipation is that it may be wrong; that may be 1 in 100 or 1 in 1,000, we cannot be too casual. History and physical examination are adequate as long as they are properly performed. As far as management, doing nothing is often best. Placing children on home management with harsh enemas cannot only lead to metabolic disorders but general unhappiness and difficulty in establishing a normal bowel pattern.

It is impossible to make parents believe that a normal stool every 2–3 days is just fine and that children do not need to have a daily bowel movement to obtain admission to Harvard. Of note, repeat vital signs show that the heart rate has improved, though his respiratory rate is higher.

III. The Bounceback (5 hours, 58 minutes after ED discharge)

Chief Complaint (2348): no BM

- Vital signs: T 39.9, HR 173, RR 40, BP unable x3, Pain 8/10
- RN Triage notes (23:55):
  - o Grunting, nasal flaring, pale, normal temperature, regular pulse, normal skin turgor, no edema, sticky MM. Lethargic, poor air entry bilateral lungs. (++) distended abdomen. Cool extremities, distal pulses present.
  - o Pt brought into Bed A via triage. Skin cool/cap refill 5-6 sec. (+) grunting, pox 85% on 15 L NRB. Abd distended. (+) BM loose in diaper. Dr. X at bedside. IV NS bolus running.
- Attending Note: 2yo F in extremis, distended abd, hypoxia, and fever. Seen earlier for constipation→fleets given x2. IVF's
- (0004) Dr Y intubated with 4.5 cuffed ETT, verified with ETCO2 @25. BP 59/30.
- (0015) Attending Note: Abx, surgery consult, x-rays, EKG, labs done. Concern for sepsis, abd catastrophe. Unclear source of chronic constip. PICU admit.
- (0025) HR 150, BP 86/62. 3rd NS bolus running.

Test results

- o VBG/iSTAT lytes: VBG : pH 7.26, PCO2 30, PO2 40, Base deficit -12, HCO3 14. Hgb 13.9 Na 140, K 4.1, glucose 95. Ionized Ca2+: 1.4 (!L!)
- o Phosphorus (45.3!), magnesium (2.7).

- EKG: sinus tachycardia with a normal QRS duration (70msec) and normal PR interval (100msec)
- Calcium gluconate given, started on dopamine. As GI and bladder decompression continued, abdominal girth lessened and the vent settings were reduced. O2 saturations improved. Pt transferred to PICU.
- Other results:
  - KUB/X-table lateral: No free air or pneumatosis. Large amounts of stool throughout dilated large intestine, and small bowel dilation. (+)air fluid levels. No gas in rectum.
  - UA (cath): No glu, small ketones, small blood, No LE, No nit, Sp grav 1.030
  - CBC: WBC 8.5 (29% segs, 14% bands, 38% lymphs, 9% monos), Hgb 12.4, Hct 36.3, platelets 298
  - PT 15.6, INR 1.6, PTT 41, D-dimer (+), fibrinogen 371
    - Na 146, K 3.6, Cl 94, HCO3 13, Anion gap 21,BUN 30, Cr 0.6, glu 95, Alb 3.3 total protein 5.5, total bili 0.5, AST 48, ALT <6, alk phos 122, amylase 110, lipase 95
    - TSH 0.22 (low), Free T4 1.49 (normal)

ED ADMITTING DIAGNOSES:

1. Hypocalcemia
2. Sepsis
3. Hyperphosphatemia- iatrogenic
4. Respiratory Failure
5. Chronic constipation

Hospital Course:

- He remained in the hospital for 17 days to wean off the ventilator and vasopressors, correct his electrolyte abnormalities, and workup his chronic constipation.
- His thyroid studies were normal, blood and urine cultures were (-).
- Rectal disimpaction in the OR by pediatric surgery was performed, along with colonic biopsy for Hirschsprung's disease which was negative
- Urine toxicology was (+) for cocaine after a social history revealed the father to be incarcerated for drug use and dealing. The department of child and family services (DCFS) was called and the pt was removed from the home, and parents detained for dealing drugs/ exposing child to cocaine.
- He was discharged on polyethylene glycol electrolyte solution, senna and bisacodyl in good condition

FINAL DIAGNOSIS: Constipation secondary to cocaine toxicity with iatrogenic hyperphosphatemia secondary to enema administration

PART 2—THE ANALYSIS

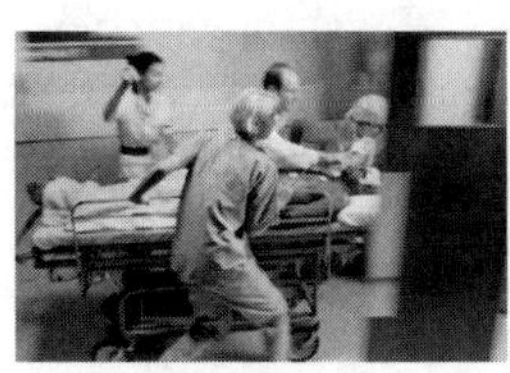

EVALUATION AND EMERGENT MANAGEMENT OF CONSTIPATION IN CHILDREN

Solomon Behar, MD, FACEP, FAAP
Assistant Professor of Emergency Medicine and Pediatrics
Los Angeles County Medical Center and Children's Hospital Los Angeles
Keck School of Medicine at the University of Southern California

Introduction

Constipation is the most common discharge diagnosis in children seen in the ED for abdominal pain.[1] It is characterized by infrequent, hard or incomplete evacuation of stool from a child's bowels. ER visits and outpatient medical resource utilization is higher in patients with constipation than those patients without constipation.[2] You will be seeing these patients in your ED!

Definition of functional constipation in children

Diagnostic criteria for functional constipation were most recently delineated in 2006 (so called Rome III criteria)[3] which include 2 or more of the following symptoms:

1. Two or fewer stools per week,
2. At least 1 episode of fecal incontinence per week,
3. History of retentive posturing or excessive volitional stool retention,
4. History of hard or painful bowel movements,
5. Presence of a large fecal mass in the rectum,
6. History of large diameter stools that may obstruct the toilet

Our patient meets these criteria by not having stool for 1.5 weeks, and by having hard stool in his rectum on exam. The parents have tried glycerin, Miralax) but he seems to have had constipation resistant to these treatments. It is unclear whether 1.5 weeks is the norm for our patient or if this is a prolonged amount of time even for him.

Epidemiology

Between 0.7–29% of all children in the pediatric population are affected by constipation.[4] Peak age for functional constipation in children is 1–4 years. There are three peaks during which onset of constipation is common:

1. When starting solid foods from breast milk or formula (age 4-6 months), particularly if the infant is started on rice cereal too early (some parents will place cereal in the bottle to make their "baby sleep through the night!")
2. During potty training (usually 2–3 yrs of age)

3. When the child starts school and does not want to use the bathroom at school (age 4–5 years)[5]

The prevalence of ED visits for constipation in children is about 0.3%.[6] Our patient has had constipation for one year, falling into a less common age group (age 1–2 yrs) for which one usually sees constipation arise. He was not being potty trained yet, and had been eating a mostly liquid diet by history. Perhaps an organic cause should have been suspected given the severity and timing of his constipation.

History and differential diagnosis of constipation

Birth history should be obtained, inquiring about passage of meconium within the first 48 hours of life. Failure to pass meconium in a timely fashion may indicate the presence of a pathologic condition such as Hirschsprung's disease (intestinal aganglionosis) or meconium ileus associated with cystic fibrosis. Onset of true constipation before 1 month of life should raise your suspicion for organic disease. In exclusively breast-fed children, it can be normal for the child to not pass stool for up to 7 days, but the stool should be soft, and there should be no associated vomiting or abdominal distention. There was no mention on the initial visit of the stool history immediately after birth.

Parental description of the stools can be helpful. Ribbon-like stools implies a stenotic anal opening. Other anatomic abnormalities of the lower GI tract include:

- Perineal fistulae
- Anterior displaced anus
- Anal stenosis
- Fistulae between the lower GI tract and urinary system
- Rectovaginal fistula in females.

Patients may report passage of stool from the urinary tract when GI/GU fistulae are present. Neural tube defects such as spina bifida can lead to bowel dysfunction as the nerves controlling bowel function are located at the abnormally formed sacral level.

Other history should include exposure to medications or toxins, which can lead to slow GI motility. The list of medications that can lead to colonic pseudo-obstruction are myriad and include: opiates, phenothiazines, atropine and other anticholinergics, nifedipine, procainamide, tricyclic antidepressants, amphetamines, barbiturates, clonidine, ipecac, and verapamil.[7]

Botulism can occur in the young patient (<1 year old) exposed to spores in honey or soil, and severe constipation is one of the earliest presenting symptoms. Lead or other heavy metal poisoning may present with constipation. Clearly, given the rarity of childhood exposure to cocaine, no one suspected occult cocaine exposure.

There is an association of dysfunctional voiding behaviors and child maltreatment,[8] so this avenue should be explored in children with unexplained longstanding constipation or recent change in bowel habits (e.g., new encopresis in a previously potty trained child).

Cow's milk-protein allergy is associated with constipation[9,10] in the infant newly starting on cow's milk (or cow's milk based formula, i.e. most standard infant formulas). Common symptoms of this condition are chronic diarrhea, bloating, fussiness, flatulence, anal fissures, urticaria, rhinorrhea, wheezing, with occasional vomiting or frank blood in the stool with an otherwise well-appearing infant.

Family history should be obtained for gastrointestinal diseases (inflammatory bowel disease, celiac disease, food sensitivities or allergies) or other systemic diseases (thyroid, parathyroid, renal disease, cystic fibrosis) that may be a factor in the child's constipation.

Functional constipation makes up the vast majority of causes diagnosed in the ED. Inadequate water and fiber intake, diets rich in starch and junk food are the usual suspects. Symptoms begin after age 4–6 months when infants are introduced to solid food.

Physical exam

Physical examination in longstanding constipation should include inspection of the anus and a rectal examination. An empty rectal vault, caused by failure of the distal portion of the large intestine to relax due to absence of myenteric innervation is typically seen in Hirschsprung's, whereas a full vault is more consistent with functional constipation. Digital rectal examination (DRE) may detect anal stenosis or other pelvic mass. Note that DRE is not needed to make the diagnosis of functional constipation.[11]

Findings of a patulous or bruised anal area or one with multiple fissures should lead to suspicion of sexual abuse. The sacrum of the child should be inspected for sacral dimples or hair tufts indicative of an underlying possible neural tube defect. Evaluate the child's lower limb neuromuscular tone, deep tendon reflexes and anal tone to evaluate abnormalities of the lumbar/sacral nerve plexus. Check the child's weight to make sure they are not failing to thrive (<3rd percentile for age), common in cystic fibrosis.

Hypothyroid infants may have relative bradycardia, puffy face, large and protruded tongue, large anterior fontanelle that remain open longer than expected (> age 1 year), poor growth leading to short stature and developmental delay. Severe constipation followed by descending paralysis and bulbar palsies should raise suspicion for botulism toxin. In our patient, no mention is made of abnormalities in the perineal or sacral anatomy. There is a note on the first visit of decreased rectal tone without explanation of the reason behind this finding. Perhaps this could have been interpreted as a sign of physical/sexual abuse or underlying neurologic issue.

Diagnostic testing for constipation

Physical exam and history alone are usually adequate to make the diagnosis of functional constipation. However, imaging is occasionally used to confirm the diagnosis or make an alternative diagnosis. Various authors have attempted to devise constipation scores based on abdominal radiographic findings to diagnose functional constipation (using the clinical definition as the gold standard), but most have wide ranges of sensitivities (60–80%), and specificities (43–90%).[12-16] In routine cases of functional constipation, without evidence of "red-flag" symptoms and exam findings as listed above, an x-ray or testing for other underlying conditions (e.g. thyroid testing, electrolytes, milk protein allergy tests) is not necessary.

Management of constipation

The age of the child often dictates the mode of treatment. The first step is disimpaction of hard, backed up stool. Polyethylene glycol (PEG) given orally or as an enema (1.5 g/kg/day) is equally efficacious and safe in kids older than 2 years,[17] but oral medications are preferable for use in children since rectal administration may cause undue distress.

Once you've cleaned out the old poop, your goal is to keep things flowing smoothly, i.e., maintenance dosing. This can be accomplished in a number of ways. PEG (a lower dose than in disimpaction phase—0.4 mg/kg/day[18]), and milk of magnesia are osmotic laxatives than are effective in keeping stool soft in the child older than 2 years.

Lactulose (1–2 g/kg daily or BID) is another osmotic laxative that can be used in kids as young as 1 month. Glycerin suppositories are commonly used in neonates and young infants with a good safety profile, but should not be used for more than 3 days consecutively, mostly to avoid missing a serious medical diagnosis.[19]

Stool softeners such as mineral oil work but should be avoided if developmental delay or swallowing dysfunction is present[20] due to aspiration risk. Stimulant laxatives such as bisacodyl (approved for children older than 3 years), and senna (older than 2 years) also do the job, but cause more side effects of abdominal pain and bloating. Many enemas (e.g. bisacodyl, sodium docusate, NaCl, molasses, saline, mineral oil) are available, but are probably best avoided in the maintenance phase.

Maintenance therapy should last for 2 months; follow-up with the primary care doctor is a must. Modification of the diet to increase fiber intake and bowel training (asking the children to sit on the toilet at the same time every day) with positive rewards are important for long-term management and prevention.

So, what are you supposed to do with the child younger than 2 years who has constipation? First and foremost, don't hurt them with your therapies. As in our case, sodium phosphate enemas can be downright dangerous. There are case reports demonstrating the risks (including death[21,22]) in young children,[21-24] those with renal issues,[25] and even in the older pediatric patient with delayed GI motility.[26] In the infant on a cow's milk containing formula with constipation, hydrolyzed protein formula may be tried for 2–4 weeks, though this is not based on strong evidence. Despite a lack of good evidence for fiber and fluid intake, consensus experts do recommend a normal intake of these, while probiotics are not recommended.[11]

✔ Teaching points

- Suppository dependent kids? → Think organic pathology
- Constipation since birth or age less than 1 month? → Think organic pathology
- Longstanding, unexplained constipation? → Think organic causes and/or evaluate for possible abuse/neglect
- Review meds (even OTC and illicit drugs) for possible cause of constipation
- First do no harm: Avoid phosphate enemas in children <3 year old, and patients with renal disease. Distinguish between pediatric and adult enemas prior to administration

References

1. Caperell K, Pitetti R, and Cross KP. Race and acute abdominal pain in a pediatric emergency department. Pediatrics. 2013;131(6):1098–106.
2. Choung RS, Shah ND, Chitkara D, et al. Direct medical costs of constipation from childhood to early adulthood: a population-based birth cohort study. J Pediatr Gastroenterol Nutr. 2011; 52(1):47–54.
3. Rasquin A, DiLorenzo C, Forbes D, et al. Childhood functional gastrointestinal disorders: child/adolescent. Gastroenterol. 2006; 130(5):1527–37.
4. van den Berg MM, Benninga MA, Di Lorenzo C. Epidemiology of childhood constipation: a systematic review. Am J Gastroenterol. 2006; 101(10):2401–9.
5. Hyman PE, Milla PJ, Benninga MA, et al. Childhood functional gastrointestinal disorders: neonate/toddler. Gastroenterol. 2006; 130(5):1519–26.
6. Diamanti A, Bracci F, Reale A, et al. Incidence, clinical presentation, and management of constipation in a pediatric ED. AM J of Emerg Med. 2010; 28(2):189–94.
7. Cappell M. Colonic toxicity of administered drugs and chemicals. Am J of Gastroenterol. 2004; 99(6): 1175–90. Carlson TL, Plackett TP, Gagliano RA, et al. Methamphetamine induced paralytic ileus. Hawaii J of Med and Pub Health. 2012; 71(2)244–5.
8. Rajindrajith S, Devanarayana NM, Lakmini C, et al. Association between child maltreatment and constipation: a school based survey using Rome III criteria. J Pediatr Gastroenterol Nutr. 2014; 58(4): 486–90.
9. Iacono G, Carrocio A, Cavotaio FA, et al. Chronic constipation as a symptom of cow's milk allergy. J Pediatr. 1995; 126(1)34–9.
10. Iacono G, Cavotaio FA, Montalto G, et al. Intolerance of cow's milk and chronic constipation in childhood. N Engl J Med. 1998; 339(16) 1100–04.
11. Tabbers MM, DiLorenzo C, Berger MY, et al. Evaluation and treatment of functional constipation in infants and children: evidence-based recommendations from ESPGHAN and NASPGHAN. J of Pediatr Gastroenterol Nutr. 2014 58 (2): 258–74.
12. Barr RG, Levine MD, Wilkinson RH, et al. Chronic and occult stool retention: a clinical tool for its evaluation in school-aged children. Clin Pediatr (Phila).1979;18(11): 676–9.
13. Benninga MA, Buller HA, Staalman CR, et al. Defecation disorders in children, colonic transit time versus the Barr-score. Eur J Pediatr 1995, 154, 277–84.
14. Leech SC, McHugh K, Sullivan PB. Evaluation of a method of assessing faecal loading on plain abdominal radiographs in children. Pediatr Radiol. 1999, 29, 255–8.
15. de Lorijn F, van Rijn RR, Heijmans J, et al. The Leech method for diagnosing constipation: intra- and interobserver variability and accuracy. Pediatr Radiol. 2006;36:43–9.
16. Blethyn AJ, Verrier Jones K, Newcombe R, et al. Radiological assessment of constipation. Arch Dis Child. 1995;73:532–3.
17. Bekkali NL, van den Berg MM, Dijkgraaf MG, et al. Rectal fecal impaction treatment in childhood constipation: enemas vs high doses oral PEG. Pediatrics. 2009;124(3):1108–15.
18. Nurko S, Youssef NN, Sabri M, et al.PEG3350 in the treatment of childhood constipation: a multicenter, double-blinded, placebo-controlled trial. J Pediatr. 2008;153(2):254–61.

19. Blackmer AB, Farrington EA. Constipation in the pediatric patient: an overview and pharmacologic considerations. J Pediatr Health Care. 2010;24(6):385–99.
20. Bandla HP, Davis SH, Hopkins NE. Lipoid pneumonia: a silent complication of mineral oil aspiration. Pediatrics. 1999;103(2): E19.
21. Ismail EAR, Al-Mutairi G; Al-Anzy H. A fatal small dose of phosphate enema in a young child with no renal or gastrointestinal abnormality. J Pediatr Gastroenterol Nutr. 2000;(30)2:220–21.
22. Martin RR, Lisehora GR, Braxton M Jr, et al. Fatal poisoning from sodium phosphate enema. Case report and experimental study. JAMA. 1987; 257(16):2190–2.
23. Marraffa JM, Hui A, Stork C. Severe hyperphosphatemia and hypocalcemia following the rectal administration of a phosphate-containing pediatric enema. Ped Emerg Care. 2004;(20)7:453–6.
24. Sotos JF, Cutler EA, Finkel MA, et al. Hypocalcemic coma following two pediatric phosphate enemas. Pediatrics. 1977; 60(3):305–7.
25. Chesney RW, Haughton PB. Tetany following phosphate enemas in chronic renal disease. Am J Dis Child. 1974;127(4):584–6.
26. Biebl A, Grillenberger A, Schmitt K. Enema-induced severe hyperphosphatemia in children. Eur J Pediatr. 2009;168(1):111–12.

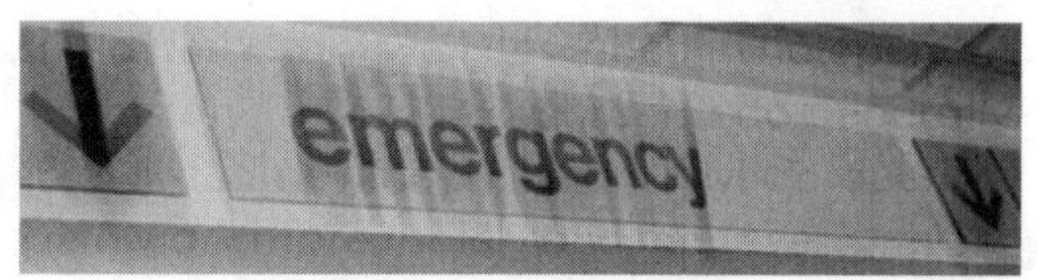

CASE 13

21-MONTH-OLD WITH FEVER

Genevieve Santillanes, MD
Assistant Professor of Clinical Medicine
LAC + USC Medical Center
Keck School of Medicine at USC
Pediatric Emergency Medicine

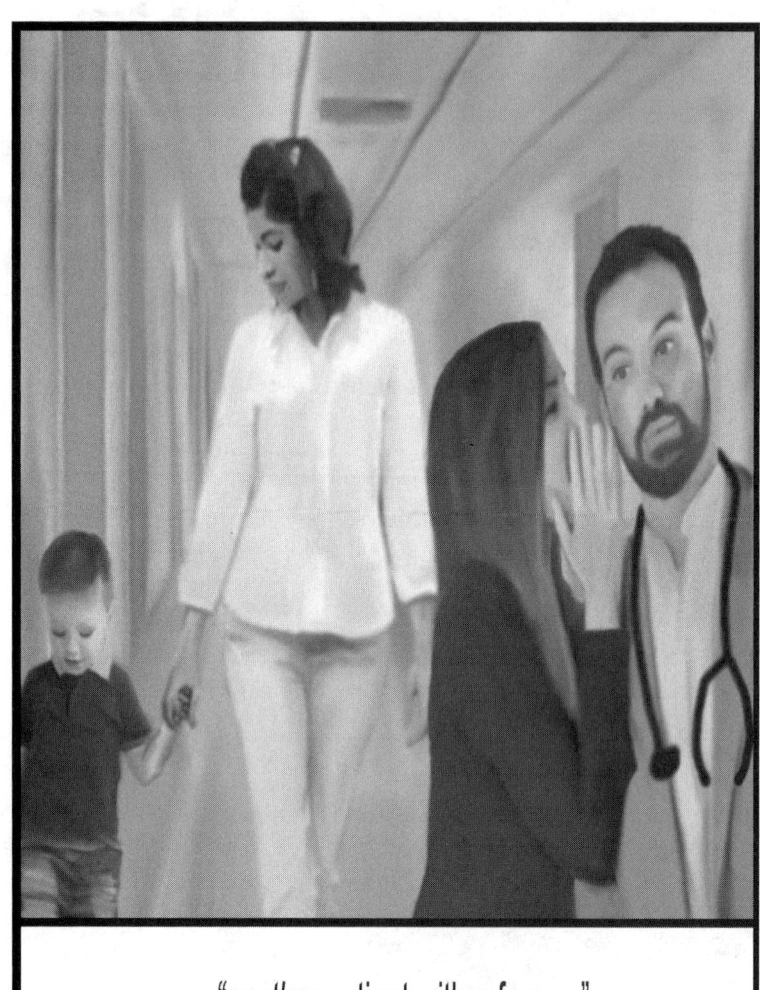

"*another* patient with a fever..."

CASE 13

21-MONTH-OLD WITH FEVER

PART 1—MEDICAL

I. The Doctor's Version (the following is the actual documentation of the provider)

Chief complaint (9:21): Fever

Nurse note (09:34): Pt here for above c/o x 5 days (on and off). Temp 102F + cold today. Rubs his head. Bump to RT side of neck. Rash to feet and legs started today. + emesis 3 days approx. 2x day, Decrease appetite.

HISTORY OF PRESENT ILLNESS (Per resident @ 10:02): 21 month old male with fever x 5 days. Tmax 104 yesterday. Fever today of 102 gave Motrin prior to ER. Responds to Motrin, but returns throughout the day. Has also had emesis, nonbilious, nonbloody, about 1/day during this time, usually after drinking his bottle. Has had decreased oral intake of solids and liquids with decreased urine output as well. No diarrhea. Reports congestion and rhinorrhea, no ill contacts. Mother notes swelling of neck with overlying redness yesterday, notes redness has resolved but swelling continues.

PAST MEDICAL HISTORY: (left blank)

NKDA
MEDICATIONS: Motrin
PMH: None

EXAM:

VITAL SIGNS

Time	Temp(F)	Rt	Pulse	Resp	Syst	Diast	Sat
09:28	98.5	TM	158	25	BP not checked because "Pt is moving"		100%

General: well nourished, alert, crying but easily consoled by mother, +tears
Head: NCAT, no swelling/tenderness. Neck with swelling on R and matted lymph noted, no overlying erythema
Eyes: Pupils equal and round, conjunctiva clear
ENT: Oropharynx clear, no erythema, neck supple, B TM without erythema/bulging/fullness
Heart: RRR, no murmur
Lungs: clear, no increased WOB, good aeration
Abd: soft, no tenderness
Ext: no edema
Skin: warm, dry, maculopapular rash on feet and trunk with mild erythema of palms and soles

Neuro: Responds appropriately, motor grossly intact

ED COURSE:

10:33 **Medical decision making (MDM)**: 21 month old male with 5 days of fever, 1 day rash and neck swelling likely viral infection with early lymphadenitis. Despite 5 days fevers and palmar changes, Kawasaki less likely given lack of conjunctival and mucosal involvement. Will have mother return in 48 hours or visit PMD in 48 hours for recheck. Will send home with Augmentin for early lymphadenitis and watch PO before sending home.

10:43: **Attending note.** Case presentation, assessment and plan discussed with resident.

11:15 Patient is taking juice and tolerating, mother reassured of diagnosis and agrees to return early Monday morning for recheck or earlier if she has concerns.

DIAGNOSIS: (1) URI (2) Lymphadenitis (3) Viral Exanthem

➢**Author's note (MW):** Though "we all would have sent this patient home and there was no way to make the final diagnosis" may be true, we are attempting to transcend "standard of care" and searching for *excellence* in care. The comments below speak not only to the medical management, but how it is documented in the medical record.

II. The Errors—Risk Management/Patient Safety Issues

Risk management/patient safety issue #1:

Error: Incomplete documentation of history and physical.

Discussion: The HPI reads like a ROS with a list of symptoms, some of which are not further explored. The nurse's note mentions complaints of rash and head rubbing but these are not addressed in the HPI. The medical decision making note mentions that conjunctivitis and mucous membrane changes are not present, but there is no indication that parents were asked about history of hand or foot swelling or conjunctivitis prior to emergency department presentation.

On the physical exam, swelling without erythema of the right neck was noted, but there was no documentation of the size of the lymph node or whether it was warm, indurated or fluctuant. A diagnosis of lymphadenitis was made and the patient was told to return for follow-up, but without documentation of the size and consistency of the node, the physician seeing the patient for follow-up would not know if the patient had improved.

✔ **Teaching point:** When a specific diagnosis is in question (in this case, Kawasaki disease), pertinent positives and negatives should be documented in the HPI, ROS, and PE.

Risk management/patient safety issue #2:

Error: Ignoring information that doesn't support the discharge diagnosis.

Discussion: It is tempting to make a diagnosis and focus only on the data supporting that diagnosis. However, if other data points do not fit in, the diagnosis should be reconsidered. In this case, erythema of the palms and soles was noted and the resident even mentioned this in the medical decision making note when she wrote "despite the...palmar changes." The diagnosis of Kawasaki disease clearly crossed the physician's mind and she mentioned a key finding in favor of Kawasaki disease, but she dismissed the finding without further explanation.

✔ **Teaching point:** If features of the history or physical exam aren't consistent with the discharge diagnosis, reconsider the diagnosis before discharging the patient.

Risk management/patient safety issue #3:

Error: Making multiple, unrelated diagnoses without considering a single unifying diagnosis.

Discussion: This patient was given three acute diagnoses: URI, bacterial lymphadenitis and viral exanthem. Viral exanthems and bacterial lymphadenitis generally do not co-exist.

✔ **Teaching point:** When patients present with multiple acute complaints, strong consideration should be given to diagnoses that can explain all findings.

Risk management/patient safety issue #4:

Error: It is unclear if the attending examined the patient

Discussion: This was a patient in whom the resident considered a serious, time-sensitive diagnosis (Kawasaki disease). The documentation only states that the attending discussed the case but no documentation of examination.

✔ **Teaching point:** When a serious diagnosis is entertained, the attending should strongly consider examining the patient (and documenting the exam).

Risk management/patient safety #5:

Error: Unexplained tachycardia.

Discussion: Abnormal vital signs may be an indicator of serious underlying pathology. One study of unanticipated deaths after an emergency department visit found that abnormal vital signs, most commonly tachycardia, at the initial visit were common in patients who died unexpectedly within a week.[1]

Pediatric patients have many reasons to be tachycardic, but ignoring abnormal vital signs is perilous. If the clinician is confident of the reason for the abnormality, it should be noted in the chart ("Patient is mildly tachycardic likely due to fever/pain/crying"). Vital signs can be repeated after the child defervesces or stops crying. If it is unclear whether tachycardia is due to crying or anxiety or if it is a sign of more serious pathology such as sepsis, significant dehydration or myocarditis, a more accurate heart rate can be obtained by leaving the child on a cardiac monitor or pulse oximeter while the clinician is out of the room. Once the child is alone with the parents and calms down, a resting heart can be obtained. Although the patient presented was not dramatically tachycardic, his heart rate was elevated for age and he did not have a fever at the time of triage to explain the tachycardia.

✔ **Teaching point:** Abnormal vital signs must be addressed.

Risk management/patient safety issue #6:

Error: "Mother reassured of diagnosis."

Discussion: From the charting, it sounds like the resident herself was not completely reassured about the diagnosis! While diagnostic uncertainty is common and treating the likely diagnosis is reasonable, the patient or parents should understand that diagnostic uncertainty exists so they understand the importance of follow-up. A better approach would have been to explain to the mother that the most likely diagnosis was bacterial lymphadenitis, but that other diseases can present similarly so a follow-up exam would be important. A parent who understands that diagnostic uncertainty exists is more likely to return for follow-up care.

✔ **Teaching point:** Reassuring a parent of a diagnosis when the diagnosis is uncertain is risky. If diagnostic uncertainty exists, patients and parents should be aware so they understand the importance of follow-up care.

III. The Bounceback—At 22:04 the same day as the ED discharge

- **HPI:** (22:04 the same day) - Parents complain that rash has extended to cover his whole body and that the right neck swelling has increased. He has continued having fevers that they are treating with ibuprofen. Pt very fussy.
- **PE:** Afebrile but tachycardic to 145, have dry cracked lips with mild erythema of the tongue, mild edema of the feet, a diffuse maculopapular rash on his torso and extremities.
- **MDM (resident):** Symptoms concerning for Kawasaki disease. Pt also dehydrated on exam and tachycardic. Will give 20cc/kg bolus and get following labs for Kawasaki workup: CBC, CRP, ESR, CMP, UA with micro (bag specimen)."
- **Labs:**
  - WBC: 19.6 (N 72, L 18, M 8, E 1, B 1), Hgb: 10.5/Hct 31.4
  - CMP: Na 139 K 4.5 Cl 99 Bicarb 16 BUN 10 Cr 0.23 Glu 86 Ca 9.7
  - Alk Phos 214 TP 6.9 Alb 4.4 AST 25 ALT 14 T Bili 0.6
  - CRP: 12.9 mg/dL, ESR: 83
  - UA significant for moderate leukocyte esterase with 11-30 WBC/hpf
- **Disposition:** The patient was admitted to pediatrics with a diagnosis of Kawasaki disease.
  - Echocardiogram shows prominent coronary arteries, increased perivascular brightness of the coronary arteries and a possible lack of tapering.
  - IVIG and aspirin are started.
  - **Follow up:** In cardiology clinic 1 week after discharge, a repeat echocardiogram was normal with resolution of the prominence of the coronary arteries.

FINAL DIAGNOSIS: Kawasaki disease

PART 2—THE ANALYSIS

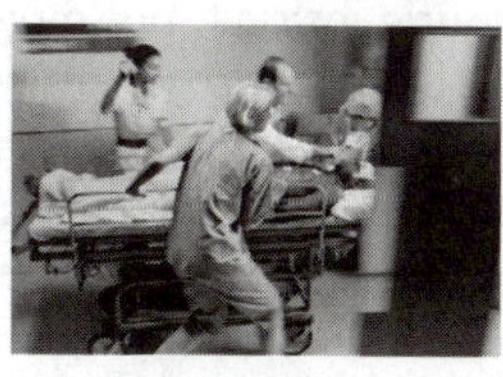

EVALUATION OF FEVER AND RASH, DIAGNOSIS OF KAWASAKI DISEASE

Genevieve Santillanes, MD
Assistant Professor of Clinical Medicine
LAC + USC Medical Center
Keck School of Medicine at USC
Pediatric Emergency Medicin

Evaluation of the pediatric patient with fever and rash

The approach to the pediatric patient with fever varies based on age of the patient, co-morbidities, duration of fever and other signs and symptoms of illness. In general, most pediatric patients can be evaluated with a detailed history and physical examination. Laboratory work-up (other than perhaps a urinalysis in young children) is often unnecessary unless petechiae are present below nipple line, typically starting in the genital area as can occur with meningoccemia. Petechiae above the nipple line can be due to forceful cough or vomiting.

In this case, we have an otherwise healthy 21 month-old boy with a chief complaint of fever to 104° F. A viral infection is the most likely etiology of the fever, but the differential diagnosis is broad. Urinary tract infections are unlikely in circumcised boys over six months of age and uncircumcised boys over a year of age, so a urinalysis to evaluate for urinary tract infection in the absence of a persistent high fever is unnecessary without other symptoms. Meningitis should be clinically apparent in a child of this age, so a lumbar puncture is unnecessary unless the physical exam is concerning. Depending on the season, likely viral infections include influenza and enterovirus. Roseola is another common cause of a high fever. Pneumonia and otitis media may complicate upper respiratory tract infections, but should be evident on physical exam. As duration of fever increases beyond what would be expected with most viral infections, other etiologies should be considered including:

1. Epstein-Barr virus
2. Cat scratch disease
3. Systemic juvenile idiopathic arthritis (formerly known as systemic juvenile rheumatoid arthritis)
4. Other rheumatologic diseases
5. Leukemia
6. Myocarditis and endocarditis
7. Osteomyelitis
8. Intra-abdominal abscesses

Rash is another common chief complaint with a broad differential diagnosis. Common causes of rash include viral exanthems, contact dermatitis and systemic allergic reactions (urticaria). In this 21-month-old male with a complaint of rash on the feet and legs, Henoch-Schonlein Purpura (HSP) is in the differential. HSP classically presents as purpuric lesions, but may present with macules, papules or urticaria, especially early in the illness. Lesions are generally maximal on the lower extremities and buttocks in ambulatory children. Many viral illnesses present with rash and diagnosis is based on the morphology of the rash and associated symptoms. Although most rashes presenting to the emergency department are benign, serious causes of rash include:

1. Stevens-Johnson syndrome
2. Meningococcemia
3. Kawasaki disease
4. Toxic shock syndrome
5. Staphylococcal scalded skin syndrome

Putting it all together to make a diagnosis

This patient is presenting with both rash and fever, narrowing the differential diagnosis. Although the patient has an enlarged lymph node and fever, bacterial lymphadenitis is less likely given the co-existent rash. HSP is also unlikely given the height of the fever and the cervical lymph node. HSP can present with low-grade fever, but a temperature of 104° F would be unusual. Scarlet fever is a common cause of fever and rash, and streptococcal disease is associated with enlarged cervical lymph nodes, but the typical rash is a sandpapery, not maculopapular, rash maximal on the upper torso.

Scarlet fever is also more common in somewhat older children. Adenovirus and enterovirus can both cause fever and a rash, but would not be associated with a single enlarged cervical node. Roseola does cause a maculopapular rash, but the fever is resolved by the time the rash appears. Toxic shock and Staphylococcal scalded skin syndromes are both associated with diffuse erythroderma, not maculopapular rashes.

In this 21-month-old patient with 5 days of fever, rash, unilateral enlarged cervical lymph node and erythema of the palms and soles on the first ED visit, incomplete Kawasaki disease is high on the differential diagnosis and should be further investigated.

Kawasaki Disease and differential diagnosis

Kawasaki disease was mentioned, but dismissed, in the medical decision making note. Kawasaki disease should be considered in every child presenting with five or more days of fever. It is a time-sensitive diagnosis because patients who are treated earlier in the course of illness have a lower incidence of coronary artery abnormalities,[2-6] the most common serious complication of Kawasaki disease.

Kawasaki disease is diagnosed when a patient has five days of fever and at least four of the five following principal features:

1. Extremity changes—In the acute phase, erythema or edema of palms and soles and in the subacute phase, peeling of fingers and toes
2. Polymorphous exanthem

- Most commonly diffuse maculopapular, but other rashes may be seen
- Rash is not vesicular or bullous

3. Bilateral non-exudative bulbar conjunctivitis with limbic sparing
4. Lip and oral cavity changes—Erythema, lip cracking, strawberry tongue or injection of the oral and pharyngeal mucosa
5. Cervical lymphadenopathy greater than 1.5 centimeters (generally unilateral in the anterior cervical triangle)

However, the diagnosis is often not so simple. The most recent recommendations by the American Heart Association state that the diagnosis of Kawasaki disease can be made on day four if patients have at least four of the five principal features listed above,[7] so the first criteria we associate with Kawasaki disease (five days of fever), is not required to make the diagnosis.

Why was this diagnosis missed?

The diagnosis does seem reasonably straightforward in toddlers presenting with five days of fever and four principal features. However, it can be overlooked even in classic cases. One reason is that the features are nonspecific and the presentation can overlap with other common illnesses. Scarlet fever, for example, has many features in common with Kawasaki disease (rash, fever, mucosal changes, peeling of fingers and toes).

Many Kawasaki features such as conjunctivitis and rash are seen with common viral illnesses like adenovirus. If the clinician is not thinking about the diagnosis of Kawasaki disease, it is very easy to attribute signs and symptoms to other common childhood illnesses. In the case presented, the clinicians focused on the lymphadenopathy and made a diagnosis of bacterial lymphadenitis. There is no definitive test for Kawasaki disease and the features are nonspecific and sometimes subjective, so diagnosis requires a high index of suspicion.

Another factor in some missed cases of Kawasaki disease is presentation in patients outside of the classic age range. Kawasaki disease typically occurs in toddlers with most cases occurring in children under age five.[4,7] However, it can occur at any age and has even been reported in adults.[8] In patients older or younger than the typical Kawasaki patient, the diagnosis may not be on the clinician's differential. Infants and older children have a higher incidence of coronary artery abnormalities,[6,9] possibly due to delayed diagnosis.

Incomplete Kawasaki Disease

It is even easier to miss the diagnosis in children with incomplete Kawasaki disease. Complete Kawasaki disease is defined as five or more days of fever with at least four of the principal criteria. On the first emergency department visit, our patient had incomplete Kawasaki disease. Up to 28% of patients ultimately diagnosed with Kawasaki disease will have an incomplete presentation.[10-12] Incomplete Kawasaki disease is five or more days of fever with fewer than four of the principal features and echocardiographic or laboratory findings consistent with the disease. Not surprisingly, the diagnosis is more commonly delayed in patients with incomplete disease.[11]

AHA recommendations for diagnosis of patients with *possible* Kawasaki disease

Because the classic criteria miss a significant number of cases of Kawasaki disease, the American Heart Association published recommendations to guide the work-up of patients with possible

Kawasaki disease (See Figure below). The recommendations are to consider the diagnosis in patients with five days of fever and at least two of the principal features not otherwise explained by another illness.

In these cases, if the ESR or CRP is elevated, further laboratory testing is recommended. Laboratory values consistent with Kawasaki disease include hypoalbuminemia, anemia, thrombocytosis, elevated white blood cell count, elevated ALT, and sterile pyuria.[7] Patients with three laboratory findings supporting the diagnosis should be presumptively treated and patients not meeting the laboratory criteria should be further worked up with an echocardiogram. The algorithm is complicated and unwieldy, but can be looked up if patients present with prolonged fever and several Kawasaki symptoms.

Evaluation of suspected incomplete Kawasaki disease (KD)[1]

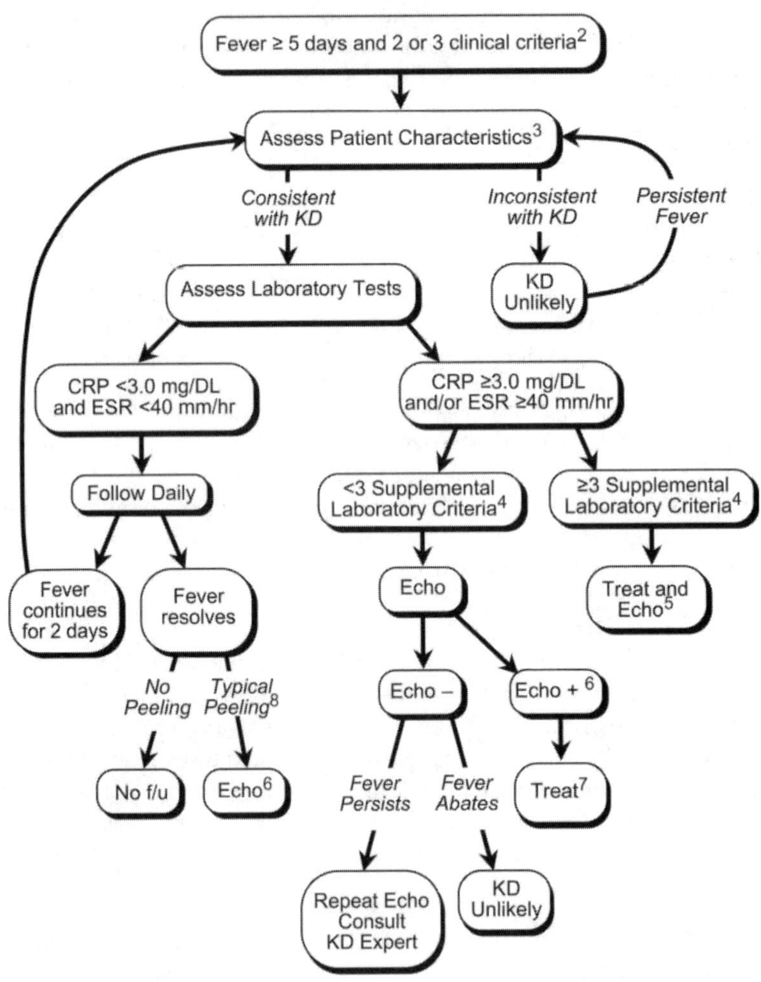

(1) In the absence of gold standard for diagnosis, this algorithm cannot be evidence based but rather represents the informed opinion of the expert committee. Consultation with an expert should be sought anytime assistance is needed.
(2) Infants ≤ 6 months old on day ≥7 of fever without other explanation should undergo laboratory testing and, if evidence of systemic inflammation is found, an echocardiogram, even if the infants have no clinical criteria.
(3) Patient characteristics suggesting Kawasaki disease are listed in Table 1. Characteristics suggesting disease other than Kawasaki disease include exudative conjunctivitis, exudative pharyngitis, discrete intraoral lesions, bullous or vesicular rash, or generalized adenopathy. Consider alternative diagnoses (see Table 2).
(4) Supplemental laboratory criteria include albumin ≤ 3.0 g/dL, anemia for age, elevation of alanine aminotransferase, platelets after 7 d ≥450 000/mm3, white blood cell count ≥15 000/mm3, and urine ≥10 white blood cells/high-power field.
(5) Can treat before performing echocardiogram.
(6) Echocardiogram is considered positive for purposes of this algorithm if any of 3 conditions are met: *z* score of LAD or RCA ≥ 2.5, coronary arteries meet Japanese Ministry of Health criteria for aneurysms, or ≥ 3 other suggestive features exist, including perivascular brightness, lack of tapering, decreased LV function, mitral regurgitation, pericardial effusion, or *z* scores in LAD or RCA of 2–2.5.
(7) If the echocardiogram is positive, treatment should be given to children within 10 d of fever onset and those beyond day 10 with clinical and laboratory signs (CRP, ESR) of ongoing inflammation.
(8) Typical peeling begins under nail bed of fingers and then toes.

Newberger JW, Takahashi M, Gerber MA, et al. Diagnosis, treatment and long-term management of Kawasaki disease: a statement for health professionals from the Committee on Rheumatic Fever, Endocarditis, and Kawasaki Disease, Council on Cardiovascular Disease in the Young, American Heart Association. Pediatrics. 2004;114(6):1708–33. Figure 1 at 1709.

Infants under six months of age have particularly high rates of incomplete presentation and are more likely to have a delayed diagnosis[11] and coronary artery involvement.[13] Because infants under six months of age can present with prolonged fever without any other features of the disease, the American Heart Association recommendations are to consider echocardiography in young infants with seven or more days of fever and laboratory evidence of systemic inflammation that is otherwise unexplained.[7]

More pitfalls in the diagnosis of Kawasaki Disease

We all learn that patients with Kawasaki disease present with five days of fever plus rash, conjunctivitis, mucosal changes, extremity changes and lymphadenopathy. Further complicating the diagnostic picture is that many patients with Kawasaki disease present with additional nonspecific complaints. Our patient had rhinorrhea, vomiting and decreased oral intake, which aren't classically associated with Kawasaki disease. This led the clinicians to make a diagnosis of URI. In reality, these symptoms are common in patients with Kawasaki disease. One recent study found that 61% of patients had at least one gastrointestinal symptom (vomiting, diarrhea or abdominal pain), and 35% of patients had at least one respiratory symptom (cough or rhinorrhea).[14]

Other features including myocarditis, pericarditis, gallbladder hydrops, arthralgias and hyponatremia are well described and may further complicate the diagnostic picture.[7] Irritability is very common.[14] Sterile pyuria and pleocytosis are sometimes seen and can lead to a diagnosis of urinary tract infection or meningitis. Do not be surprised if patients with Kawasaki disease have signs and symptoms that don't fit the classic teaching!

How To avoid missing the diagnosis

Because it is easy to overlook the diagnosis and patients receiving earlier treatment have a lower incidence of developing coronary aneurysms, it is good practice to consider the diagnosis of Kawasaki disease in every child with a fever lasting five days or longer. Look for and ask about the five principal features of Kawasaki disease. Some features may be transient. Patients do not have to have all features present on exam at the time of diagnosis, so the history is important. And since toddlers generally have pudgy hands and feet, it may be difficult to appreciate edema, but parents generally know if their child is swollen. If you are in the habit of documenting presence or absence of each feature of Kawasaki disease every time you evaluate a child with prolonged fever, you are less likely to miss a case.

Patients do not have to meet the criteria for complete Kawasaki disease; at the initial visit, our patient had five days of fever plus lymphadenopathy, extremity changes and rash. Although additional features of conjunctivitis and mucous membrane changes are very common in Kawasaki disease, neither is required to make the diagnosis. Five days of fever and three principal features should have prompted a laboratory work-up for Kawasaki disease.

Treatment

All children with suspected Kawasaki disease should be admitted to a pediatrics ward with capability of performing a pediatric echocardiogram. Depending on the hospital, the patient may be managed by general pediatrics or infectious disease or rheumatology. First line treatment is intravenous gamma globulin (IVIG) and high dose aspirin.

Chapter Summary

Kawasaki disease can be a tricky diagnosis. The signs and symptoms are nonspecific and overlap with other common illnesses. Many patients do not meet criteria for complete Kawasaki disease. Consider further work-up of infants and children with five days of fever and two principal features and consider echocardiography in infants with seven days of unexplained fever and signs of systemic inflammation.

References

1. Sklar DP, Crandall CS, Loeliger E, et al. Unanticipated death after discharge home from the emergency department. Annals Emerg Med. 2007;49:735–45.
2. Baer AZ, Rubin LG, Shapiro CA, et al. Prevalence of coronary artery lesions on the initial echocardiogram in Kawasaki syndrome. Arch Pediatr Adolesc Med. 2006;160:686–90.
3. Tse SML, Silverman ED, McCrindle BW, et al. Early treatment with intravenous immunoglobulin in patients with Kawasaki disease. J Pediatr. 2002;140(4):450–5.

4. Tacke CE, Breunis WB, Pereira RR, et al. Five years of Kawasaki disease in the Netherlands: a national surveillance study. Pediatr Infect Dis J. 2014;33(8):793–7.
5. Kim T, Choi W, Woo CW. Predictive risk factors for coronary artery abnormalities in Kawasaki disease. Eur J Pediatr. 2007;166(5):421–5.
6. Callinan LS, Tabnak F, Holman RC, et al. Kawasaki syndrome and factors associated with coronary artery abnormalities in California. Pediatr Infect Dis J. 2012;31(9):894–8.
7. Newberger JW, Takahashi M, Gerber MA, et al. Diagnosis, treatment and long-term management of Kawasaki disease: a statement for health professionals from the Committee on Rheumatic Fever, Endocarditis, and Kawasaki Disease, Council on Cardiovascular Disease in the Young, American Heart Association. Pediatrics. 2004;114(6):1708–33.
8. Gomard-Menneson E, Landron C, Dauphin C, et al. Kawasaki disease in adults: report of 10 cases. Medicine (Baltimore). 2010;89(3):149–58.
9. Belay ED, Maddox RA, Holman RC, et al. Kawasaki syndrome and risk factors for coronary artery abnormalities. United States, 1994–2003. Pediatr Infect Dis J. 2006;25(3):245–9.
10. Giannouli G, Tzoumaka-Bakoula C, Kopsidas I, et al. Epidemiology and risk factors for coronary artery abnormalities in children with complete and incomplete Kawasaki disease during a 10-year period. Pediatr Cardiol. 2013;34(6):1476–81.
11. Minich LL, Sleeper LA, Atz AM, et al. Delayed diagnosis of Kawasaki disease: What are the risk factors? Pediatrics. 2007;120:e1434–40.
12. Yellen ES, Gauvreau K, Takahashi M, et al. Performance of 2004 American Heart Association recommendations for treatment of Kawasaki disease. Pediatrics. 2010;125(2):e234–41.
13. Chang FY, Hwang B, Chen SJ, et al. Characteristics of Kawasaki disease in infants younger than six months of age. Pediatr Infect Dis J. 2006;25(3):241–4.
14. Baker AL, Lu M, Minich LL, et al. Associated symptoms in the ten days before diagnosis of Kawasaki disease. J Pediatrics. 2009;154(4):592–95.

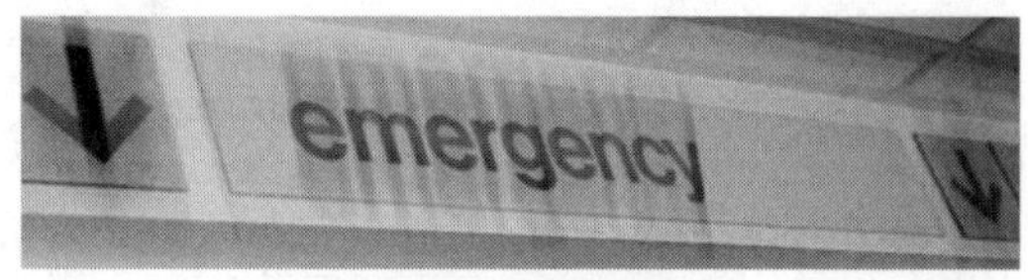

CASE 14

FEVER, COUGH, AND DYSPHAGIA IN A 14-YEAR-OLD ADOLESCENT

Madeline Matar Joseph, MD, FAAP, FACEP

Professor of Emergency Medicine and Pediatrics
University of Florida College of Medicine–Jacksonville

Ryan McKenna, DO

Emergency Medicine Resident
University of Florida College of Medicine-Jacksonville

Nizar Maraqa, MD

Assistant Professor, Pediatric Infectious Diseases
Department of Pediatrics, University of Florida College of Medicine-Jacksonville

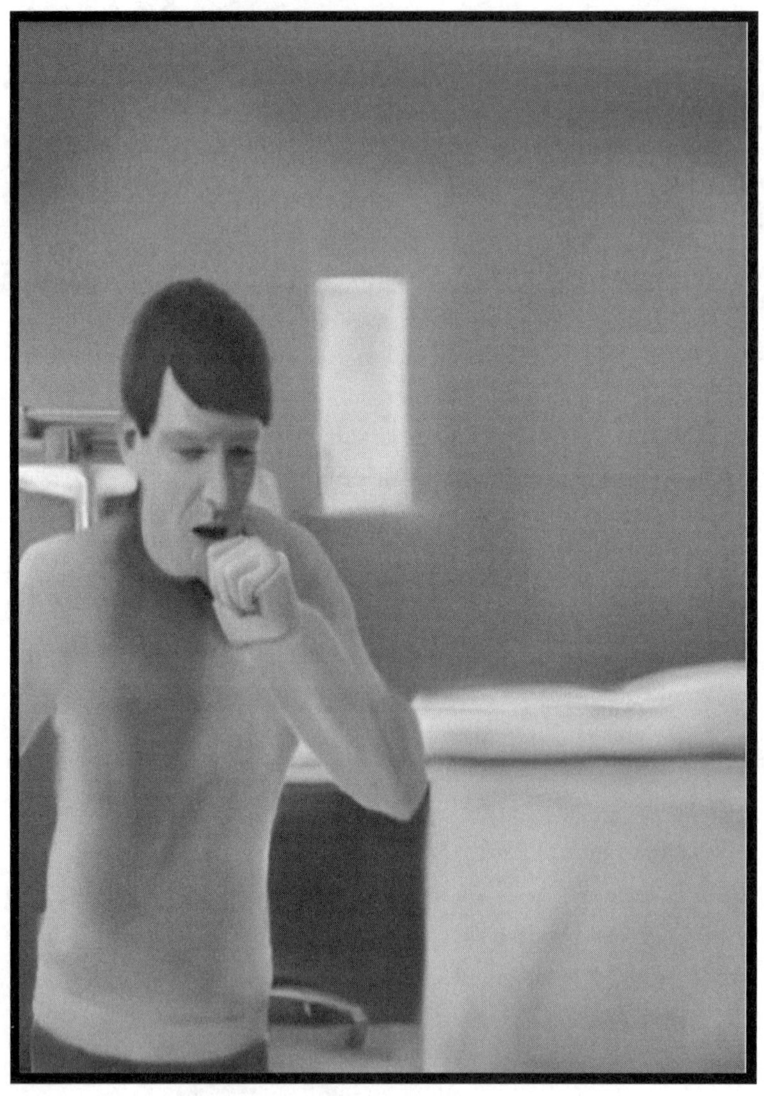

CASE 14

FEVER, COUGH, AND DYSPHAGIA IN A 14-YEAR-OLD ADOLESCENT

PART 1—MEDICAL

I. The Doctor's Version (the following is the actual documentation of the provider)

Chief Complaint: Cough, Fever

Nurse note: Patient awake, alert, ambulatory to triage with mom. C/o headache today. Also c/o fevers off and on for a week. Patient reports sore throat and upper back pain. Patient stated that he was walking to bed today and passed out on bed. He felt real dizzy prior to passing out.

HPI: 14 y/o AAM [African-American male] with no PMH presents with 1 week history of fevers (the highest 101), congestion, clear nasal discharge, and nonproductive cough (worse at night). Patient also felt SOB during his football practice yesterday. Patient also reports 3 week of history of retrosternal burning chest pain radiating to his back worse with eating and dysphagia. Patient notes that the retrosternal pain started after swallowing an "over the counter tablet". Patient denies any pain currently. Patient reports decreased appetite. Patient also notes getting up from his chair too quickly, feeling dizzy and then falling asleep. ROS: + cough, - confusion, LOC, n/v/d, abd. pain, myalgias, gait disturbance, lymphadenopathy, polydipsia/ polyphagia

PAST MEDICAL HISTORY: None

NKDA

Social History: Non-smoker, denied drugs or alcohol use

VITAL SIGNS

Time	Temp(F)	Pulse	Resp	Syst/Diast	Sat	Weight
13:57	99.6po	95	18	126/71	99%	58.6kg

PHYSICAL EXAM

Constitutional: He is oriented to person, place, and time. Well-developed and well-nourished.

HEENT: Head: TM's right and left ear normal. No oro-pharyngeal exudates. Eyes: Conjunctivae and EOM are normal. Pupils are ERRL.

Neck: Normal range of motion. Neck supple. No thyromegaly present

Cardiovascular: Normal rate, regular rhythm and normal heart sounds. Exam reveals no gallop and no friction rub. No murmur heard.

Pulmonary/Chest: Effort normal and breath sounds normal. No stridor. No respiratory distress. No wheezes or inspiratory rales.
Abdominal: Soft. No distension or tenderness. There is no rebound and no guarding.
Genitourinary: Penis normal. No penile tenderness.
Musculoskeletal: Normal range of motion. He exhibits no edema.
Lymphadenopathy: He has no cervical adenopathy.
Neurological: He is alert and oriented to person, place, and time. No cranial nerve deficit. Coordination normal.
Skin: Skin is warm. He is not diaphoretic. No rash noted.

DIFFERENTIAL DDX: URI, GERD, Pill Esophagitis, Peptic ulcer disease

ED COURSE:

Point of care test (POCT) Rapid Strep A – Negative, POCT urinalysis WNL, Chest X-ray: NAD
Patient was given GI cocktail and was able to tolerate PO and doesn't complain of any abdominal or retrosternal pain currently. He reports improvement of throat pain, and is able to drink entire bottle of Gatorade. Discussed with mom. Plan to start on zantac and prn Maalox. Patient will need PCP follow-up ASAP for GI referral and possible endoscopy. Recheck in the ED in 24 hours

DIAGNOSIS:

URI (upper respiratory infection)
Dysphagia/GERD
Burning chest pain

DISPOSITION: Discharge

II. Risk Management/Patient Safety Discussion

➢**Author's note (MW):** This patient has no shortage of complaints to pick from:

- Fever
- Syncope
- Sore throat
- Back pain
- Congestion
- Headache
- Retrosternal chest pain
- Dysphagia

He is truly a multiple complaint patient! Kudos to the concern of the emergency physician to recognize that *something* was going on with this patient; they asked him to return the next day for a recheck, an effective technique when faced with diagnostic uncertainty.

Far be it for us to insinuate that a better history and exam would have made this diagnosis on the first visit —more can always be done, especially with the range of complaints listed above. The teaching points with this case are the expanded differential considerations as well as a discussion (below) about evaluation of some of these presenting complaints and what turned out to be the final diagnosis.

As emergency providers, we serve many functions in the ED, including diagnosis and emergent management, providing therapy for nonemergent condition, reassurance, and to help arrange follow up to monitor progression of disease. With a concerning story to inability to make a specific diagnosis, ED follow up in 24 hours is often the best option.

III. The Bouncebacks

Second Visit: (in 24 hours)

- **Chief Complaint:** Chest pain, recheck
- **Nurse note:** Child brought to ED by mom for recheck. Feeling a little better, but still having pain with deep breaths. Denies fevers. Child c/o feeling light headed.
- **HPI:** Also c/o several days of upper back pain that is pleuritic in nature since recent URI. Cough that is not productive, did have fever several days ago. Now main complaint is of upper abdominal pain, worse with fasting, better with food.
- **VS:** Temp 99.5, pulse 89, Resp 20, BP 111/60, sat 99%, Wgt 57.15
- **PE:** No significant change from previous P
- **ED Course:** EKG: NSR, normal intervals
- **MDM:** Agree with yesterday's assessment of GI origin. Patient feeling better with GI cocktail, tolerating PO, will have patient f/u with PCP for GI referral.
- **Diagnosis:** Chest pain, GERD, Back Pain
- **Disposition:** Discharge

Third Visit: (2 weeks later)

- **Chief Complaint:** Diarrhea, Fever
- **Nurse note:** Max fever of 103 for the past 3 days, last Tylenol given was the night prior to ED visit.
- **HPI:** Presents with malaise, fatigue, lightheadedness, fevers TMax of 103 x3 days, weight loss 14 lbs in last 3 weeks, decreased po intake, worsening of dysphagia, headaches, nausea, loose stools non-bloody, and night sweats. Cough. No vomiting. Seen at PCP for same complaints.
- **Chief Complaint:** Chest pain, recheck
- **VS:** Temp 98.4, pulse 72, resp 16, BP 104/57, sat 100%, Wgt 54.8
- **PE:** No change
- **Differential DDx:** Malignancy, infection, endocrine disorder, psych/eating disorders, other
- **ED Course:** CBC: WNL, BMP: WNL, TSH: WNL, LFT: WNL, Urinalysis WNL
  - Chest X-Ray: Widening of the upper mediastinum with new prominence of the right para-tracheal region and increased prominence of the right perihilar region suggestive of adenopathy which may represent infectious versus inflammatory process versus lymphoma
  - CT Chest: Mediastinal and hilar lymphadenopathy with pulmonary nodules along the minor fissure and right lower lobe. Ddx infectious process or lymphatic proliferative disorder such as lymphoma.

- **Disposition:** Patient was admitted for evaluation of possible infectious etiology of weight loss, fever, and lymphadenopathy, infectious vs. lymphoma.
- **Inpatient course:** Patient underwent bronchoscopy with BAL, which demonstrated necrotic lymph nodes; Sputum AFB smear was positive, confirming a diagnosis of tuberculosis.
- **FINAL DIAGNOSIS:** Tuberculosis

PART 2—THE ANALYSIS

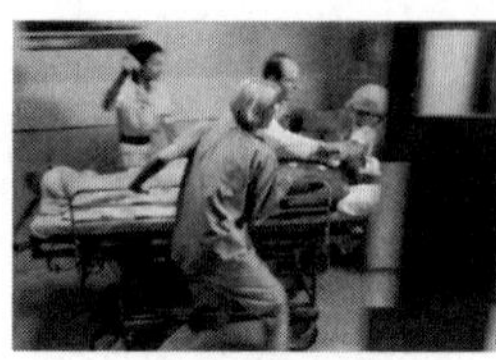

EVALUATION OF DYSPHAGIA, HILAR ADENOPATHY, AND TUBERCULOSIS

Madeline Matar Joseph, MD, FAAP, FACEP
Professor of Emergency Medicine and Pediatrics
University of Florida College of Medicine–Jacksonville

Ryan McKenna, DO
Emergency Medicine Resident
University of Florida College of Medicine-Jacksonville

Nizar Maraqa, MD
Assistant Professor, Pediatric Infectious Diseases
Department of Pediatrics, University of Florida College of Medicine-Jacksonville

Initial presentation:

The patient presented with URI, fever, cough, and SOB during his football practice. He also had retrosternal burning chest pain radiating to his back, worse with eating and dysphagia, uncommon complaints in children. At this point, it is reasonable to first think of common diseases such pneumonia, which was ruled out by the clinical examination and a negative chest x-ray; of note, there was no cardiomegaly. The patient reported decreased appetite but was still eating.

The impression was complicated GERD due to the presence of dysphagia or esophagitis from the "swallowed pill." Strep was ruled out with a negative rapid test. At this point, is it reasonable to initiate the treatment for GERD with follow up? Proton Pump Inhibitors (PPIs) and histamine type 2 receptors antagonists are safe, well tolerated and effective in the treatment of complicated GERD (with erosive esophagitis) in children and adolescents, but also require a close follow up.[1]

Was the dizziness (+/- syncope) secondary to dehydration from decreased oral input? The patient's vitals and physical examination did not support such a diagnosis. The patient did feel better after the GI cocktail and drank an entire bottle of Gatorade. The question at this point is did let our guard down too quickly?...

Causes of dysphagia

A. Life-threatening causes of "dysphagia" include:

- Esophageal FB: A stuck pill would be expected to pass with eating.
- Caustic ingestion: Non-accidental ingestion is uncommon in this age group.
- Infection: Retropharyngeal abscess (common in toddlers), epiglottitis (the patient is not ill looking, and has no drooling), and CNS infection (no headache or meningeal signs).

B. Common non-life-threatiening etiologies for dysphagia include:

- Stomatitis: none on exam
- Pharyngitis: rapid strep was obtained
- Peritonsillar abscess: no evidence on exam
- Esophagitis (possibility): The most common cause of esophageal injury is GERD, however other less recognized causes may affect the esophagus. Esophageal infections are less frequent since HIV infection has become better controlled with antiviral therapies. The most emergent "allergic" disease of the esophagus is eosinophilic esophagitis, which has become increasingly recognized in children and adults over the last decade. Eosinophilic esophagitis is a clinical pathologic disorder characterized by a dense esophageal eosinophilia generally occurring in association with upper gastrointestinal symptoms, primarily intermittent dysphagia, and refractory to proton pump inhibitor therapy.[2]
- Dystonic reaction (unlikely)
- Oropharyngeal trauma (negative history and exam)
- Achalasia (possibility): typically associated with failure to thrive

C. "Zebras" include diseases that cause impairment of swallowing:

- Rare infections such as tetanus, diphtheria, and poliomyositis
- CNS tumors
- Esophageal perforation (unlikely in our patient since he was eating!)

The second visit:

In addition to the various multiple complaints from the first visit, the patient is now complaining of abdominal pain. If the differential diagnosis includes the possibility of hepatitis, appendicitis, pancreatitis or myocarditis, further workup is needed. This would include CBC, electrolytes, LFTs, Lipase, troponin, AST, CK-MB, or imaging as indicated clinically. Bottom line, the thought process should be followed through to rule out life threatening pathology. ECG alone does not rule out myocarditis.

The third visit: *Now the patient is reading the book... or is he?*

Three weeks after the initial ED visit, the patient continued to have high fever, cough, decreased appetite, worsening dysphagia, significant weight loss, night sweats, and diarrhea.

The combination of these symptoms indicates a real pathology including infection, inflammation or malignancies. Obtaining laboratory workup of CBC, Diff, LFTs, electrolytes and even thyroid testing is appropriate.

Of note, the chest x-ray revealed widening of the upper mediastinum with new prominence of the right para-tracheal region and increased prominence of the right peri-hilar region suggestive of hilar adenopathy.

Differential Diagnosis for hilar adenopathy on Chest X-Ray includes:

1. Infection
   - Tuberculosis
   - Mycoplasma
   - Histoplasmosis
   - Coccidiodomycosis
2. Malignancy
   - Lymphoma—more common in Hodgkin lymphoma than non-Hodgkin lymphoma
   - Carcinoma—bronchogenic, occult malignancy/metastatic disease
3. Inorganic dust disease
   - Silicosis
   - Berylliosis
4. Sarcoidosis

Epidemiology. Worldwide, tuberculosis (TB) is second only to HIV/AIDS as the greatest killer due to an infectious agent. It is estimated that one-third of the world's population is infected with TB (~1.7 billion) and it is responsible for over 1.3 million deaths annually. Despite the fact that 95% of TB deaths occur in low and middle-income countries, TB still causes significant morbidity and mortality in the developed world. In the US, a national average of 3.2 TB cases per 100,000 population occur annually, most of which are reported from the Northeast, Florida/Georgia, Texas and California. More than 60% of TB cases in the US are detected in foreign-born individuals and the majority occur among adults and the elderly. Children under 15 years of age account for 5% of TB cases with half of those occurring in those 1 to 4 years of age.[3]

In healthy individuals, infection with TB carries an average 10% lifetime risk of progression to TB disease if untreated. This risk is highest in the first 1–2 years following the acquisition of *M. tuberculosis*. Progression from infection to TB disease is especially high in younger children (4 years or younger) and the immunocompromised.[4]

Clinical Manifestations. Most infections with *M. tuberculosis* in US children are detected through active measures (TB contact investigations or screening high risk individuals) as opposed to symptomatic disease. In a US study of pediatric TB cases between 2008 and 2010, one-third were symptomatic and 75% had an international connection (foreign-born, foreign-born parent or residence outside the US). Of the foreign-born TB cases, more than half were teens that lived in the US for over 3.5 years before diagnosis.[5]

The most common site of childhood TB disease is the lung (~80%) and the most likely extra-pulmonary TB manifestation is sub-acute/chronic lymphadenitis (67%) followed by meningitis (13%, mostly in infants and toddlers), pleural TB (6%), miliary TB (5%), skeletal TB (4%) and others (chronic otitis/mastioditis, renal, gastrointestinal, and genitourinary). The risk of extra-pulmonary TB is higher among children with immune suppression. Children with pulmonary TB disease are less likely than adults to infect others due to the pauci-bacillary nature of the illness and their less effective coughing. Patients with Extrapulmonary TB are usually non-infectious, unless there is concomitant pulmonary TB or an infection of the oral cavity and larynx.[6]

Pulmonary TB (intra-thoracic adenopathy and parenchymal disease) can be a primary infection, progressive primary infection or reactivation disease.

- **Primary** pulmonary TB occurs 5–10 years after infection in infants and adolescents who present with cough, low-grade fever and rarely, weight loss. Symptoms and signs may develop due to hilar or mediastinal adenopathy that compresses adjacent structures, collapses a terminal bronchus or causes collapse consolidation of the lung.
- The disease may become **progressive** and lead to lung destruction and cavity formation with possible extension to the pleural space or the pericardium.
- **Reactivation** pulmonary TB disease is more common in adolescents and presents with constitutional symptoms (fever, weight loss, night sweats and malaise) and cough (sometimes with hemoptysis). Physical findings may be unremarkable at times and radiologic findings overlap considerably with primary or progressive primary TB (unlike in adults where reactivation TB affects the apices while primary TB affects the lower bases of the lungs).

Chest imaging is reliable for the diagnosis of pulmonary TB with the presence of suspicious symptoms. The most common picture is persistent opacification together with enlarged hilar or subcarinal lymph nodes (which may not always be discernible).[7]

TB lymphadenopathy tends to occur in children older than children with non-tuberculous mycobacterial lymphadenopathy. Anterior cervical nodes (scrofula) are more commonly involved than posterior cervical, submandibular or supraclavicular nodes. The nodes are typically 2–4 cm in diameter with a violaceous discoloration and lack the inflammatory findings of pyogenic nodes. Systemic symptoms are present in only half the patients and an abnormal CXR is found in less than a third of them. Left untreated, these nodes may caseate, ulcerate, spread to contiguous structures or create a disfiguring draining sinus.

TB infection of the nervous system occurs rarely, especially in children under 2 years old and presents as a sub-acute **meningitis** or a tuberculoma. Children usually experience nonspecific constitutional symptoms with prominent headache, a cranial nerve palsy, profound altered mental status or hydrocephalus.

Pleural TB disease is usually encountered in the older child or adolescent with or without parenchymal pulmonary disease. Patients present with chest pain, fever, cough, dyspnea and anorexia. Unilateral disease is more common and pleural effusions are usually lymphocytic with high protein, low glucose and elevated adenosine deaminase content. Acid fast stain of the effusion is positive in about 33% of cases and a pleural biopsy has a higher diagnostic yield.

Miliary TB is a severe form of TB disease that occurs as M. *tuberculosis* disseminates lymphohematogenously, especially in the very young and the immunocompromised. Fever and constitutional symptoms are usually present and hepatosplenomegaly may be found on examination. Affected children may have a negative PPD skin test due to anergy caused by the overwhelming infection.

Skeletal TB is generally a disease of older children (except for spinal disease which may occur at any age). Spondylitis, arthritis or osteomyelitis may be seen. Solitary bone lesions occur in healthy children and present with local signs of inflammation. Systemic symptoms may be present in one third of cases. Dactylitis is more commonly encountered in the infants or young child. Up to 50% of patients with skeletal TB may have an abnormal chest X-ray.

Treatment. Prompt administration of a multi-drug anti-tuberculous regimen via direct observed therapy after establishing a presumptive diagnosis is associated with a favorable outcome. A definitive diagnosis is usually based on culture results (which are not uncommonly negative in young children with paucibacillary TB disease). Six months of therapy is usually sufficient for pulmonary TB, which may be extended depending on the illness severity and response to treatment. Extrapulmonary TB treatment duration is dependent on the site involved (e.g., 6 months for TB lymphadenopathy and 12 months for TB meningitis). Susceptibility testing may further help direct therapeutic options. Consulting a TB expert is recommended when faced with multi-drug resistant TB disease.[4,6]

✔Teaching Points

- The child's prolonged and persistent constitutional symptoms, especially the anorexia and, eventually, night sweats and significant weight loss should raise suspicion for the possibility of tuberculosis.
- Dysphagia is an unusual complaint is children and adolescents. In our case, the patient stated that it started after "swallowing a pill," which was distracting to the treating physician. Ultimately, dysphagia in this case was most likely due to nodal compression on intra-thoracic structures.
- Not every TB case will have the classic high-risk epidemiologic factors in their history. Our patient had no exposure to the homeless, incarcerated, HIV-infected, IV drug users and had not travelled outside the US recently. However, his mother was foreign-born and he had resided outside the US (albeit in Canada) during his lifetime.
- TB should be strongly considered in any child with pneumonia (consolidation on chest x-ray) not responding to appropriate antibiotic therapy, especially if a patient is foreign-born or has an "international connection."

References

1. Gold BD. Gastroesophageal reflux disease in infants, children and adolescents. Adv Stud Med. 2003;3(3A):S117–S122.
2. Geagea A, Cellier C. Scope of drug-induced, infectious and allergic esophageal injury. Curr Opin Gastroenterol. 2008;24(4):496–501.
3. Alami NY, Yeun CM, Miramontes R, et al. Trends in tuberculosis-United States, 2013. MMWR. 2014 Mar 20;63(11):229–33. Pubmed PMID: 2467398.
4. Cruz AT, Starfke JR. Pediatric Tuberculosis. Pediatr Rev. 2010;31:13–27.
5. Winston CA Menzies HJ. Pediatric and adolescent tuberculosis in the United States, 2008–2010. Pediatrics. 2012;130(6):e1425–32.
6. Pickering LK, ed. American Academy of Pediatrics. Red Book: 2012 Report of the Committee on Infectious Diseases. 29th ed. Elk Grove Village, IL. 2012:741.
7. Marais BJ, Gie RP, Schaaf HS, et al. Childhood pulmonary tuberculosis: old wisdom and new challenges. Am J Resp Crit Care Med. 2006;173:1078–90.

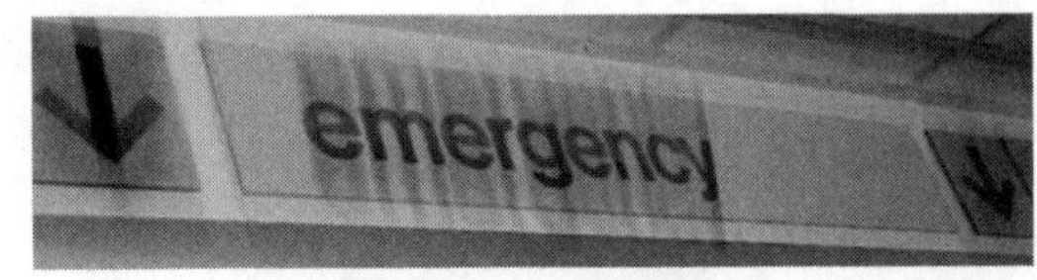

CASE 15

14-YEAR-OLD GIRL WITH A SUICIDE ATTEMPT —PLUS—PEDIATRIC TOXICOLOGY "SHORTS"

Sean Patrick Nordt, MD
Associate Professor of Clinical Emergency Medicine
Attending Physician and Director of the Section of Toxicology
Department of Emergency Medicine
Keck School of Medicine of USC

Mike Unger, MD
Psychiatrist
A.C.T. Team Psychiatrist for the Cobb & Douglas County Svcs. Board, Atlanta, GA

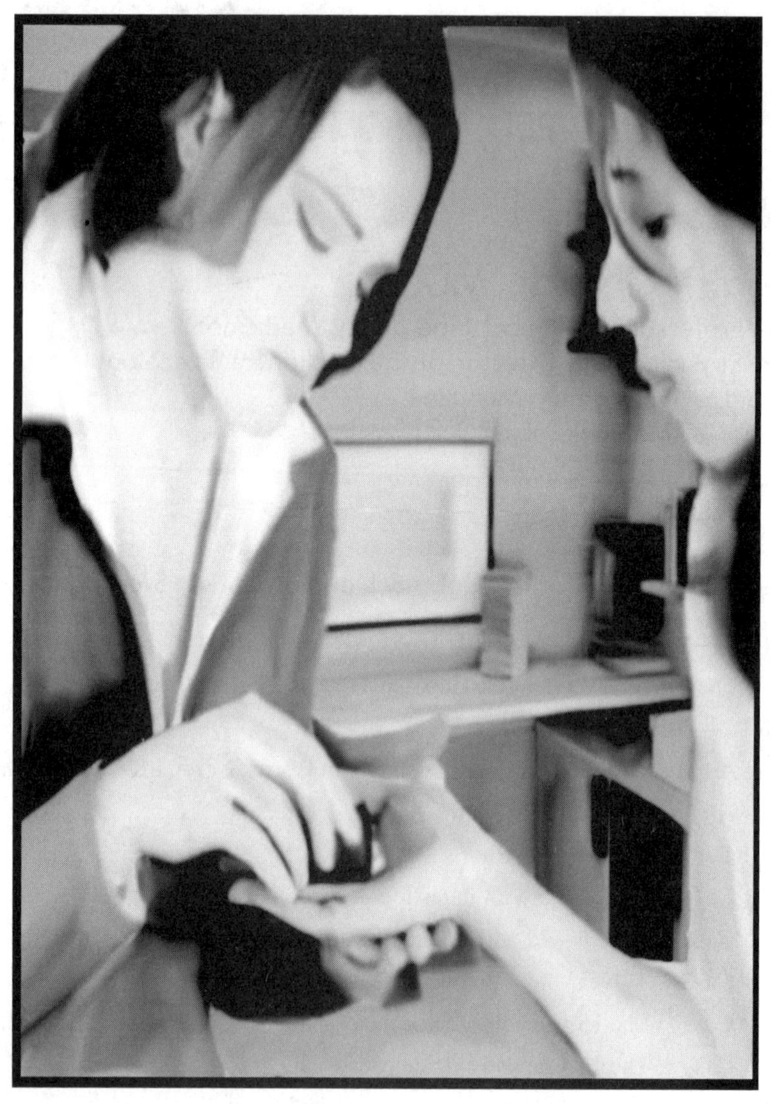

CASE 15

14-YEAR-OLD GIRL WITH A SUICIDE ATTEMPT—PLUS—PEDIATRIC TOXICOLOGY "SHORTS"

➢**Author's note:** The assessment of a child with an overdose requires two evaluations: medical as well as mental-health. The first step is to stabilize the patient; determine the type of overdose (if possible) and provide emergent interventions. Sean Nordt, board certified in emergency medicine, toxicology and pharmacology (yes, he is an over-achiever!) guides us through a general approach, then throws us pearls on some specific overdose scenarios with four tox shorts. The chapter ends with a discussion by Mike Unger, psychiatrist, who weighs in on assessing the suicidal teen and providing tips on who needs to be admitted.

CASE 1: 14-YEAR-OLD GIRL WITH OVERDOSE AND SUICIDE ATTEMPT

The Doctor's Version (the following is the actual documentation of the provider)

CC: Overdose

History of Present Illness (Mid-level provider): 14-year-old white female with past history of ADHD and in otherwise good general health presents today via EMS for evaluation of an overdose/ suicidal attempt. Patient states approximately 1 hour prior to arrival she took five 30 mg Vyvanse in an attempt to end her life. States that she has been off again/off again with her boyfriend for the last year and broke up 2 months ago. Since the breakup she has been having thoughts of suicide, but denies suicidal attempts prior to today. Today while she was at school she found out that her ex-boyfriend is not "in love with her" which caused her to have a "breakdown" (crying) and her school counselor drove her home. When she got home, she went to her room and took the pills, her mother upon further investigation realized she took the medication and called EMS. Patient denies any nausea, vomiting, abdominal pain, chest pain, shortness of breath or headache. Patient states that she has cut herself in the past, but prior to today has not really "attempted" to end her life. She denies homicidal ideation. No fever, chills, nausea vomiting. No chest pain or shortness of breath. No abdominal pain.

PAST MEDICAL HISTORY:

NKDA
Meds: Vyvanse (Lisdexamfetamine for ADHD)
PMH: ADHD
SH: Not recorded
FH: Not recorded

VITAL SIGNS							
Time	Temp(F)	Pulse	Resp	Syst	Diast	O2 Sat	O2%
13:08	98.8	79	16	139	70	100	RA

PHYSICAL EXAMINATION

Constitutional: 14-year-old white female sitting up in bed. Patient is alone. She is alert and oriented X3, well-nourished, well appearing, tearful but in no apparent distress

Eyes: PERRLA. EOM intact. No scleral icterus or injection.

Neck: No cervical lymphadenopathy. Neck supple without nuchal rigidity.

Resp: Breath sounds clear and equal bilaterally; no wheezes, rhonchi, or rales

Card: Regular rhythm, without murmurs, rub or gallop.

Abd: Non-distended; non-tender, soft, without rigidity, rebound or guarding. No masses or organomegaly

Ext: Pulses are 2+ and equal in upper and lower extremities bilaterally. No calf pain or swelling.

Neurological: Patient is alert and oriented times three. Cranial nerves III-XII are intact. Sensory and motor functions are intact. Strength is 5/5 for flexion and extension in all 4 extremities. Patellar DTR's are equal and intact. No pronator drift. Finger to nose and heel to shin are equal and intact bilaterally.

be consistent

TESTING (inc. XR, iv, lab, ECG): CBC, BMP, drug of abuse screen, alcohol and serum tox - all within normal levels

Medical Decision Making

I reviewed the nurse's notes. Patient evaluated by social worker and patient/family members are agreeable to placement for psychiatric evaluation. Patient has been stable and pleasant in the ED thus far. I did discuss the patient's case with the attending doctor who will complete the patient' s case. This provider has ended her shift. Care transitioned to attending physician Dr. Ringer.

Impression and Plan

DIAGNOSIS:

Suicidal ideation
Overdose

William Ringer, PA-C

ED Attending Note

Patient had c/o pain with her canker sore. Viscous lidocaine was applied with a q-tip. She has had no other complaints through the evening. Parents have been at bedside. Patient continues to await placement at Mental Health Facility.

Disposition: Patient is transferred to a mental health facility

Patrick Murray, MD

I. APPROACH TO THE OVERDOSE PATIENT

Sean Patrick Nordt, MD

Associate Professor of Clinical Emergency Medicine
Attending Physician and Director of the Section of Toxicology, Department of Emergency Medicine, Keck School of Medicine of USC
Former Chair, Medication Safety Committee, Los Angeles County-USC Medical Center
Board-certified emergency physician, board-certified medical toxicologist, pharmacist

➢**Author's note:** The following is an approach to evaluation of the overdose patient. It begins with a general approach then is focused to this specific case. The chapter continues with 4 additional cases with tips for each specific type of overdose, ending with the *"grand finale"* case; a suicide-pact between two 16-year-old girls, both overdosing on Wellbutrin and Adderal and presenting with seizures and tachycardia.

Dr. Nordt's initial approach can be applied to all of the following cases.

A GENERAL APPROACH TO THE OVERDOSE PATIENT

The Nordt 'Four-step': The following is my 4-step approach to "every" acute poisoning, particularly in attempts at self-harm:

1. Assessment of ABCs
2. EKG
3. Electrolytes and anion gap
4. Drug levels (acetaminophen, salicylates, ethanol)

Step #1: ABC's on a crashing patient are handled on an emergent basis with intubation, fluid resuscitation, and maintenance of circulation

Step #2: EKG—Focus on:

- "Too fast or too slow"
- Any interval changes, specifically widening especially of the QRS, particularly in sodium channel blocking agents such as cyclic antidepressants, cocaine, diphenhydramine, many antidepressant and antipsychotic medications
- QTc prolongation—The QTc may be prolonged but this is generally less of a clinical consequence than a widened QRS ≥ 0.12 seconds, which can precede ventricular tachycardia and ventricular fibrillation.
- Any high atrioventricular blocks (e.g. Mobitz Type I or II or third-degree block)
- The axis: Specifically a rightward axis (particularly concerning is a RSR′ in aVR), which can be seen in sodium channel blocking agents.

Step #3: Serum electrolytes should be ordered and an anion gap should be calculated. Of all the mnemonics ever taught, MUDPILES holds up fairly well and will allow for a rapid toxicological differential diagnosis:

M – Methanol, metformin
U – Uremia
D – Diabetic ketoacidosis
P – Phenformin
I – Iron
L – Lactate
E – Ethanol ketoacidosis, ethylene glycol
S – Salicylates

Step #4: Drug levels

- Acetaminophen toxicity can be clinically silent early in poisoning.
- Salicylate toxicity can be protean and subtle early in poisoning. May be confused with DXA or sepsis.
- Urine toxicology is generally unhelpful as there is cross-reactivity, false negatives, or may remain positive for several days following last use.
- Perform a urine pregnancy test in any female of childbearing potential.

TOXIDROMES

Most acute poisonings can be narrowed down to a handful of toxidromes; a constellation of signs and symptoms commonly manifested in poisonings.[1] These include:

- **Sympathomimetic** (cocaine, amphetamines, bath salts)
  - o Tachycardia
  - o Hypertension
  - o Hyperthermia
  - o Diaphoresis
  - o Mydriasis
  - o Agitation/violent behavior

- **Anticholinergic** (think: the 4 "anti's"—antihistamines, antipsychotics, antidepressants, anti-parkinsonian drugs + jimson weed, atropine, benztropine)
  - o Dry as a bone (dry flushed skin)
  - o Mad as a hatter (delirium, hallucinations, *not* violent)
  - o Hot as a hare (hyperthermia)
  - o Blind as a bat (mydriasis, blurred vision)
  - o Red as a beet
  - o Decreased or absent bowel sounds and urinary retention
  - o Note: There is some overlap with sympathomimetic, e.g., tachycardia, mydriasis, and hyperthermia may be seen from lack of ability to sweat. *A key difference is that anticholinergic poisoned patients are confused but not violent

- **Cholinergic**—(think organophosphates, nerve agents such as Sarin, Soman, Tabun, VX, and carbamates such as pilocarpine, physostigmine, malathion) are the *opposite* of anticholinergic with:
  - o S – Salivation
  - o L – Lacrimation
  - o U – Urination

- o D – Defecation
- o G – GI effects
- o E – Emesis

o Most concerning are the "Killer B's":
- Bronchoconstriction
- Bradycardia
- Bronchorrhea

- **Opioid** (Morphine, codeine, hydrocodone, oxycodone, methadone, hydromorphone, heroin, fentanyl, meperidine)
  - o Often miosis but some opioids can mydriasis (e.g. meperidine)
  - o Respiratory depression/possibly apnea
  - o Somnolence/ coma and most often miosis

- **Sedative-hypnotics**
  - o Benzodiazepines, barbiturates, ethanol, Gamma-hydroxybutyrate/GHB) present with:
    - Somnolence
    - Coma
    - Often there are fairly normal vital signs but respiratory depression can be seen, particularly with co-ingestants such as ethanol.

APPROACH FOR THIS PATIENT

ADHD is a common and increasing diagnosis encountered in both pediatric and adult patients. The approach requires an understanding of which medication classes are used to treat ADHD, while remembering that many patients may have been on alternative agents previously, but remain accessible to patient in suicide attempt.

Classes of ADHD meds[2]

- Stimulants: The majority of these agents are "stimulants" including amphetamine derivatives e.g., Adderall, Vyvanse causing norepinephrine, serotonin and dopamine release or methylphenidate-like agents e.g., Focalyn, Ritalin, which inhibit the reuptake of dopamine and norepinephrine. These classes present similarly with a "sympathomimetic" toxidrome of tachycardia, hypertension, agitation, diaphoresis.
- Newer agents that are "non-stimulants" include: Stattera, which can present with sympathomimetic features but also somnolence.
- Various antidepressants are used to treat ADHD including: cyclic antidepressants, which can cause seizures and QRS widening and ventricular dysrhythmias and bupropion, which causes seizures commonly and occasionally ventricular dysrhythmias.
- Alpha-2 agonists, e.g., clonidine, guanfacine, which can cause an opioid-like respiratory depression and somnolence as well as bradycardia and hypotension.

II. Questions and answers with Dr. Sean Nordt!

Q: *How do you initially approach this patient?*

A: For this case we go back to the basics as outlined above. Order an EKG, continuous cardiac monitoring, serum electrolytes, urine pregnancy test, and acetaminophen and salicylate levels.

Q: *Should activated charcoal be used, as she presents within 1 hour of ingestion?*
A: One of the risks of sympathomimetic poisoning is seizures. I would not give activated charcoal as the risk of aspiration outweighs the questionable potential benefit.

Q: *Is alcohol testing needed?*
A: Ethanol is not indicated based on history and the fact that the patient is not somnolent.

Q: *What am I looking for on her ECG?*
A: The cardiovascular toxicity anticipated from a single ingestion Lisdexamfetamine (Vyvanase) poisoning would be sinus tachycardia and hypertension. However, ADHD is often treated with multiple classes of medications including antidepressants, which may be discovered, solely by a widened QRS or ventricular dysrhythmias evident on ECG or continuous cardiac monitoring. Patients with intentional self-harm may purposefully omit a history of concomitant ingestions.

Q: *The patient's heart rate is normal and blood pressure is only minimally elevated. Are benzodiazepines indicated?*
A: Benzodiazepines have tremendous breadth and benefit in various poisonings. Benzodiazepines can effectively treat most drug-induced seizures. In addition, their anxiolytic properties can be advantageous in acutely agitated or violent patients. Furthermore, benzodiazepines are effective sympatholytics following acute sympathomimetic poisonings treating tachycardia, hypertension and even the hyperthermia. However, as our patient is not manifesting a severe sympathomimetic poisoning and is alert and awake, I would not recommend a benzodiazepine as it would not be expected to have a therapeutic benefit and may preclude or delay the psychiatric evaluation.

Q: *How does an overdose in a suicidal patient differ from inadvertent overdose?*
A: Self-harm poisonings are often more severe poisonings, a result of the amount and type of agent ingested, a delay in presentation, frequent poly-drug poisonings, and the inability to obtain an accurate history, particularly if the patient is actively suicidal.

Q: *What is haloperidol (Haldol) and what is the preferred route of administration and dose?*
A: Haloperidol is a dopamine antagonist and is useful for the acutely psychotic and/or agitated patient. Haloperidol is only FDA approved for intramuscular use, however, years and years of clinical use support IV administration. The route of administration should be chosen based on intravenous access; often patients are too agitated to safely establish intravenous access requiring an IM injection. Intravenous haloperidol works more rapidly and is the preferred route of administration. The initial dose of IV haloperidol is 2.5 mg to 10 mg for an adult.

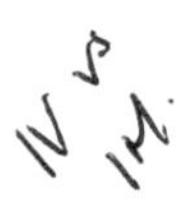

Q: *Are there any scenarios when we would NOT want to use haloperidol?*
A: Haloperidol is a generally very safe and can be used in the vast majority of patients. Avoid with a true allergy, though many of the patient-reported "allergies" are previous dystonic reactions. If a patient has a prolonged QTc[3] or known congenital prolonged QTc syndrome, it is probably best to avoid, however, this is often not known in the acutely agitated patient and haloperidol may be required for the patient's safety to allow initial stabilization of the acute poisoned patient.

Though reported to lower the seizure threshold, this is not well described in haloperidol and would not preclude its use, even with a history of seizure disorder. I do generally recommend that a benzodiazepine be given at the same time as the anxiolytic properties often complement the haloperidol, helping it to work more rapidly and may even prevent a seizure from occurring.

Q: *Which other meds may be used in agitated patients?*

A: Benzodiazepines, particularly midazolam and lorazepam work faster than haloperidol and result in somnolence and blunt the sympathetic drive. The addition of diphenhydramine has a two-fold benefit by initially causing somnolence from the antihistaminic effects and may also prevent a dystonic reaction.

Bounceback Visit to Same ED 13 Days Later

- Brought in by police after threatening to harm herself
- Pt. says she did not do anything and does not want to harm herself
- Denies ingestion of drugs
- No specific complaints
- Home meds: Lexapro (escitalopram) and **Vyvanse** (Lisdexamfetamine)
- PE: Pulse 82, Respir 16, BP 112/60, sat 100%
- General appearance of emotional distress, otherwise physical exam normal
- Labs normal including acetaminophen, salicylate, alcohol level
- **Diagnosis:** Suicidal ideation
- **Disposition:** Pt. transferred back to psych facility

III. PEDIATRIC TOXICOLOGY SHORTS

CASE 2: 2-YEAR-OLD WITH INGESTION OF CALAMINE LOTION

The Doctor's Version (the following is the actual documentation of the provider)

- **22:15 – HPI (physician):** At 945 PM tonight, pt. drank 3 oz of Calamine lotion with no emesis afterwards. [Mother] spoke with Poison Control who advised that it contains Pramoxine and was told to go to ED. Child acting appropriate
- **PE:** WNL
- Testing: ECG, cardiac monitor, methemoglobin level
- **2230:** [I] spoke with poison control, recommend evaluating for prolonged QT, methemoglobinemia, bradycardia, hypotension.
- **Results/MDM:** I feel patient will be fine, methemoglobin level is very low but not "WNL." No hypotension, no bradycardia, no QT prolongation
  - 0025: Spoke with poison control, recommended repeat level in 4 hours.
  - 0030: Poison control called back, states discussing case with fellow prior to transfer or recheck.
  - 0050: Fellow advised to transfer and recheck.
  - Spoke with Children's Hospital ED attending, recommended transfer for f/u methemoglobin level at the advice of poison control. Pt will be transferred

- **Diagnosis:** Ingestion calamine lotion

Questions and answers with Dr. Sean Nordt:

Q: *When should poison control be called?*

A: For the vast majority of poisonings, consult your staff toxicologist or your local poison control center. A consultation can rapidly alleviate fears and misconceptions of the provider as well as the patient or family. In addition, this may afford some medico-legal "protection" if a case does poorly. Though it may take some time to call, in the long run a toxicologist and/or poison center often helps to minimize costs by guiding appropriate laboratory analysis and obviating unnecessary and potentially dangerous therapies such as gastric lavage or activated charcoal.

Q: *How should we approach a calamine lotion/pramoxine ingestion?*

A: The history of 3 ounces ingested is probably incorrect but has to be assumed to be true. Another poison center or toxicologist may have recommended observation at home with poison center follow up, however, if there is ever concern of worsening at home, transport to a healthcare facility is advised. Calamine lotion is non-toxic[4] and no therapy or observation is necessary, but the toxic potential and probable reason for healthcare center evaluation is the pramoxine. Pramoxine is also known as pramocaine, an ester local anesthetic. The major toxicities with ester anesthetics are seizures and methemoglobinemia.[5,6]

- Seizures generally are not seen with oral ingestions unless massive, but if they do occur would be treated with a benzodiazepine or barbiturate.
- Persons with methemoglobinemia do not become cyanotic until the methemoglobin level is ≥ 1.5 g/dL methemoglobin, which is approximately 10 % assuming a normal serum hemoglobin of 15 g/dL. Toxicity is generally not seen until the methemoglobin level is ≥ 30%. Monitoring for cyanosis not responsive to oxygen and/or respiratory distress is paramount. Place methylene blue at the bedside if needed.

Q: *Why was an ECG and cardiac monitoring recommended?*

A: Cardiovascular collapse and dysrhythmias can occur following local anesthetic poisonings although they are unusual following oral ingestions. However, I do agree with continuous cardiac monitoring and a baseline EKG in this case. In addition, continuous pulse oximetry should be performed, but note that the reading may not be accurate as methemoglobin can give aberrant pulse oximetry readings in the 85% range. Monitoring may alert the staff of a seizure.

Q: *Other thoughts? Could we be missing anything?*

A: Though the history is a calamine and pramoxine ingestion, unless we can confirm this is correct product, i.e., parents bring bottle in, there is possibility of another calamine-containing product being ingested such as Caladryl, which contains calamine and diphenhydramine. Diphenhydramine may case anticholinergic poisoning with seizures and a widened QRS and ventricular dysrhythmias similar to that seen with cyclic antidepressants.[7]

CASE 3: 12-YEAR-OLD WITH SUICIDAL OVERDOSE

The Doctor's Version (the following is the actual documentation of the provider)

HPI: Arrival per EMS. I did see the patient immediately upon arrival. She presents after she took what she says were 109 clonidine 0.1 mg that she normally takes for ADD and she took these in a suicide attempt at home at 9:30 this evening. No vomiting. No history of visual or auditory hallucinations. She does have a history of cutting. Has never tried to end her life in the past. History is from the patient. I also did speak with the mother

VITAL SIGNS		
Pulse	Respir.	BP
58	16	144/84. Recheck 154/109

Testing:

Sodium Level	136 mMol/L
Potassium Level	4.0 mMol/L
Chloride Level	105 mMol/L
Carbon Dioxide Level	26 mMol/L
Anion Gap	5.0 mMol/L LOW
Glucose Level	169 mg/dL HI
Acetaminophen (Tylenol) Level	<10 mcg/mL
Alcohol (Ethanol) Level	<0.01 gm/dL
Salicylate Level	<4.0 mg/dL

MDM: EKG does show normal sinus rhythm with a rate of 62. As the pt did take a large amt of clonidine, I did call and speak with the Poison Control Center who agrees that lavage and charcoal are not necessary at this time. They did recommend consideration of Narcan if vital signs decompensate. The patient will be transferred to Children's Hospital for admission and further observation. It is questionable how many pills the patient took. The mother thought the bottle was almost empty but the patient does give a specific number - she says she has not been taking her pills and has been saving them up

Diagnosis: Overdose clonidine, suicide attempt

Questions and answers with Dr. Sean Nordt:

Q: *What is your specific approach to a clonidine overdose?*

A: Clonidine is a unique anti-hypertensive in that it causes not only cardiovascular toxicity e.g., bradycardia and hypotension, but also specific central nervous and respiratory system effects as it can mimic acute opioid poisoning causing somnolence, coma, respiratory depression, apnea and pinpoint pupils.[8]

Q: *Why was her blood pressure so high given that she ingested a medicine, which causes hypotension?*

A: An interesting phenomenon that can be seen early is hypertension. This results from direct stimulation of alpha 1 receptors. This is generally brief and self-limiting not requiring any therapy but can be followed by profound hypotension.

Q: *What at the most common cardiovascular effects from clonidine ingestion?*

A: Bradycardia and hypotension are the most common cardiovascular effects. If hypotension does occur, intravenous crystalloid boluses should be given and if refractory a direct activating alpha agonist (e.g. norepinephrine, phenylephrine) should be used. An ECG should be obtained and continuous cardiopulmonary monitoring should be employed. Rarely clonidine can cause atrioventricular conduction abnormalities e.g., second and third degree heart block, however, if this does occur I would consider co-ingestion of other cardiovascular agents such as a beta antagonist or calcium channel antagonist.

Q: *How is central nervous system and respiratory depression treated?*

A: Usually tactile stimuli alone, e.g., sternal rub, will reverse these events, however, there are case reports of naloxone being effective.

Q: *Should active charcoal be used?*

A: Clonidine is rapidly absorbed with a risk of decreased level of consciousness, therefore activated charcoal should be avoided.

Q: *How long should a patient with clonidine ingestion be watched?*

A: Clonidine is rapidly absorbed from the gastrointestinal tract and clinical manifestations of toxicity should be seen within one to two hours. If a patient is asymptomatic at six hours can be cleared from the clonidine standpoint.

CASE 4: 17-YEAR-OLD WITH OVERDOSE OF SEROQUEL AND IBUPROFEN

The Doctor's Version (the following is the actual documentation of the provider)

HPI: 17yo WF +smoker comes to the ED with report of overdose. Patient notes that she was trying to kill herself. She took 6 Seroquel (quetiapine) and ibuprofen. Denies taking any drugs, Tylenol or aspirin. She also was sipping on Nyquil since 10pm. She has had 2 previous suicide attempts in the past. She notes on arrival that she is 'feeling pretty good' and that she has no pain, nausea. Patient reported to me that she just wanted to be with her mother in heaven.

VITAL SIGNS

Pulse	Respir.	BP
126	28	124/84

MDM: Patient has become combative in the ED with attempt at NGT for charcoal. She has required 4-point leather restraints for her safety and for staff safety. In an attempt to remove the restraints, patient became combative again. Patient's airway is safe at this time. She does have a gag. She is very sleepy and so I believe that she may require admission. As she is 17yo, I am unable to admit her to this hospital. I spoke with ED physician at Children's and will transfer.

Diagnosis: Medication overdose, altered mental status

Bounceback Visit to Same ED 13 Days Later

Pt returns 2½ months later after ingestion of 2 Xanax the previous night. Stated she felt irritated and suicidal. She no longer feels suicidal. After assessment and social work consultation, patient is discharged and asked to follow up with the family practice clinic in 1-2 days.

Questions and answers with Dr. Sean Nordt:

Q: *How does Seroquel work?*

A: Seroquel (quetiapine) is an atypical antipsychotic with various pharmacologic effects at multiple receptors (dopamine 2 antagonism, serotonin 5HT-2 antagonism) accounting for much of its beneficial clinical effects. It also has antihistaminic properties causing sedation, anticholinergic properties causing agitation, and alpha-adrenergic blockade properties causing hypotension and miosis. These effects are exaggerated in large acute poisonings, affecting two major systems: the central nervous system and cardiovascular system.[9]

Q: *How do patients present clinically?*

A: Following acute quetiapine poisoning patients often present with somnolence, which can be coupled with agitation. Progression to coma is not uncommon and intubation may be required for airway protection. Though quetiapine has anticholinergic effects, miosis from alpha-adrenergic blockade is more common than mydriasis. Seizures have been reported and should be treated with benzodiazepines, however, consider potential co-ingestions if seizures are seen. From a cardiovascular standpoint, tachycardia from anticholinergic effects and hypotension from alpha-adrenergic blockade are most common.

Q: *How should the tachycardia, hypotension, and ECG changes be managed?*

A: The tachycardia does not generally require any therapy. Hypotension should be treated with intravenous crystalloid boluses and if refractory, a direct-acting alpha agonist such as norepinephrine or phenylephrine. QTc prolongation is common with quetiapine both in clinical use and following acute poisonings. However, this is rarely of clinical consequence. QRS prolongation has also been reported following quetiapine poisoning and should be treated with boluses of sodium bicarbonate intravenously with consideration of co-ingestion.

Q: *What is your approach to ibuprofen overdose?*

A: Ibuprofen, a propionic acid non-steroidal anti-inflammatory, is a common agent used in acute poisonings due to its widespread use and availability. Ibuprofen is generally well tolerated with no or minimal toxicity following acute poisonings. Much of the toxicity associated with NSAIDs is from their chronic use; gastrointestinal bleeding, renal insufficiency, and cardiovascular events, but this is not generally relevant following acute poisonings.[10]

Q: *What are the most serious findings in a large ibuprofen ingestion?*

A: Occasionally severe toxicity can be seen including somnolence, which can rarely proceed to coma or severe lactic acidosis.

Q: *How is ibuprofen toxicity managed?*

A: Hemodialysis while not generally thought to be effective or clinically indicated for the majority of ibuprofen poisonings has been reported to be effective in cases of coma, persistent lactic acidosis, particularly in the setting of renal insufficiency. However, the vast majority of ibuprofen poisonings can be managed supportively and often require no specific therapy.

Q: Is GI decontamination indicated in quetiapine or ibuprofen overdose?

A: No, it is not routinely recommended as quetiapine can cause decreased level of consciousness and ibuprofen rarely causes any clinically significant effects. Of note, restraining or otherwise "forcing" a patient to take activated charcoal is not recommended.

Q: OK. Rubber meets the road: Has activated charcoal ever been shown to decrease moridity?

A: On a general note, single dose activated charcoal has not been shown to have a mortality benefit following *any* acute poisonings.

Q: *Is any testing indicated?*

A: No specific testing for either quetiapine or ibuprofen is indicated. Routine acetaminophen, salicylate, serum electrolytes, ECG, cardiac monitoring, and urine pregnancy testing as described above, should be obtained. Physostigmine, an acetylcholinesterase inhibitor used as an antidote for anticholinergic poisoning should *not* be used to reverse the antimuscarinic effects seen following quetiapine poisoning and may worsen toxicity by potentiating other effects, e.g., further prolongation of QTc due to slowing cardiac rate. Of note, quetiapine can cross react with some urine toxicology screens giving false positive results for cyclic antidepressants and methadone illustrating a major limitation of urine toxicology screening.

CASE 5: THE 16-YEAR-OLD SUICIDE PACT—PATIENT #1

The Doctor's Version (the following is the actual documentation of the provider)

HPI: The story is that the patient has depression. She has been living with a friend since June because of an altercation at home and today was scheduled to go back to live with her mother. At an unknown time she took Wellbutrin 150 mg and Adderall 25 mg XL. The prescriptions were filled for #90 Wellbutrin (bupropion) and #30 Adderall (amphetamine and dextroamphetamine) three days ago and there were only 1-2 pills left in each bottle. The patient is unable to give an adequate history secondary to her altered consciousness. Per paramedics the patient had a seizure at home prior to their arrival. They say she has expressed suicidal intent. The mother did later arrive and I spoke with her - says the patient has never had a suicide attempt but was called (she was not at home) so does not have any additional history.

Meds: Adderall XR 25mg, Wellbutrin XL 150mg

VITAL SIGNS				
Temp	Pulse	Resp	BP	Sat
98.4 F	147	20	98/60	91%RA

PE: The patient does respond to verbal stimulation by saying some words but these are minimal. I do not see any bite marks on the tongue. She is not seizing when I'm in the room. I don't find any evidence of trauma. No neck pain. Otherwise normal

MDM (10:03): I did see the patient immediately upon arrival. I reviewed her EKG showing what appears to be a sinus tachycardia with a rate of 135. There is QT prolongation with a rate of 627 so I did call pharmacy and they sent magnesium 1 g down right away that we administered over an expedited protocol of 15 minutes. I also gave her 1 mg IV Ativan to prevent further seizures. The paramedics had given her Narcan. The mother later arrived and I did go back and check on the patient again also spoke with the mother but not significantly increased amount of information. The caregiver that she has been staying with is reportedly on the way here but has not arrived at this time. I did speak with poison control. I did also speak with Children's Hospital who accepts the patient for transfer to the emergency department and will likely be admitted to the intensive care unit care. We are at this time calling for critical care transport. The children's transport team was not available at this time. Pt is protecting her airway.

Labs (1053):

Sodium Level	146 mMol/L HI
Potassium Level	**3.0 mMol/L LOW**
Chloride Level	108 mMol/L HI
Carbon Dioxide Level	**14 mMol/L LOW**
Anion Gap	**24.0 mMol/L HI**
Glucose Level	**158 mg/dL HI**
BUN	8 mg/dL
Alcohol (Ethanol) Level	<0.01 gm/dL
Pregnancy Test POCT	Negative

MDM (11:25): I did review the initial lab results. The patient was hypokalemic and this will be replaced IV. She is significantly acidotic with bicarbonate level 14 and will continue to receive IV fluids with another bolus. This could be from lactic acidosis from seizure or from the ingestion. She did receive magnesium and I will repeat her EKG to reassess the QTc interval. Foley catheter is in place with only very small amount of urine. I did call the number of the woman who is currently watching her since June and her name is Stacy - there was no answer and I did leave a message but did they have not called back. We do not have a definitive time of ingestion.

MDM (11:36): I spoke with Stacy (caregiver) who tells me she does not know the time of ingestion. Her daughter Brianna will also come in shortly for an overdose also. She is 16 years old. Thinks her daughter took the meds last night but is "out of it".

MDM (11:43): Repeat EKG shows that the tachycardia is improved at 129. The QTC interval is improved 474. Transport is currently here to take the child to Children's Hospital.

DIAGNOSIS: Overdose Wellbutrin and Adderall, suicide attempt, seizures, altered level of consciousness.

Questions and answers with Dr. Sean Nordt:

Q: *How does Bupropion work and how does it present with overdose?*

A: Bupropion, a unicyclic antidepressant, predominantly inhibits the reuptake of dopamine but also inhibits reuptake of serotonin and norepinephrine to some extent. In addition to managing depression and ADHD, it is also used in the treatment of smoking cessation, marketed as Zyban. Many bupropion pharmaceutical preparations are sustained-release preparations (e.g., Wellbutrin XR). Seizures are common following bupropion poisoning and occur at relatively low dosages, e.g., 500 mg. Bupropion also can present identically to cyclic antidepressants with not only seizures, but also QRS widening and ventricular dysrhythmias.[11]

Q: *How do we approach this patient?*

A: The QRS widening and ventricular dysrhythmias should be treated with boluses of sodium bicarbonate to narrow and to keep serum pH in the 7.45 to 7.55 range. As there are many sustained release preparations, both activated charcoal and whole bowel irrigation may be beneficial, however, airway protection with endotracheal intubation prior to administration should be considered as rapid mental status deterioration and seizures may result in aspiration. More recently lipid fat emulsion therapy or Intralipid given intravenously has been reported to be beneficial in severe bupropion poisonings.[12] Toxicology consultation with a toxicologist or poison control center is recommended if consider lipid fat emulsion therapy.

Q: *Is the seizure treated any differently because it is from an overdose?*

A: Poisoned patients presenting with seizures should be initially approached similar to any seizing patient with proper positioning, oxygen, suction, finger stick glucose and benzodiazepine or barbiturate. Once stabilized, potential toxicological etiologies can be considered.

Q: *Which other overdoses case cause seizures?*

A:
- Sulfonylureas and insulin can cause seizures from hypoglycemia.
- Bupropion, as in this case commonly causes seizures.
- Cyclic antidepressants, phenothiazines, propoxyphene, and diphenhydramine can all cause seizures that often precede widening of the QRS and should be anticipated.
- Isoniazid (with pyridoxine intravenously as antidote)
- Theophylline (no specific antidote but aggressive benzodiazepine and/or barbiturates and consideration of emergent hemodialysis).
- Severe salicylate poisoning may cause seizures from cerebral edema and should prompt emergent hemodialysis.
- Amphetamine and cocaine poisoning can cause seizures and when occur should raise concern of possible intracranial hemorrhage. Therefore, emergent intubation and CT scan of head would be indicated.

Of note, routine antiepileptics (e.g., phenytoin, levetiracetam, valproic acid) have no role for toxin-induced seizures but can be given if an etiology other than toxin is in differential or if toxin resulted in intracerebral hemorrhage.

Q: *Can you explain more about QT prolongation?*

A: QT prolongation is rarely of severe clinical consequence following acute poisonings. QT prolongation is more concerning with prolonged medication administration from drug-drug interactions or congenital prolonged QT syndrome or organic heart disease and also electrolyte abnormalities.[13] Many toxins that cause QT prolongation following acute poisonings also cause sinus tachycardia (e.g., cyclic antidepressants). This has a beneficial effect as the faster the rate, the shorter the QT (in relation to the cardiac rate).

Q: What is the most serious effect of QT prolongation and how is it managed?

A: Clinicians should be concerned if there is bradycardia or even slow normal cardiac rate with prolonged QTc as this increases the risk of Torsade de pointes. As such, avoid treating sinus tachycardia if possible. Magnesium sulfate 1 to 2 gram intravenous infusion can be given for a prolonged QTc. If Torsade de pointes does occur intravenous magnesium should be given in addition to overdrive cardiac pacing with either transthoracic or transvenous cardiac pacing. Isoproterenol can be given intravenously for chemical overdrive pacing.

Q: Why was her anion gap elevated?

A: This patient has an elevated anion gap and low serum bicarbonate. This was most likely secondary to the seizure activity but the differentia diagnosis should include "MUDPILES" (see page 222) as a potential etiology. The hypokalemia is of unclear etiology as we would expect a normal or elevated potassium from shift to extracellular space in the setting of acidemia with the increased anion gap. I agree with the administration of potassium repletion as the serum potassium would be expected to further decrease as pH normalized.

Q: How do you approach the "crashing" overdose patient with unknown overdose?

A: The initial approach to the "crashing" poisoned patient is similar to any other unstable patient. Rapid assessment of ABCs and emergent resuscitation are paramount.

- However, specific therapies should be considered.
- For ventricular dysrhythmias, consider aggressive sodium bicarbonate boluses.
- When beta antagonist or calcium channel antagonist poisoning is suspected, consider glucagon and intravenous calcium if refractory high dose insulin and epinephrine or norepinephrine infusions.
- For cardiac glycoside sympathomimetic poisonings, use digoxin-specific Fab fragment antibodies.
- For any "crashing" patient from cyclic antidepressants, beta antagonist or calcium channel antagonist, or local anesthetic toxicity, consider lipid fat emulsion "rescue" therapy.

Q: Which patients should be emergently dialyzed?

A: Poisonings from:

- Ethylene glycol
- Theophylline
- Methanol
- Salicylates

Consider in:

- Severe lithium poisoning, particularly in setting of renal failure

May have role in:

- Massive valproic acid poisonings
- Phenobarbital poisonings

➢**Author's note:** As the patient is leaving with Children's hospital transport, the physician hears EMS encoding "we are 5 minutes out with a 16-year-old girl who is actively seizing. There is a history of overdose."

CASE 5: THE 16-YEAR-OLD SUICIDE PACT—PATIENT #2

The Doctor's Version (the following is the actual documentation of the provider)

HPI (11:56): The patient presents after taking 40 Wellbutrin at an unknown time. I did see the patient immediately upon arrival and also spoke with the paramedics who tell me that they arrived at the patient's home, which was a poor state of repair, and they did inform children services. I should also note that the patient's friend who is 16 years old just arrived a little over one hour ago with an overdose of Wellbutrin and Adderall and was just transferred to Children's Hospital. The patient is not responding to questions. I did speak with the paramedics who tell me that when they arrived the patient was speaking and did express suicidal intention. When they attempted to start the IV the patient had a 20 second generalized tonic-clonic seizure. No incontinence or biting of the tongue or blood in the mouth that they are aware.

PE: Patient is warm and pink, not diaphoretic, looking around the room, does not respond to verbal questions. She does have a slight gag reflex with tongue depressor. Is protecting her airway.

MDM (1200) - I did review the EKG showing sinus tachycardia with a rate of 159 with a prolonged QT of 543 and I did call and spoke with the pharmacist and they will send 1 g of magnesium to be administered in an expedited manner over 15 minutes. The patient also received 1 L IV fluid bolus. I ordered 1 mg intravenous Ativan; she is not seizing at this time. I was just informed the patient's mother has arrived. Orders for overdose labs, social worker consult, suicide precautions and seizure precautions are in place.

MDM (12:28) - I did go back and see the patient and also spoke with the mother. The patient is able to speak now but she does have a very thick tongue. She is protecting her airway, and her tachycardia has improved with the IV fluids. The mother said that the patient's friend [patient #1] was a victim of abuse from the mother's girlfriend in June and they did file a report with children's services and for that reason she came to live with them. The patient took the pills last night and these were out of the pill bottle from her friend. It was 40 Wellbutrin 150 mg. Denies taking any pills today. She will be transferred to Children's Hospital for further management. The patient's initial oxygen saturation on room air was 85%, which increased to 96% on a non-rebreather mask so we'll try again for a nasal cannula and monitor the oxygen level.

MDM (1407) - I did review the patient's lab results showing leukocytosis, elevated blood sugar and positive urine toxicology screen for amphetamines. The patient did receive a second gram of magnesium. Was transferred to Children's Hospital. She is more alert but was still groggy and slightly confused.

Results (1311)

- Urine tox – Negative except for amphetamines
- Labs:

Sodium Level	142 mMol/L
Potassium Level	**3.4 mMol/L LOW**
Chloride Level	105 mMol/L
Carbon Dioxide Level	**11 mMol/L LOW**
Anion Gap	**26.0 mMol/L HI**
Glucose Level	**187 mg/dL HI**
BUN	9 mg/dL
Creatinine	1.11 mg/dL
Acetaminophen level	<10 mcg/mL
Alcohol (Ethanol) Level	<0.01 gm/dL
Salicylate Level	<4.0 mg/dL

DIAGNOSIS: OD, suicide attempt, alt LOC, tachy, hypoxic

Questions and answers with Dr. Sean Nordt:

Q: *Is there any difference in management between these 2 patients?*

A: The management approach is similar with these two patients. These patients both presented from bupropion poisoning with seizures, altered mental status and somnolence. Paramedics gave report of "suicidal intent" although mother reports no previous suicide attempts. Though this case appears "pure tox" clinicians should always keep the differential broad with consideration of other etiologies of seizures such as meningitis, or carbon monoxide poisoning, or trauma. In this case, arrival of the second patient supports a toxicological process.

Q: *Why was she hypoxic on arrival?*

A: This patient may have been hypoxic for many reasons: non convulsive or minimally convulsive seizures, airway obstruction from obtundation, co-ingestion of respiratory depressant agent, pulse oximeter without good waveform, e.g., nail polish in a young female. Consider placing an end tidal CO2 monitor. Many toxins are respiratory depressants that can cause hypercarbia, which may go unnoticed with high flow supplemental oxygenation maintaining a normal oxygen saturation and giving a false sense of security.

Q: *Why was the urine tox screen positive for amphetamines?*

A: Bupropion can cross react with amphetamines as a class on urine toxicology screens.[14] However, amphetamines on a urine toxicology screen is the least helpful of all classes of drugs as many medications cross react and have a positive result for amphetamines including pseudoephedrine, amantadine, promethazine, trazodone, and labetalol. In addition, urine toxicology screens for amphetamine can be positive for approximately 48 hours since last use and do not equate with ongoing toxicity. Clinically significant sympathomimetic poisoning generally will be obvious on physical examination with the expected toxidrome.

Q: *Final thoughts?*

A: The toxicological approach to poisonings is often described as "supportive care alone." However, the better term is "early goal-directed supportive care." Toxicology, with some exceptions, is generally an exaggeration of normal pharmacologic actions. Therefore, a good basic knowledge of the pharmacologic actions can assist the clinician to anticipate the clinical course of the acutely poisoned patient. Early toxicology consultation can assist in rapidly narrowing the toxicological differential, judicious use of laboratory testing and gastrointestinal decontamination techniques, expedite disposition and expand the differential to non-toxicological etiologies which can mimic poisonings.

IV. CHILD SUICIDE RISK ASSESSMENT IN THE ED

Mike Unger, MD

Psychiatrist

A.C.T. Team Psychiatrist for the Cobb & Douglas County Svcs. Board, Atlanta, GA.

Q: How do you assess pediatric suicide risk in the ED?

None of us can predict the future behavior of children, but asking the right questions in a nonjudgmental manner and coordinating care with a multispecialty approach can keep children safe and avoid unnecessary interventions.

The child is usually the best source of information, and this data is best obtained when the child is interviewed separate from the parents or legal guardian. Correlating the seriousness of the injury with their history can help to determine if they are telling an accurate story.

- When obtaining the HPI, screening questions like "'Do you feel like crying a lot?" or ''Do you ever feel sad enough that it makes you want to go away and not come back?" may help the child disclose important thoughts and feelings.[15]
- Be cautious about beginning the interview with questions about "suicide," which can be a leading question if the child is somewhat suggestible.[15]
- Interview the parents/guardian separately.
- Parents may underestimate the level of suicidality in their child. In one study, 75% of parents of were unaware of suicidal ideation in their 8-year-olds.[15]

Anyone under the age of 18 presenting with suicidal ideation or attempt should be placed on 1:1 observation in the emergency department. The child's belongings and clothing should be searched for any potential suicide instruments such as pills, sharp objects, or firearms.

Try to ascertain if the child truly has thoughts of "wanting to be dead." What does "being dead" mean to them? Younger children think more concretely, whereas older children may be able to employ abstract thinking, consider existential issues, or think about the effects their actions will have on others.[15]

Q: What are high risk factors for suicide?

Although no tool is validated, "SADPERSONS" is a mnemonic that includes several risk factors for suicide:[17]

- Sex (male higher risk)
- Age (15 and older are at greater risk)
- Depression(or any existing psychiatric dx)
- Previous suicide attempt
- Ethanol or drug abuse
- Rational thinking loss (psychosis)
- Social supports lacking (living environment)
- Organized plan for suicide
- Negligent parenting or family history of suicide
- School problems(victim of bullying, history of violence or aggressive behaviors)

There is a scoring system that attempts to equate with low, moderate or high risk.[18]

Q. Does self-mutilation (cutting) equate with a suicide attempt?

I have treated many people that self-mutilate by cutting superficially or burning themselves in non-lethal areas of the body (surface of thighs, forearms). This can be common in children and young adults that have experienced trauma, abuse, and/or neglect. The child may be walled off from their own emotions—feeling emotionally mute. The act of cutting is often described as being a helpful way to "feel again," "end the numbness" or "release pent up stress or emotion," and the person denies having suicidal thoughts. I almost never admit patients for this, as long as I have excluded the intention of "cutting in order to bleed out and die."

Q. Does an overdose always require an admission?

Sometimes an overdose is accidental and there are no medical complications. For example, a child who took a parent's Ativan to help fall asleep and was unaware it could lead to serious sedation or a child who took too much of a medicine to "get high." In the case of an accidental overdose, there will be an absence of recent stressors, clinical depression and intent of harm. If the behavior looks suspicious, err on the side of safety.
Factors against admission include:

- No clear plan
- Hope for the future and things to look forward to
- Supportive, responsible care-giver that is willing to monitor them and take them to outpatient f/u appointments

Q. How do you manage a suicidal child when the parents refuse admission?

Laws regarding the involuntary commitment of minors vary from state to state. In general, try to work with the parents or legal guardian and explain that hospitalization is the best, safest choice for their child. This is usually effective, but if not, consult with the hospital attorney, a child psychiatrist on call, or a patient advocate/ethics personnel regarding options. In some instances, a child may have to be placed in a more restrictive setting than medically indicated if the caregiver cannot or will not supervise the child, follow up with recommendations, or is threatening toward the child.

References

1. Erickson TB, Thompson TM, Lu JJ. The approach to the patient with an unknown overdose. Emerg Med Clin North Am. 2007;25:249–281.
2. Antshel KM, Hargrave TM, Simonescu M, et al. Advances in understanding and treating ADHD. BMC Med. 2011;9:72.
3. Glassman AH, Bigger JT. Antipsychotic drugs: prolonged QTc interval, torsade de pointes, and sudden death. Am J Psych. 2001;158:1774–82.
4. McGuigan MA. Guideline for the out-of-hospital management of human exposures to minimally toxic substances. J Toxicol Clin Toxicol.1992;21:907–17.
5. Ash-Bernal R, Wise R, Wright SM. Acquired methemoglobinemia: a retrospective series of 138 cases at 2 teaching hospitals. Medicine. 2004;83:265–73.
6. Dahshan A, Donovan GK. Severe methemoglobinemia complicating topical benzocaine use during endoscopy in a toddler: a case report and review of the literature. Pediatrics. 2006;117:e806–9.
7. Clark RF, Vance MW. Massive diphenhydramine poisoning resulting in a wide-complex tachycardia: successful treatment with sodium bicarbonate. Ann Emerg Med. 1992;21:318–21.
8. Nichols MH, King WD, James LP. Clonidine poisoning in Jefferson County, Alabama. Ann Emerg Med. 1997;29:511–7.
9. Ngo A, Ciranni M, Olson KR. Acute quetiapine overdose in adults: a 5-year retrospective case series. Ann Emerg Med. 2008;52:541–7.
10. Holubek WJ. Nonsteroidal anti-inflammatory drugs. In: Nelson LS, et al, eds. Goldfrank's toxicologic emergencies. 9th ed. 528–36. McGraw Hill: New York NY.
11. Balt CR, Lynch CN, Isbister GK. Bupropion poisoning: a case series. Med J Aust. 2003;20:61–3.
12. Sirianni AJ, Osterhoudt KC, Calello DP, et al. Use of lipid emulsion in the resuscitation of a patient with prolonged cardiovascular collapse after overdose of bupropion and lamotrigine. Ann Emerg Med. 2008;51:412–5.
13. Yap YG, Camm AJ. Drug induced QT prolongation and Torsade de pointes. Heart 2003;89:1363–72.
14. Phan HM, Yoshizuka K, Murray DJ, et al. Drug testing in the workplace. Pharmacotherapy 2012;32:649–56.
15. Tishler CL, Staats Reiss N, Rhodes, AR. Suicidal behavior in children younger than twelve: a diagnostic challenge for emergency department personnel. Acad Emerg Med. 2007;14(9):810–8. doi: 10.1197/j.aem.2007.05.014.
16. Goldstein AB, Findling RL. Assessment and evaluation of child and adolescent psychiatric emergencies. Psychiatric times. August 01, 2006. http://www.psychiatrictimes.com/articles/assessment-and-evaluation-child-and-adolescent-psychiatric-emergencies. See more at: http://www.psychiatrictimes.com/articles/assessment-and-evaluation-child-and-adolescent-psychiatric-emergencies#comment-form.

17. Faille L, Clair M, Penn JV. Special risk management issues in child and adolescent psychiatry. Psychiatric times. July 1, 2007. http://www.psychiatrictimes.com/articles/special-risk-management-issues-child-and-adolescent-psychiatry
18. SADPERSONS mnemonic comes from:
    Patterson W, Dohn H, Bird J, Patterson G. Evaluation of suicidal patients: The SAD PERSONS Scale. Psychosomatics. 1983;24:343–9.
    Juhnke GE. SAD PERSONS scale review. Measurement & Evaluation in Counseling & Development. 1994; 27:325–8.
    Juhnke GE. The adapted SAD PERSONS: an assessment scale designed for use with children. Elementary School Guidance & Counseling, 1996;119:252–8.

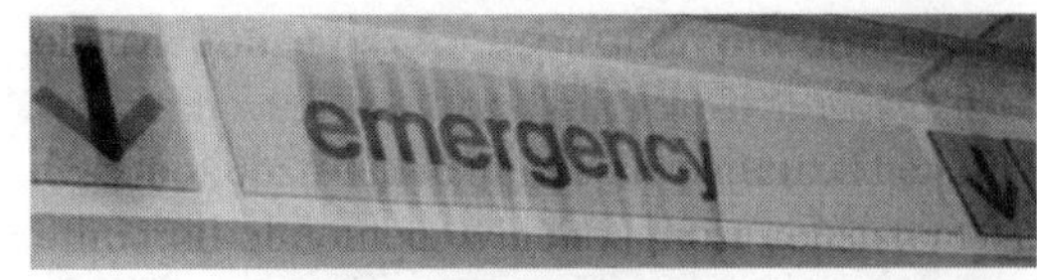

CASE 16

25-DAY-OLD NEONATE WITH FEVER

Bennie D. Rush II, MD PGY-2
EM resident
Department of Emergency Medicine
University of Texas Health Science Center at San Antonio

Gillian Schmitz, MD, FACEP
Associate Program Director
Department of Emergency Medicine
University of Texas Health Science Center at San Antonio

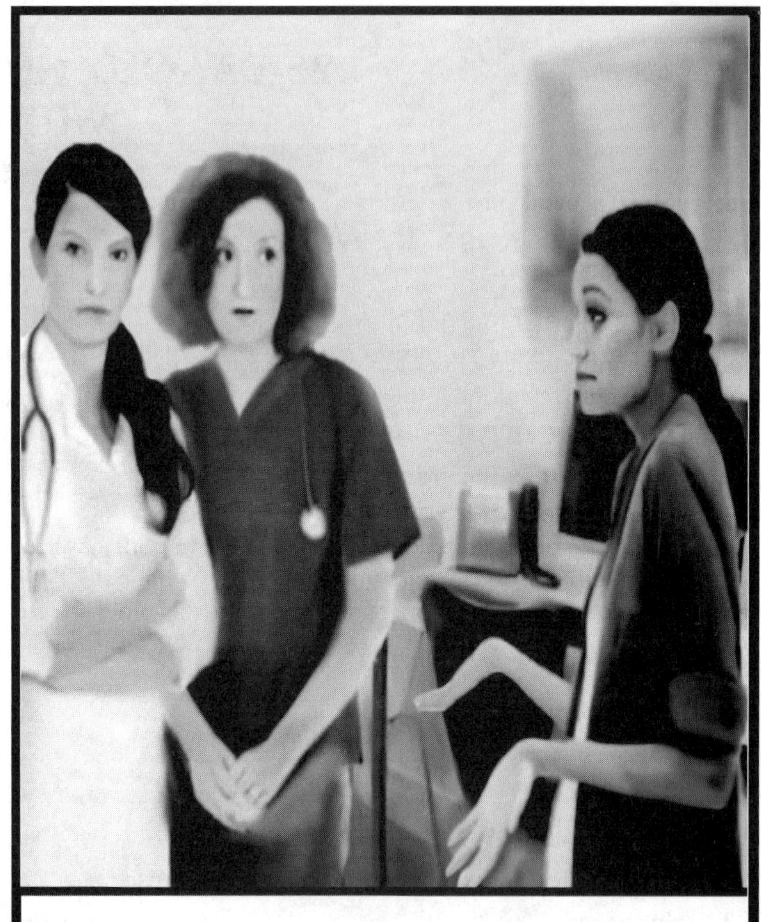

"You really don't need to tap this kid!"

CASE 16

25-DAY-OLD NEONATE WITH FEVER

PART 1—MEDICAL

I. The Doctor's Version (the following is the actual documentation of the provider)

Date: December 28, 2014 at 11:48

Chief complaint: Fever. Patient's statement of chief complaint, neonatal fever 100.4 rectal at home.

Nurse note: Source is per care provider: Fever 100.3 rectal at home.

HPI: (History obtained from mother and father by ED resident) 25 day old neonate, vaginal delivery without complications or prolonged hospital stay after delivery, per mother she was Group B Strep positive, but the infant tested negative after delivery. No medical problems since birth, the baby has been feeding well with no vomiting and no change in stool, regular frequency of feeds/stools/wet diaper changes with no blood noted in the stool or urine/diaper, no increased fussiness, good muscle tone, non-toxic appearing. He has a sibling who had some runny nose and congestion and then after that the baby developed some nasal congestion and the mother thought he was hot last night and took a rectal temperature that was 100.4 per mom (history given at triage noted temperature reported as 100.3), but he received no Motrin or Tylenol and he is afebrile now, he has a rash on his back.

REVIEW OF SYSTEMS: Except marked as positive all other systems reviewed and found negative.

GENERAL: (+) Fever, weight gain, (-)no chills, no sweating, no persistent crying, no decreased activity, no poor feeding, no weight loss
SKIN: (+) erythema, patchy erythema
EARS: (-) no earache, no pulling at ears, no ear discharge, no hearing loss
NOSE: (+) Nasal discharge, nasal congestion (-) no nasal obstruction, no sneezing
RESPIRATORY: (-) no productive cough, no wheezing, no dyspnea, no tachypnea

PAST MEDICAL HISTORY:
Allergies: NKDA
Medications: No current mediations
PMH: Mother with birth history significant for GBS positive during pregnancy s/p abx, negative cultures at birth. Full term vaginal delivery.
Social History: Pt lives at home with mother and brother

EXAM: Reference Range for normal vitals in infants < 3 months old[1]

VITAL SIGNS							
Time	Temp	Src	Pulse	Resp	Syst	Diast	Sat
11:58	99.3	rectal	170	53	105	39	100%
			(100-150)	(30-35)	(65-85)	(35-55)	

PE:

General appearance: active, playful, smiles, alert, good eye contact, consolable
Head: Normocephalic, anterior fontanel normal, symmetrical
Neck: supple, range of motion painless, trachea midline
Skin appearance: Macular rash trunk, lower extremity left and right, lower back
Eyes: lids normal, no discharge, pupils equal, round and reacting to light
Ears: external normal, tympanic membranes not visualized
Nose: nasal cavity normal, mucous membrane normal, no discharge
Respiratory system: breath sounds normal, no respiratory distress, no added respiratory sounds
Cardiovascular system: heart rate normal, heart sounds normal, rhythm regular
Gastrointestinal system: soft, abdomen normal, nontender, no distention
Genitourinary system: external genitalia normal, uncircumcised male

RESULTS:

UA- negative for nitrites or leukocytes,
4 WBC (0-5)
1+ blood (0 blood)
epithelial cell 7, bacteria 8 (0 epithelial cells, 0 bacteria)
CXR: normal
BABYGRAM: IMPRESSION: Single AP view of the chest and abdomen, within normal limits.
CBC: WBC 17.7, Hb 13.0, plt 321
Blood cultures: Pending

REPEAT VITAL SIGNS					
Time	Pulse	Resp	Syst	Diast	Sat
14:19	155	60			100%

MEDICAL DECISION MAKING (ED Faculty Note)

DDx - viral URI vs bacterial infection (very low suspicion)
Condition - stable, well appearing, nontoxic

TREATMENT PLAN - Would not do LP at this time given the patient is afebrile and well appearing with hx of sick sibling and eating well, ? of temperature actually above cutoff for fever (100.3 vs 100.4), will consult pediatrics for evaluation, consider ceftriaxone 50-100mg/kg

PEDIATRIC RESIDENT CONSULT NOTE: 25 day old infant presenting with reported fever and congestion, likely consistent with viral URI. No concerning findings on labs, cultures pending. No need to perform LP and do not recommend Rocephin. Rash on exam consistent with erythema toxicum, a common newborn rash. Mother given strict precautions including return with fever to 100.4 or greater, change in activity, decrease in PO intake, lethargy.

ED ATTENDING PROGRESS NOTE: Peds recommendation appreciated. Will cover with 1 dose of Rocephin 100 mg/kg and follow up with pediatrician in 24 hours.

DIAGNOSIS: Fever

DISPOSITION: Discharge after 1 dose of Rocephin 100 mg/kg to be given in ED. Follow up with pediatrician in 24 hours. If you experience recurrent fever, nausea, vomiting, or any other concerning sign or symptoms please return to the ED.

II. Greg Henry Comments

"Nothing undermines the confidence in the healthcare system like open disagreement."

The well appearing infant with a minimal fever has been a quandary since the beginning of time ... which is about when I started practice! In the past, 90 days was the cut off; 3-month-old children who were looking perfectly normal were tortured with IV lines, antibiotics, endless blood studies, and lumbar punctures. Over the years this number has dropped precipitously.

The question as to where the standard of care lies in such children is unclear. Even in those less than 28 days, since the wide spread use of immunizations, bacterial meningitis is vanishingly rare. Still, due to the severe sequelae of the disease, the 28-day cut-off is not a bad one. The nice thing about small babies is that they are easy to tap ... and I've never had one object!

The patient's discharge instructions in this particular case may have been somewhat difficult. Does the patient return with a temperate of 100.4 degrees? Seems curious as they came in with a temperature of 100.3 degrees. In truth, you don't care what the temperature is; some of the sickest children are actually hypothermic. The decision is how the child looks. Short term interval follow up is the key; my suggestion is that 8 hours is preferable to 24 hours, but there is no one set practice which constitutes the standard of care.

The interaction between a pediatric consultant and the attending emergency physician can be tense. The pediatric resident does not have the clinical experience of the ED attending when it comes to diagnosing undifferentiated patients. The conversation should be between the emergency attending and the pediatric attending. This family was made to feel very apprehensive when two doctors say that the patient does not need a lumbar puncture and one does—have these discussions somewhere else. Come to an agreement, and then present it to the family. Nothing undermines the confidence in the healthcare system like open disagreement. Nothing heightens this anxiety as much as when it is being done to one of your children.

III. The Bounceback

- After peds left, initial ED attending asked new attending at checkout (1500) to give a dose of Rocephin "just in case." There was some concern and discussion about discharging a 25 day old with a fever and about giving antibiotics without having a lumbar puncture.
- Per the 2nd ED attending: "I was not comfortable with that and had to go back, re-evaluate, check him back in and explain to mom that we needed to do LP. She was *pissed* because 2 doctors, both ED and peds, had told her baby did *not* need an LP. After 30 minutes of discussion, she agreed and consented to LP."
- Family was checked back in and reassessed. Family was notified of the risks and benefits of lumbar puncture with CSF analysis and had the procedure performed (results below).

Results: Time: 1713

CSF Analysis

Tube number	1	4
CSF color	Red	Red
CSF Appearance	Bloody	Bloody
CSF RBC count	Clotted (0-0)	41000
CSF Total Cell Count	Clotted (0-30)	84
CSF Segmented Granulocytes	77 (0-8%)	55
CSF Lymphocytes	12 (5-35%)	34
CSF Monocytes	2 (50-90)	9
CSF Eosinophils	9 (%)	2

Glucose CSF 41 (40-75)
Protein CSF 110 (15-45)
Gram Stain Report: Many Leukocytes, Many Erythrocytes (RBC), No bacteria seen
CRP 11.10 (0-10.0)

- Pediatrics was re-consulted for admission, antibiotics (ceftriaxone) and observation.

Final Disposition

- Patient was admitted to the hospital and remained afebrile. Acyclovir was ordered in ED but held by pediatrics.
- **Results:**
  - o Virology Report: Positive Rhinovirus/Enterovirus Group Detected by PCR.
  - o Micro: No growth at 72 hours
  - o Blood Cultures: no growth at 48 hours
  - o Urine Cultures: no growth at 48 hours
- Pt was discharged the next day with scheduled follow up in clinic.
- **Follow up:** The remainder of clinic notes indicate the child has been doing well, has remained non-toxic and has reached all appropriate milestones.

PART 2—THE ANALYSIS

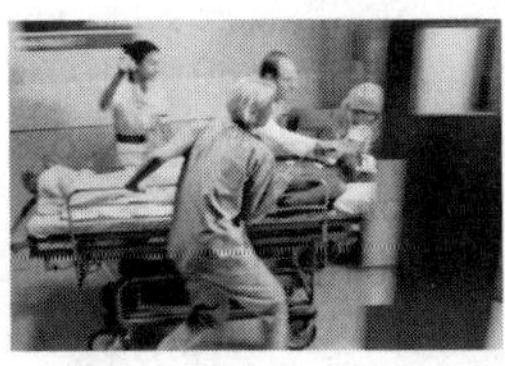

EVALUATION OF FEVER IN NEONATES

Bennie D. Rush II, MD PGY-2
EM resident
Department of Emergency Medicine
University of Texas Health Science Center at San Antonio

Gillian Schmitz, MD, FACEP
Associate Program Director
Department of Emergency Medicine
University of Texas Health Science Center at San Antonio

What is the required evaluation in a febrile infant < 28 days of age?

Most guidelines suggest that febrile neonates younger than 28 days should have blood cultures, urine analysis and cultures, CBC, and CSF analysis and cultures. Neonates should be empirically treated with antibiotics. In addition, those patients with tachypnea, crackles, retractions, nasal flaring, cyanosis, or oxygen saturation < 95%, should have a CXR and viral cultures. Stool cultures may be reserved for those infants with diarrhea.[2-5]

Neonates with fever can "look good" and still have underlying serious bacterial illness (SBI). The correlation between patient appearance and underlying SBI is very poor correlation; physicians are generally unable to tell by physical exam alone which babies have a serious source of underlying fever.[3, 4]

What is a fever in an infant?

Fever is defined as $\geq$ 38.0°C (100.4 F) for infants 0–3 months.[2-4]

In this case, it was unclear whether the mother actually measured a fever of 100.3° F, or 100.4° F, as both are documented slightly differently from RN notes and MD note. Given the serious risk of missing a SBI, however, it would be reasonable to assume the higher temperature and practice conservatively.

What if the infant is bundled in warm blankets?

A temperature over 38°C for infants 0–90 days should be considered a fever, regardless of their clothing.[4] Bundling of infants creates confusion because it may raise the skin temperature but not rectal temperature.[6]

Is mom's report of a fever accurate?

Caretakers who are reliable and report a subjective or objective fever must be taken seriously and should be treated as if it were measured in the department.[5,7] Six of 63 patients with bacteremia or bacterial meningitis in a large office-based study of young febrile infants were found to be afebrile in physicians' offices but were febrile at home.[8]

What if there is an "obvious source" (i.e., viral illness) in a baby < 28 days old? Are viral infections such as Respiratory Syncytial Virus (RSV) bronchiolitis considered sources?

In neonates < 28 days, the presence of signs suggestive of viral illness does not negate the need for a full diagnostic evaluation.[3,5,10] Unlike older children, in whom documented respiratory syncytial virus (RSV) infections decrease the likelihood of serious bacterial illness, RSV-infected neonates have the same rate of SBI compared with RSV-negative neonates.[10]

One study in infants 3–36 months old demonstrated that patients with recognizable viral syndromes (croup, varicella, stomatitis) had lower rates of serious bacterial infections than those without obvious sources.[9] Other studies have demonstrated a reduced rate of bacteremia in febrile children over 2 months with symptoms of bronchiolitis, but recognizable symptoms did not absolutely exclude bacteremia or a urinary tract infection.[4]

What do you do with a traumatic tap?

Some guidelines suggest ways to estimate the predicted CSF white blood cell count (WBC) in a traumatic tap. One method is to divide the number of red blood cells (RBCs) in the CSF by 500 and subtract that number from the reported WBCs in the CSF.[11] Other references suggest that a WBC: RBC of ≤1:100 in a traumatic tap can identify a large group of patients without meningitis.[12] Yet other studies demonstrated that adjustment of CSF white blood cell count to account for increased red blood cells in a traumatic tap did not aid in the diagnosis of bacterial and fungal meningitis. The bottom line is that the adjustment of WBC counts decreases the sensitivity of detecting meningitis in the setting of a traumatic tap with only a marginal gain in specificity and does not improve diagnostic utility.[13]

Can I give antibiotics without doing the lumbar puncture?

Lumbar puncture should be performed in all febrile children < 28 days and strongly considered in all children < 90 days who receive antibiotics.

The physician has a certain window to perform the LP after antibiotics have been given to have accurate results with as little as 15 minutes to sterilization of CSF in some cases.[14] Administration of antibiotics should not be delayed for the lumbar puncture, especially in an ill appearing child.[15]

In our case, there was some discussion of not performing the lumbar puncture, but covering the neonate with antibiotics "just in case." This practice is highly discouraged as it clouds the clinical picture when the patient returns with a fever on day 2 or 3, making It impossible to tell if the child has partially treated meningitis. Clinical practice guidelines recommend performing a lumbar puncture in febrile infants < 28 days and administration of antibiotics.

CSF culture will not result for 24–48 hours. Admission is recommended for babies < 28 days with a fever for observation.[2-4]

What antibiotics should I use in a febrile infant < 28 days of age?

Patients are typically treated with a third-generation cephalosporin or gentamicin PLUS ampicillin.

- Cefotaxime, 50 mg/kg intravenously (IV) (100 mg/kg if there is a concern for meningitis based on CSF results)—or—Gentamicin, 2.5 mg/kg IV **PLUS**
- Ampicillin, 50 mg/kg IV (100 mg/kg IV if there is a concern for meningitis) is recommended for the empiric treatment of these patients to cover *Listeria monocytogenes*.
- Additional antiviral or antibiotic coverage with acyclovir or vancomycin can be considered respectively in patients considered at risk for neonatal herpes or *S. aureus* infection such as patients with a scalp abscess.
- Note: Ceftriaxone is not recommended for neonates who have jaundice because of the concern for inducing unconjugated hyperbilirubinemia.[2,3,4,5]

What about fevers in children > 28 days and < 90 days of age?

There is more controversy in well appearing infants in this age group.

The Boston, Rochester, and Philadelphia Criteria have all attempted to create screening criteria that were sensitive, specific, and had high negative predictive values (NPV). Though they vary in protocol and recommendations, they all focused on stratifying febrile infants into high and low risk categories. Low risk infants could be justifiably sent home with close follow up. In order to utilize these criteria, patients must meet *all* of the criteria to be considered low risk and close follow up must be assured.

So, what to do with those pesky febrile 28–90 day olds?

One conservative approach would be to perform blood, urine and CSF studies in infants between 28 days and 60 days (who are low risk by Rochester criteria), cover with ceftriaxone, and discharge them with 24 hour follow up. For well appearing low risk infants between 60 days and 90 days, it is reasonable to perform blood and urine studies only. If the child is already being treated with antibiotics, a lumbar puncture is generally recommended. Close follow up and return precautions are required in all cases discharged from the emergency department.[3]

✔ Teaching Points

- Trust the parent when they report a fever at home.
- A well-appearing neonate with an "obvious viral source" does not exclude meningitis.
- Missed meningitis in a neonate is a HUGE risk and opens up the potential for adverse outcomes including seizures, death and severe disability. It is uncommon but can't be missed.
- There is a lot of controversy in fever management between 28 and 90 days, but the <28 days should be a no brainer. Work up (even if fever is reported only) includes:
  - o CBC w/diff
  - o Blood cultures
  - o Urinalysis and urine culture
  - o CSF studies and culture including viral cultures (herpes, enterovirus, etc.)

- Chest x-ray if appropriate
- Start antibiotics and admit to the hospital until cultures are negative

References

1. Dieckmann R, Brownstein D, Gausche-Hill M, eds. Pediatric Education for Prehospital Professionals. Sudbury, MA: Jones & Bartlett, Am Acad Pediatr. 2000, 43–5.
2. Wang VJ. Fever and serious bacterial illness: Sec. 12, Ch. 113 at 752. In Tintinalli's Emergency medicine: a comprehensive study guide. 7th ed. 2010. New York: McGraw-Hill.
3. Baraff L. Management of fever without source in infants and children. Ann Emerg Med. 2000; 36(6):602–14.
4. Steere M, Sharieff GQ, Stenklyft PH. Fever in children less than 36 months of age: questions and strategies for management in the emergency department. J Emerg Med. 2003; 25(2):149–57.
5. Ishimine P. Fever without source in children 0 to 36 months of age. Pediatr Clin N Am. 2006;53(2):167–94.
6. Grover G, Berkowitz CD, Lewis RJ, et al. The effects of bundling on infant temperature. Pediatrics. 1994;94:669–73.
7. Claudius I, Baraff LJ. Pediatric emergencies associated with fever. Emerg Med Clin N Am. 2010;28(1):67–84.
8. Pantell RH, Newman TB, Bernzweig J, et al. Management and outcomes of care of fever in early infancy. JAMA. 2004;291:1203–12.
9. Greenes DS, Harper MB. Low risk of bacteremia in febrile children with recognizable viral syndromes. Pediatr Infect Dis J. 1999;18(3):258–61.
10. Levine DA, Platt SL, Dayan PS, et al. Risk of serious bacterial infection in young febrile infants with respiratory syncytial virus infections. Pediatrics. 2004;113(6):1728–34.
11. Bonsu BK, Harper MB. Corrections for leukocytosis and percent of neutrophils do not match observations in blood contaminated cerebrospinal fluid and have no value over uncorrected cells for diagnosis. Pediatr Infect Dis J. 2006;25(1): 8–11.
12. Mazor SS, McNulty JE, Roosevelt GE. Interpretation of traumatic lumbar punctures: who can go home? Pediatrics. 2003;111(3):525–8.
13. Greenburg R, Smith B, Cotton M, et al. Traumatic lumbar puncture in neonates: test performance of the cerebrospinal fluid white blood cell count. Pediatr Infect Dis. 2008;27(12):1047–51.
14. Kanegaye J, Soliemanzadeh P, Bradley J. Lumbar puncture in pediatric bacterial meningitis: defining the time interval for recovery of cerebrospinal fluid pathogens after parenteral antibiotic pretreatment. Pediatrics. 2001;108(5):1169–74.
15. Talan DA, Hoffman JR, Yoshikawa TT, et al. Role of empiric parenteral antibiotics prior to lumbar puncture in suspected bacterial meningitis: state of the art. Rev Infect Dis. 1988;10:365–76.

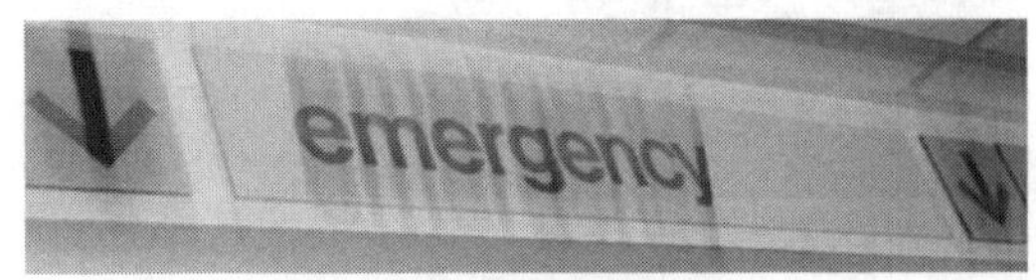

CASE 17

1-YEAR-OLD BOY WITH VOMITING AND DIARRHEA

—The double bounce—

Andrew Sloas, DO, RDMS, FAAEM
Assistant Professor of Adult and Pediatric Emergency Medicine
Department of Emergency Medicine
University of Kentucky
Editor-in-Chief PEM ED Podcast

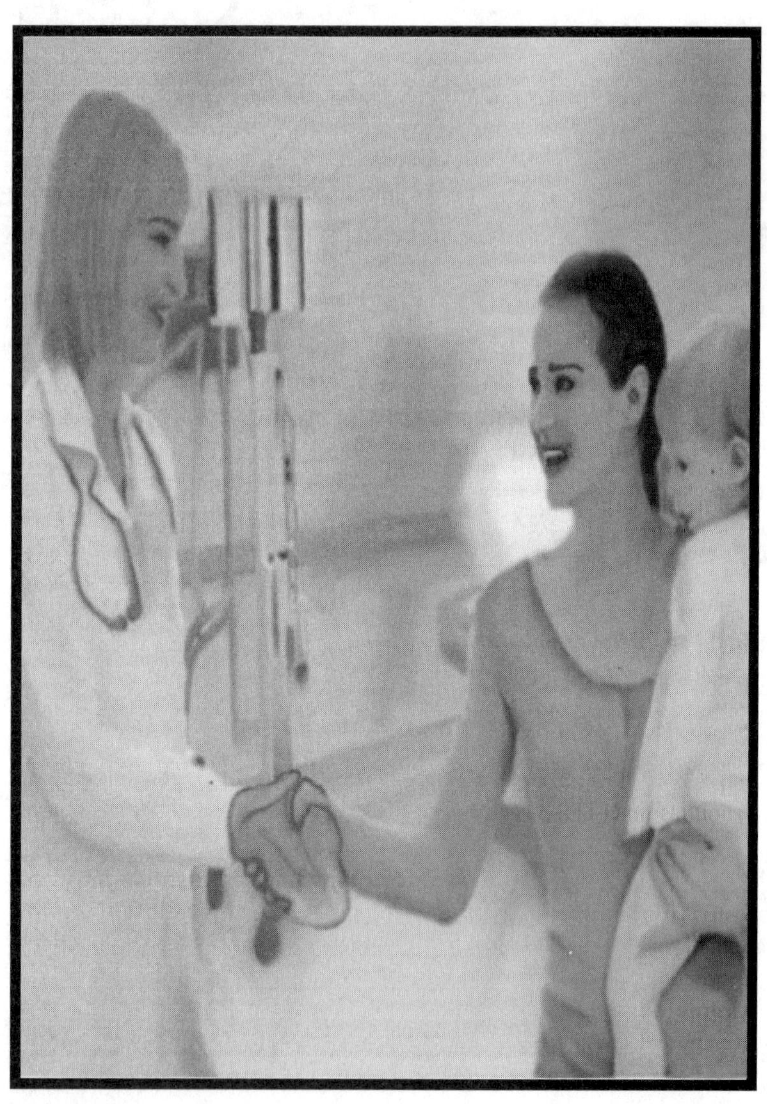

CASE 17

1-YEAR-OLD BOY WITH VOMITING AND DIARRHEA

—The double bounce—

PART 1—MEDICAL

I. The Patient's Story

John is a 1½ -year-old boy who lives in Austin, Texas. He has two working parents and a 4-year-old brother.

John is healthy, only visiting his pediatrician to receive immunizations. Six months ago, he was evaluated for Asperger Syndrome versus high functioning autism, but the specialists did not feel that he had either of these.

Just a few days after Christmas, John wakes up with cough and congestion. Right after breakfast he vomits. So, his mother decides to stay home from work.

The coughing and congestion remain mild over the next 3 days, but he continues vomiting, up to 4 times a day. His mother has been through these symptoms before with John's older brother, so she's not worried, but 2 days later, John develops copious diarrhea, and she becomes concerned about dehydration. When she notices specks of blood in the diarrhea, she decides to take John to an emergency room.

When she presents to the ER, John's mother states: "There's something not right with my child; he won't drink. I've seen him sick before, but never this sick. He usually drinks when he's sick. He loves popsicles and juice, but he won't take either."

II. The Doctor's Version (the following is the actual documentation of the provider)

Date: January 2nd, 2008 at 1100hrs
Chief complaint: Blood in stool
Nurse note: Child well appearing. Happy with mom and wants to be held. Rash on face and under Rt arm. Abdomen soft. Smiles at me once. Zofran administered. Awaiting MD review.

HISTORY OF PRESENT ILLNESS – (Per MD) : Mom reports 3 days of diarrhea and vomiting preceded by cough/congestion. Last diaper had specs of blood. In daycare with sick contacts.

REVIEW OF SYSTEMS: Unless otherwise stated in this report 10 reviewed and negative.
PAST MEDICAL HISTORY: (left blank)

ALLERGIES: NKDA
MEDICATIONS: None
PMH: None
SOCIAL HISTORY: Lives with mom and dad

VITAL SIGNS

Time	Temp(F)	Rt	Pulse	Resp	Syst	Diast
11:00	100.4	TM	188	32		

EXAM:

Constitutional: Alert and well developed
Mental status/Psychiatric: Age-appropriately responsive to mother
Head: NCAT, soft fontanelle
Eyes: PERRL, EOMI: No discharge or conjunctival injection.
Ears: TMs clear. .
Nose: Mild yellow rhinorrhea.
Throat: No lesions or erythema
Neck: FROM, No LNA.
Lungs: Clear to auscultation and breath sounds equal.
Heart: No murmur.
ABD: Soft, Non-tender to palpation, no guarding.
Neurological: Grossly non-focal.

ED COURSE:
11:15 – Zofran 2mg ODT. Tolerating po.

DIAGNOSIS: Vomiting, Gastroenteritis.

DISPOSITION (12:00): Patient was discharged home by the ED physician. Instructions: follow up with your pediatrician in 2-3 days "if continued vomiting." Condition upon discharge ____ [undocumented]. Rx for Zofran ODT. Return to ER if symptoms change.

III. The Errors—Risk Management/Patient Safety Issues

Risk management/patient safety issue #1:

Error: Incomplete evaluation.

Discussion: Gastroenteritis as a discharge diagnosis?? Why don't you just shave your nethers before taking a long relaxing cold salt water bath? Gastroenteritis is a diagnosis that should never appear on an ED chart, but could be mentioned in the differential diagnoses. Why would you give up the wiggle room your government billing agencies have allowed you to make by documenting a completely acceptable, non-specific, and yet, still accurate diagnosis of vomiting and diarrhea?

This is a plaintiff's attorney's equivalent to a pre-pubertal dream; they will gladly plant the seed of doubt in your jury's mind that whatever was missing would have not only been abnormal, it would have been the linchpin in helping you make the correct diagnosis:

- There was no rectal/diaper exam for blood, fissure, prolapse, no heme occult. Seriously? This was an academic institution.
- There is not an adequate history characterizing the patient's abdominal pain. No questions about intermittent irritability or crying or bringing legs up in a rhythmic motion (intussusception). The history does not discuss quality or frequency of blood.
- The discharge diagnosis does not mention rectal bleeding at all.

✔ **Teaching point:** The chart needs to tell a story of the patient's symptoms and a description of the findings.

Risk management/patient safety issue #2:

Error: Nurse's notes not explained—skin rash not explored in history or exam.

Discussion: In this case, one would assume the nurse's notes either weren't read by the emergency physician or he disagreed, but forgot to document why. The former is more likely than the latter given the outcome. Documentation of rash is not explored in the physician's history or exam. Was this rash tinea, urticaria, contact dermatitis or petechial? The answer could have led to the diagnosis.

✔ **Teaching point:** Read the nurses notes and check the vital signs before seeing a patient.

Risk management/patient safety issue #3:

Error: No exploration of trachycardia or fever. No documented blood pressure.

Discussion: Yeah, we've discussed this before. Unexplained tachycardia is a red flag for serious adverse outcome. What to do:

1. Recheck to see if worsening or improving
2. Give a fluid bolus or antipyretic and recheck
3. Document in a progress note why it's reasonable and safe to send the patient home with a grossly abnormal vital sign

✔ **Teaching point:** Unexplained abnormalities in vital signs need further exploration and explanation.

Risk management/patient safety issue #4:

Error: Insufficient progress note: "zofran was given and patient tolerated po."

Discussion: There was no documentation of repeated examination to demonstrate that John's clinical status was improving. Furthermore, he only stayed in the department for one hour. So, it would be hard to believe that the provider allowed a sufficient interval between treatment and re-exam for John to have improved. Not that it couldn't have happened that way, but if it did, this would have been a great time to chart the words: "rapidly improving."

Now it may seem like I'm being hard on this provider, but it's not close to what a plaintiff's attorney would do. In this day and age of customer satisfaction scores, I know that we all go back and repeat our exams, before wishing the patients a Merry Christmas and Happy New Year. However, we don't always document it. Plaintiff's attorneys love to paint the provider as sloppy and dismissive.

The progress note and Medical decision making (MDM) section is a way that you can record your thought process. At the completion of your documentation, a third party (usually a subsequent provider) should be able to understand what happened during the encounter.

✔ **Teaching point:** Documenting the repeat exam is crucial if there is an adverse outcome. When you are documenting your MDM, if you can't convince yourself of the diagnosis, reassess the patient.

Risk management/patient safety issue #5:

Error: Inadequate discharge instructions.

Discussion: Detailed discharge instructions are important to let patients know how they must participate in their own care, what you're thinking could be happening at this moment and what could potentially happen in the future. There was no specific instruction about why to return except for continued vomiting, no specific follow up date or provider.

✔ **Teaching point:** Besides MDM charting, discharge instructions are the most important piece of the ED encounter.

Risk management/patient safety issue #6:

Error: Inadequate differential diagnosis.

Discussion: It should be easy to follow the MDM thought process by reading the ED chart.

This provider may have latched onto a typical thought process: nausea, vomiting and abdominal pain begets diarrhea. Gastroenteritis is so much more prevalent than surgical abdomens, and if you play the odds, diarrhea will follow most of the time.

Unfortunately, every now and then, one of your patients is going to roll snake eyes and out pops a nausea, vomiting and abdominal pain that has a surgical abdomen. Maybe this ED provider considered surgical, medical and infectious etiologies, but the charting leads one to suppose this was thought to be just another case of viral gastroenteritis.

✔ **Teaching point:** Playing the odds *usually* works ....

IV. Greg Henry Comments

"Ill-appearing children with bloody diarrhea have a serious process occurring until proven otherwise"

Standard diarrhea, a small amount of blood from a fissure near the anus, and true bloody diarrhea, have nothing to do with each other. Standard non-hemolytic diarrhea is the usual problem for scores of our patients. Small anal fissure bleeding is common and nothing but reassurance is required. Actual bloody diarrhea is not common. Ill appearing children with bloody diarrhea have a serious process occurring until proven otherwise.

V. The Bounceback—Part 1: PCP

FOLLOW UP WITH THE PCP:

January 3, 2008—(the next day after initial ED visit) John sees his pediatrician. His mother says, "I'm telling you people there's just something not right with him. He's had three more episodes of poop with what looks to be large clots of blood. It was just specs and now it is clots. When are we going to do something about this?" Mom further reports some colicky abdominal pain and says her child was curled up in a ball just prior to presentation. Mom is also concerned that he only drank 1 ounce of juice and then vomited overnight and had no further wet diapers.

Pediatrician note:

- Vitals: HR-150, T-100.2, Sat-98%, RR-35
- **MDM:** John is mildly dehydrated, but he feels much better after Phenergan suppository and has now been drinking from his cup.
- **PE:** Abdomen is soft and non-tender. Petechiae scant on face, I believe to be secondary to vomiting
- Diarrhea noted in diaper without obvious blood.
- **Discharge instructions**: Mom instructed to call back that afternoon if John is not continuing to tolerate po with the help of Phenergan and to go to the ER if she noted any more blood in the stool or worsening abdominal pain. Rx: Phenergan suppository.

January 4, 2008— (early the next morning) John continues to have bloody diarrhea, prompting another return to the ER. His mother is now frantic. "No one is listening to me, he's really sick. It's not normal for a child to have blood in his diaper. This child got everything he wanted for Christmas and has not touched a single toy. Why won't you listen to me?"

VI. The Bounceback—Part 2: Emergency Department #2

ED RETURN #1—RN/MD notes:

RN notes:

- Sick appearing child, severely dehydrated, gross blood noticed in diaper. Temperature 102.4.
- Mom reports abdominal pain and bloody diarrhea for five days.

MD note:

- **HPI:** Mom reports child has had five days of diarrhea with blood and vomiting. Some abdominal pain, colicky in nature. Not tolerating fluids today. Seen by PCP this morning and had some juice from cup after Phenergan.
- **PE:** T-102.4, HR-190, RR-40, BP-79/45 Sat-94%. Child moderately sick appearing dehydrated, sunken eyes dry mucosal membranes. Not playful. Abdomen tender to palpation all quadrants. Gross blood in diaper with diarrhea. (No mention of petechiae).
- **ED Course:** CBC (WBC: 17, H/H: 10/31 Plt: "PND" Pending), Chemistry (Creatinine-1.2, Glucose-80), Stool sent for culture, O&P, leukocytes and C. Diff.
- 20cc/kg IV bolus x 2 administered. 2mg IV Zofran given.
- **Testing:** US (indication r/o intussusception). Result: Negative

- **MDM:** Patient improved after bolus and tolerating oral Gatorade and part of a Popsicle. Called GI to arrange outpatient follow up for continued bloody diarrhea. Nuclear Medicine Tech is on vacation and Meckel's scan can be done Tuesday. Left message for the patient's PCP to follow up stool studies.
- **Diagnosis:** Diarrhea, vomiting, abdominal pain unknown etiology
- **RN Note prior to dc:** Pt improved, tolerated part of a Popsicle and 4 oz of Gatorade. One bowel movement prior to discharge with scant blood and diarrhea. Discharge delayed 15min for bleeding at IV site, controlled with 10 min of pressure.

VII. The Bounceback—Part 3: Emergency Department #3

ED RETURN #2:

January 5, 2008 – (0900) - Just over 24hrs from previous ED discharge (different ED)

- **EMS:** John arrives via EMS intubated for respiratory failure, cyanosis, and a heart rate of 45. Compressions were started prior to arrival, but were stopped after a code dose of epinephrine was administered and heart rate increased to 85 and SBP improved from 50 to 75.
- **Physician MDM:** Initial vitals HR 65, respirations 20 (intubated), temperature 96.8 and SBP 70. A Dopamine drip is started and a second and third bolus of lactated Ringers is given.
- **Testing:**
  - o CAT scan of the brain is ordered to r/o abuse and is negative. Chest x-ray showed atelectasis and no signs of infection.
  - o ABG reveals a concomitant metabolic and respiratory acidosis thought to be from the combination of being post arrest and having had multiple days of diarrhea
  - o EKG shows bradycardia.
  - o Blood work reveals leukocytosis of 25 with a left shift, lactate of 5.6, Hb-6, Platelets-25, Creatinine-2.6, ScVO2-50 and a K-2.9.
- **ED Course:**
  - o Potassium was replaced and a NG tube was placed with gastric return
  - o There are non-blanching generalized petechiae visualized and Vancomycin and Rocephin are started for presumed meningitis
  - o The LP is deferred as the patient is too unstable post-arrest. An Artic-Sun cooling apparatus was fitted and patient was paralyzed while the hypothermia protocol was induced.
  - o Pt transferred to the ICU.

ICU course:

- Approximately two hours after admission to the ICU John arrests again. Multiple rounds of epinephrine and atropine were given for bradycardic arrest.
- Placement of arterial line and central line are performed.
- Dopamine 35mcg/kg/min and epinephrine 1mcg/kg/min are started.
- The ICU team is preparing to start Milrinone when John's heart rate rapidly trends down and then progresses to PEA followed by asystole.
- Family is brought into the room for the code.
- After 40 minutes of resuscitative efforts the code is called.

January 5, 2008- (1100) – the same day

- The lab at the original hospital calls the original ED to relay the positive culture finding of Stx2 detected and confirming O157:H7 infection.
- The resident who took the call attempted to call John's family, but got no answer (John's family is at the second ED on what would be his final visit). The resident leaves a message.

FINAL DIAGNOSIS: Hemolytic uremic syndrome/Thrombotic thrombocytopenic purpura (HUS/TTP)

PART 2—THE ANALYSIS

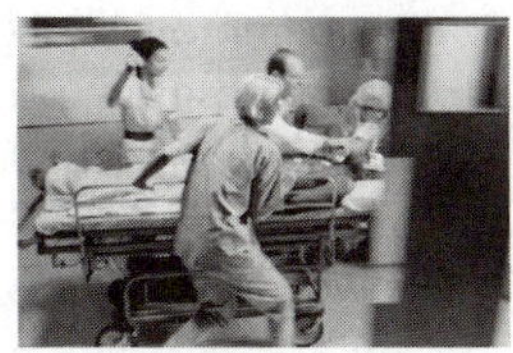

DIAGNOSIS AND MANAGEMENT OF HEMOLYTIC UREMIC SYNDROME THROMBOTIC THROMBOCYTOPENIC PURPURA (HUS/TTP)

Andrew Sloas, DO, RDMS, FAAEM

Assistant Professor of Adult and Pediatric Emergency Medicine
Department of Emergency Medicine, University of Kentucky
Editor-in-Chief PEM ED Podcast

Definition and pathophysiology of HUS/TTP

Classically, children get HUS and adults get TTP. HUS shares many features with TTP and is much more common than TTP in pediatrics, but most experts believe that these two diseases exist on a continuum.[4] Traditional HUS is defined by the triad of micro angiopathic hemolytic anemia (MAHA), thrombocytopenia and acute renal failure. HUS/TTP is characterized by endothelial cell injury, intravascular platelet—fibrin thrombi and vascular damage.[5] The continuation of neurologic changes and fever completes the pentad of TTP:

- Micro angiopathic hemolytic anemia
- Thrombocytopenia
- Acute renal failure
- Neurologic changes
- Fever

1. Types of HUS: D+, D-, familial

The classic D+ HUS [D for diarrhea or STEC-HUS from the E coli (STEC)] is caused by the deadly Shiga toxin *Escherichia coli* and is usually preceded by colitis. There are two types of Shiga Toxin, Stx1 and Stx2 (most likely to be associated with D+ HUS). At most large academic institutions, stool may be directly tested for both Stx 1 and 2 in house.[6]

The D- HUS is thought to be mediated by the complement system or other familial factors.[7] The most common D- HUS syndrome is associated with both lung and CNS infections. It is primarily caused by strep pneumonia, but drugs and sepsis[8] are also routine etiologies.[9] Other less likely, but routinely reported precipitating causes of D- HUS are surgery and DKA.[10,11] Although rare, D- HUS accounts for up to 15% of HUS[12] It falls under the category of D-disease because there are no diarrhea inducing bacterial toxins released from the dying cells, but rather the direct endothelial injury from the offending drug/illness causes a complement factor mutation resulting in aHUS and TTP.

Familial HUS is another form of atypical HUS and is caused by a genetic mutation affecting the complement regulatory proteins.[13] Upshaw-Schulmann Syndrome is an autosomal recessive disorder that results in a congenital deficiency of ADAMTS 13. It usually presents in a bimodal distribution either first as a neonate or in the pre-teenage years.

While John had both respiratory symptoms and diarrheal symptoms, the most likely cause of death would be related to D+ HUS. Although the mother reported some URI symptoms, the diarrheal component with gross blood was the common complaint throughout all the visits. John did not develop neurologic symptoms until his final presentation.

2. **ADAMTS-13**

The deficiency of the enzyme ADAMTS-13 plays a special role in TTP. The job of von Willebrand factor (vWF) is to promote platelet aggregation, while ADAMTS -13's job is to cut up vWF before it can induce unnecessary clots. With a deficiency of ADAMTS-13, many unstable platelet-based clots form. A platelet count less than 150 is suspicious for TTP, however, platelets will often be less than 40.[14]

Before these unstable clots get broken down, many will get stuck in the kidneys. This causes the acute renal failure seen in HUS/TTP. These unstable clots are also thought to be responsible for the waxing and waning neurologic disturbances seen with the disease, i.e., mini self-resolving strokes;[15] the clots momentarily obstruct cerebrovascular flow and then dissolve resting in fluctuating mental status. Colonic ischemia and perforation are also possible from these same micro emboli. In patients with symptoms of an acute abdomen, appropriate radiographic studies including a CAT scan should be performed. The clots in the vascular system are thought to cause red blood cells to fragment into schistocytes, which are pathognomonic for TTP when they are found on a peripheral smear (when TTP is overwhelmingly suspected). Patients with suspected TTP or DIC should have a peripheral blood **smear** sent to look for schistocytes.

Age of presentation and mortality

HUS and TTP can be seen at any age, but the majority of HUS cases are found between 7 months and 6 years of age. While the disease was universally fatal before 1955, the mortality rate has dropped to less than 5% during the 1990s. However, the mortality rate in underdeveloped countries remains as high as 75%. Unfortunately, the diagnosis remains difficult to make because the onset is so rapid.[5]

Of those patients infected with the 0157:H7 shiga toxin producing E. coli, HUS occurs in up to 15%. Most cases come after outbreaks in daycares, schools, or places with multiple children in close contact. The most common food-borne cause of HUS is from ingesting undercooked meat. Unfortunately, atypical HUS is caused by strains of the strep pneumonia that are not included in the 7-valent or 23-valent vaccines, such as serotype 19A.[4]

Laboratory evaluation

HUS/TTP should be considered a clinical diagnosis. Morbidity and mortality is high when missed; one should not wait for laboratory confirmation to start treatment. With that being said, a stool culture, while definitive, is usually of low yield after about seven days of diarrhea.

Whenever you are considering shiga toxin in the differential, a special MacConkey agar plate must be ordered as E. coli 0157: H7 does not grow on traditional agar plates. In those patients where familial and genetic forms of HUS are being considered, complement C3 may be decreased and should be checked. For those suspected of having HUS/TTP, ADAMTS-13 levels may be checked but a decreased level may not be enough to prove the disease.

It is also important to check ADAMTS-13 activity as well.[16] Now, those are the textbook answers, but most importantly, if you have three out of the five symptoms and schistocytes on the smear, then you have TTP and you should be on the phone with the hematologist arranging plasmapheresis. The longer the delay, the higher the mortality.

Treatment

Plasma Exchange (Plasmapheresis with Fresh Frozen Plasma exchange) is the cornerstone treatment for HUS/TTP. Fluid overload in critically ill pediatric patients can increase mortality,[17] but With HUS/TTP you cannot take that approach. Small studies indicate that prevention of oligoanuric states prevent the more serious complications of HUS/TTP. Aggressive volume expansion of IVF seems to improve outcomes and has been shown to prevent dialysis.[18] Up to 80% of affected patients with D- HUS require dialysis, compared with 40% in D+ HUS.[1]

D- HUS remains poorly understood and is very difficult to treat. Usually multiple rounds of plasma exchange are required. Obviously, reversing the potential causes of D- HUS like DKA, sepsis and offending drugs should be the primary emphasis.[9] In September 2011, Eculizumab (Soliris) was approved by the FDA in the U.S. for adults and children with D negative HUS. In small studies, those who received the drug demonstrated improved platelet counts and decreased renal failure requiring dialysis.[19]

Now let us look more specifically at our case...

Let's face it, in all that you hold in your mind to be true, you may think that you have a better chance of winning the lottery than having a pediatric patient with TTP walk into your ED on your next shift. However, remember this, nothing kills a party like a pediatric resuscitation, especially a preventable one. When you make this diagnosis, you will save a life.

In my mind, there are two types of bloody diarrhea:

1. The infectious type that could potentially cause significant morbidity and mortality.
2. All others: such as bleeding disorders, rectal prolapse, anal fissures, intussusception and others. Of note, the latter can be associated with fever if intussusception is not diagnosed promptly leading to bowel ischemia, perforation and peritonitis.

The initial ED visit

Let's start with the first emergency room visit. How many children have you seen in the last month (especially during gastroenteritis season) that have diarrhea with a little blood. For me it's a daily occurrence. It is so common we can get a little numb to the fact that something more sinister could be afoot. That is the definition of *anchoring bias*.

To be a good EM physician, one needs to be able to rapidly fit patients into the category of sick versus not sick. This is no easy task. We have developed the special gift of being able to access a patient in less than five minutes, process the sum of their complaints, sprinkle in some good ole' fashion gestalt and pop out a differential. The downside is that to do that well we have to anchor on key things the patients tell us and data that we collect. The trick is to obtain an adequate amount of data to find the correct points to anchor on.

Children are very difficult to nail down when they have nausea, vomiting and abdominal pain because they express everything through their bellies. When you think about it that way, you will be more likely to just call it what it is: nausea, vomiting and abdominal pain rather than gastroenteritis. It will also be a lot easier to defend your chart when the patient returns with appendicitis, pneumonia or even meningitis.

Unfortunately, John's evaluation did not explore these symptoms any more than just restating the nursing documentation. There is no record of frequency, quantity, exposures or travel history.

The first EP who saw John, and while I'm sure he must have considered age-appropriate illnesses involving blood in the stool, did not document the reasoning that led him away from those illnesses. A child less than two years old who has a complaint of bloody diarrhea should flag any provider to the potential causes of infectious etiologies, Meckel's diverticulum and intussusception.

There are several concerning signs that should have tipped us off to a diagnosis beyond acute gastroenteritis and even potential diagnosis of HUS/TTP. The previously mentioned fever and blood not withstanding, there was the discussion of petechiae in the nurse's notes which was also mentioned by John's mother (rash).

Given the labs from the second ED visit and the overall outcome, the presence of petechiae on John's face and axilla would have been likely. Unfortunately, that complaint was not explored, but in hindsight the combination of fever, diarrhea, and a potential blood dyscrasia prompts an expanded differential. To a pediatrician, petechiae below the level of the nipples would sound an alarm for the more common diagnosis of leukemia.

We should also take a little about the "Zo and Go" approach to vomiting and diarrhea (Zo = Zofran and Go = out of your ED) It works so well that ondansetron may give us a false sense of security. Our first provider saw it perform so phenomenally that he sent John home after only an hour of ED observation, a bite of a popsicle and some sips from his cup.

Discharge instructions

The ED was never designed to be the definitive diagnosis and treatment locale. If it works out that way then it's great, but it should not be expected. Keeping with that line of reasoning, I hammer my residents with something that I call the "eight to twelve hour belly check."

When you tell the patient, or parent, that you honestly don't know what is causing their abdominal pain and vomiting, but you doubt it's surgical and that you would need someone else to take another look in 8 to 12 hours, it is absolutely empowering for you and the patient.

If your written instructions are written above a 6th grade reading level, only 23% of your patients understand only one of the many things that are written. Comprehension of overall instructions can still be very good if simple verbal instructions are given.[1]

Persons who speak Spanish as their primary language have a far smaller chance of following up or filling the prescription unless they have a primary care provider they trust if their instructions are provided in Spanish.[2, 3] So, in my opinion, if you have a patient who you are truly concerned about, you should really take the time to make sure they understand the discharge instructions. The patient with abdominal pain of unknown etiology really needs to understand the potential for morbidity.

If we discharge our patients with very specific discharge instructions and actually go to the bedside and have a 5 to 10 minute conversation, then you are creating a virtual environment where it is safe to have the patient observed at home. Why? Because now you are empowering the patient to return to the emergency department.

✔ **Teaching point:** Abdominal pain with vomiting and diarrhea is much less likely to be a missed surgical abdomen than vomiting and abdominal pain without diarrhea. Give great discharge instructions and the truth will set you free.

In this case, the follow up with the pediatrician is a little easier to defend. The pediatrician addresses the petechiae and at least documents that they exist, but would seem to defer the rest of skin exam. I tell my residents that every preverbal child needs a head-to-toe exam. You will be astounded at what you find under the diaper.

To their credit, the pediatrician seemed to keep John in the office for a reasonable amount of time. The pediatrician is also very thorough in noting a new diaper with diarrhea that did not contain any visible blood. It would be reasonable at that point to continue John's convalescence at home.

The choice of anti-emetics may be called into question, as the child is under two years old, and Phenergan is not approved for that age group. However, after the Phenergan is administered under medical supervision in an office setting, John seems to perk up and drink a little bit; so, that my friends is the art of medicine. The pediatrician also gives reasonable discharge instructions stating that if the child does not tolerate oral fluids at home or if has any more blood in the stool then the mom should take John to the emergency department.

Later that night John returns to the same emergency department with a different provider. His mother is crying out for help. A second ED visit in two nights should prompt concern and drive you to find what others have missed. Disregard other's anchors and forge new ground to overturn the stone that everyone else missed.

The nurse's notes from that encounter reflect a sick appearing child with a fever and again mention abdominal pain and bloody diarrhea. This emergency medicine provider understands the age-appropriate diagnoses of Meckel's and intussusception and addresses them in his notes . However, the more likely infectious etiology is downplayed.

Unfortunately, in this visit all of the criteria are there to make the diagnosis, the patient has anemia, what must be a presumed bump in the creatinine (most kids this age would have a creatinine below 0.6), and an unexplained hypoxia which is never mentioned. There is a borderline hypotension that is best explained by impending TTP, sepsis and pulmonary edema (given the outcome). Don't get me wrong. This provider did not completely disregard the possibility of infection; he does send the stool cultures.

The one lab that we later find out was not back at the time of discharge was the platelet count. If you remember from the chart above they are listed as "PND" for pending. Unfortunately, those labs were never reported. At some hospitals, when platelets are critically low or high, they are listed as pending until the specimen could be re-run. This specimen was never re-run.

Given all of the data points the second ED provider had, one must wonder if they had taken the 30,000 foot view, would the diagnosis of HUS/TTP have been made? Even at the time of discharge, both the doctor and the nurse document bleeding from the IV site. Petechiae, bleeding from the site and those labs …

The most plausible explanation for not "putting it all together" is that the provider was anchoring on the potential for a mechanical causes of bleeding, given the ultrasound for intussusception and outpatient arrangements for a Meckel's scan. The provider does a nice job with the progress note when they document that John appears better and is tolerating Gatorade and a Popsicle, but there are no repeat vitals supporting his clinical observation.

John did not receive any antibiotics, but I think it is important to point out that antibiotics are a common complication that is known to potentiate HUST/TTP in children with bloody diarrhea. Many cases of HUS have been given antibiotics before they are elucidated. Antibiotics or anti-motility agents can be devastating in diarrheal illness because the antibiotics kill the bacteria at an increased rate. This results in a faster release of shiga toxin from the dying cells. Anti-motility agents slow transit times and allow the gut more time to absorb the deadly shiga toxin.

Use of antibiotics have been shown to increase the risk of HUS by 17-fold,[17] and thus, the recommendation is to avoid the use of antibiotics except in confirmed sepsis.

Chapter Summary

- The mother felt there was something wrong, and she was right.
- Petechiae, which are below the nipples, are pathological. When in this case, it was another clue to HUS/TTP.
- The second ED visit: He has now seen by an EP and the pediatrician. Come on man, the child continued to bleed, don't send that home! Admit the child to peds, and see what happens. There was gross bloody diarrhea for 5 days and you had no identified source of the fever. Did I mention his mom was uncomfortable? Get GI to lay eyes on the child. Get someone to do the proper work-up, and if you can't do all of that, then transfer them (or admit them) to someone who can.
- Multiple ED visits makes a patient more likely to have a serious disease. Look at it as a challenge and not a burden.

- Patients with HUS/TTP crump quickly, and you may be the child's last bastion. Step back and take a 30,000 foot approach when you're unsure what's going on with a patient. Phone a friend, and trust your gut. Don't be afraid to admit when your gestalt tells you to.
- A bite of a popsicle is not PO'ing. Get actively involved in the discharge. To quote the great Dr. Greg Henry, "the most important note that you write is the last note that you write."

References

1. Spandorfer JM, Karras DJ, Hughes LA, Caputo C. Comprehension of discharge instructions by patients in an urban emergency department. Ann Emerg Med. 1995;25(1):71–4. PubMed PMID: 7802373.
2. Thomas EJ, Burstin HR, O'Neil AC, et al. Patient noncompliance with medical advice after the emergency department visit. Ann Emerg Med. 1996;27(1):49–55. PubMed PMID: 8572448.
3. Crane JA. Patient comprehension of doctor-patient communication on discharge from the emergency department. J Emerg Med. 1997;15(1):1–7. PubMed PMID: 9017479.
4. Trachtman H. HUS and TTP in children. Pediatr Clin North Am. 2013;60(6):1513–26. doi: 10.1016/j.pcl.2013.08.007. PubMed PMID: 24237985.
5. Steele M, Chen HH, Steele J, et al. Thrombotic thrombocytopenic purpura in pediatric patients. Chinese J Contemp Peds. 2012;14(11):803–10. Review. PubMed PMID: 23146723.
6. Tarr PI, Gordon CA, Chandler WL. Shiga-toxin-producing Escherichia coli and haemolytic uraemic syndrome. Lancet. 2005 Mar 19–25;365(9464):1073–86. Review. PubMed PMID: 15781103.
7. Karmali MA, Petric M, Lim C, et al. The association between idiopathic hemolytic uremic syndrome and infection by verotoxin-producing Escherichia coli. 1985. J Infect Dis. 2004;189(3):556–63. PubMed PMID: 14982069.
8. Karim F, Adil SN, Afaq B, et al. Deficiency of ADAMTS-13 in pediatric patients with severe sepsis and impact on in-hospital mortality. BMC Pediatr. 2013;13(1):44. [Epub ahead of print] PubMed PMID: 23537039; PubMed Central PMCID: PMC3637410.
9. Ariceta G, Besbas N, Johnson S, Karpman D, et al. European Paediatric Study Group for HUS. Guideline for the investigation and initial therapy of diarrhea-negative hemolytic uremic syndrome. Pediatr Nephrol. 2009;24(4):687–96. doi: 10.1007/s00467-008-0964-1. Epub 2008 Sep 18. PubMed PMID: 18800230.
10. Khan MR, Maheshwari PK, Haque A. Thrombotic microangiopathic syndrome: a novel complication of diabetic ketoacidosis. Indian Pediatr. 2013;50(7):697–9. PubMed PMID: 23942435.
11. Choi EJ, Lee S. A postoperative thrombotic thrombocytopenic purpura in a cardiac surgery patient: a case report. Korean J Thorac Cardiovasc Surg. 2013 Jun;46(3):220–2. doi: 10.5090/kjtcs.2013.46.3.220. Epub 2013 Jun 5. PubMed PMID: 23772412; PubMed Central PMCID: PMC3680610.
12. Spinale JM, Ruebner RL, Kaplan BS, Copelovitch L. Update on Streptococcus pneumoniae associated hemolytic uremic syndrome. Curr Opin Pediatr. 2013 Apr;25(2):203–8. doi: 10.1097/MOP.0b013e32835d7f2c. Review. PubMed PMID: 23481474.

13. Lemaire M, Frémeaux-Bacchi V, Schaefer F, et al. Recessive mutations in DGKE cause atypical hemolytic-uremic syndrome. Nat Genet. 2013;45(5):531–6. doi: 10.1038/ng.2590. Epub 2013 Mar 31. PubMed PMID: 23542698; PubMed Central PMCID: PMC3719402.
14. Metin A, Unal S, Gümrük F, et al. Congenital thrombotic thrombocytopenic purpura with novel mutations in three unrelated Turkish children. Pediatr Blood Cancer. 2014;61(3):558–61. doi: 10.1002/pbc.24764. Epub 2013 Sep 30. PubMed PMID: 24115559.
15. Paliwal PR, Teoh HL, Sharma VK. Association between reversible cerebral vasoconstriction syndrome and thrombotic thrombocytopenic purpura. J Neurol Sci. 2014 Mar 15;338(1–2):223–5. doi: 10.1016/j.jns.2013.12.043. Epub 2014 Jan 4. pii: S0022-510X(13)03114-6. doi: 10.1016/j.jns.2013.12.043. [Epub ahead of print] PubMed PMID: 24423586]
16. Lotta LA, Wu HM, Musallam KM, Peyvandi F. The emerging concept of residual ADAMTS13 activity in ADAMTS13-deficient thrombotic thrombocytopenic purpura. Blood Rev. 2013 Mar;27(2):71-6. doi: 10.1016/j.blre.2013.01.001. Epub 2013 Feb 14. Review. PubMed PMID: 23415418.
17. Gillespie RS, Seidel K, Symons JM. Effect of fluid overload and dose of replacement fluid on survival in hemofiltration. Pediatr Nephrol. 2004;19(12):1394–9. PubMed PMID: 15517417.
18. Ake JA, Jelacic S, Ciol MA, Watkins SL, Murray KF, Christie DL. Relative nephroprotection during Escherichia coli O157:H7 infections: association with intravenous volume expansion. Pediatrics. 2005;115(6):e673 80.
19. Gulleroglu K, Fidan K, Hançer VS, Bayrakci U, Baskin E, Soylemezoglu O. Neurologic involvement in atypical hemolytic uremic syndrome and successful treatment with eculizumab. Pediatr Nephrol. 2013;28(5):827–30. doi:10.1007/s00467-013-2416-9. Epub 2013 Feb 7. PubMed PMID: 23389237.
20. Walterspiel JN, Ashkenazi S, Morrow AL, Cleary TG. Effect of subinhibitory concentrations of antibiotics on extracellular Shiga-like toxin I. Infection. 1992;20(1):25–9. PubMed PMID: 1563808.

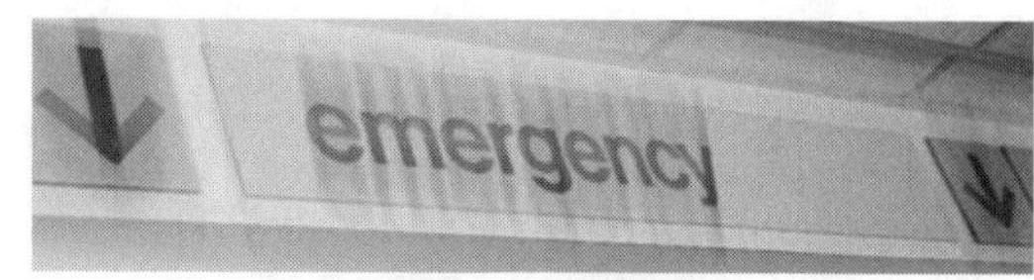

CASE 18

4-MONTH-OLD INFANT WITH VOMITING

Emily Rose, MD, FAAEM, FAAP, FACEP
Director, Pediatric Emergency Medicine MSIV Clerkship
Assistant Professor of Clinical Emergency Medicine
Keck School of Medicine of the University of Southern California
LA County + USC Medical Center

Evelyn Lee, MS, MD
Emergency Medicine PGY-2 resident
LA County + USC Medical Center, Los Angeles, CA

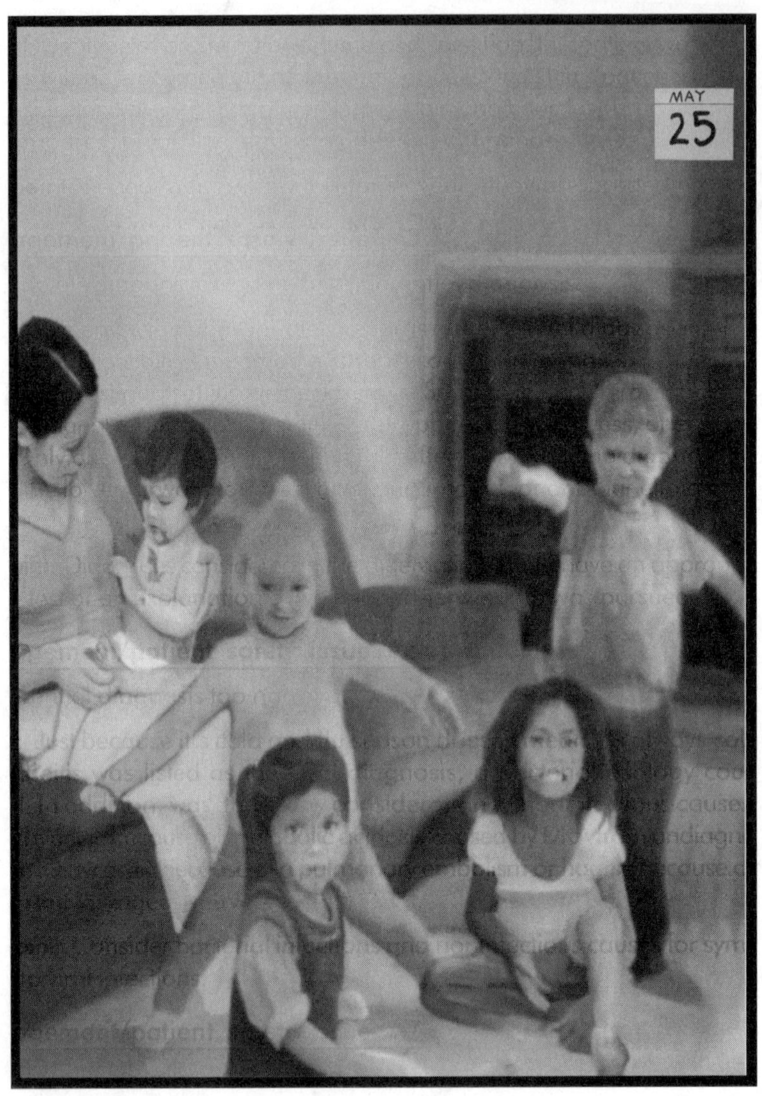
MAY
25

CASE 18

4-MONTH-OLD INFANT WITH VOMITING

PART 1—MEDICAL

I. The Patient's Story

Faith is a 4-month-old Hispanic female born to a mother with an unknown drug addiction. At one month of age, she is placed into foster care. The biological mother has unsupervised visitation rights and may regain custody. On the afternoon of May 25th, Faith began to vomit after her feedings. She is taken to the ED by the foster mother.

II. The Doctor's Version (the following is the actual documentation of the provider)

Date: 5/25/2013 8:16pm
CC: vomiting

Nursing triage note (20:16): BIB Foster Mom. +Vomiting feeding today. No fever noted. Fontanel is soft and flat mmm. No acute distress.

- Immunization_History: Routine Childhood UTD.
- Developmental_Milestones: appropriate for age, 0_to_6_months (+) regards face, (+) holds head up.

20:43: Nurse Note: Per mother, patient had another episode of emesis "all over the room". MD aware.

HPI (per resident) at 21:24: pt presents w/1 day of vomiting, 4-5x. always after feedings. taking 3-4 oz q 4hrs and almost all is coming back up. never had problems before. no diarrhea/hematochezia, normal UOP. pt crying a lot today. no contacts w/diarrhea. pt taken away from his parents due to parental drug use. no rash,

VITAL SIGNS

Time	Temp(F)	Rectal	Pulse	Resp	Syst	Diast	Sat
20:11	99.4		146	26	99	54	99%

PHYSICAL EXAM:

Vital_signs: Per Nurse's note, (+)reviewed by me
General_appearance: (peds): well_nourished, alert, (+)attentive, (+)eye contact, (+)smiling, (+)playful, no_acute_distress.
Eyes: Pupils_equal_and_round, conjunctiva_clear, tears_present
Ent: (+)oropharynx clear, mucous_membranes_moist, (+)neck supple
Lungs: no_wheezing, no_crackles
Heart: normal_rate, regular_rhythm, no_murmur
Abdomen: soft, no_abd_tenderness
Extremities: (-)obvious deformities, no_edema
Skin: warm, dry, no_rash.
Neuro: responds_appropriately, motor_grossly_intact

VITAL SIGNS							
Time	Temp(F)	Rectal	Pulse	Resp	Syst	Diast	Sat
20:53	99.6		139	24	108	58	100%

ED COURSE:

9:24pm resident note: pt w/vomiting today only. pt also vomited entire bottle while in room. will orally rehydrate and re-evaluate.

12:50am resident note: pt has been orally rehydrating for 3 hours @ 1 oz q 30min. pt now

12:57am resident note: pt vomited once in that time but is still making urine normally and clinically looks healthy and is presently sleeping well. awaiting U dip results and will d/c w/ f/u tm

12:58am Attending note: I have seen and examined the patient. I agree with the plan of care as documented in the chart. Patient is alert, smiling and interactive. Appears well hydrated with a full bag of urine on my exam

Lab Results: 1:09am: U-dip: +ketones, negative for blood/leuks/nitrites/bili/glucose/protein

DISCHARGE DIAGNOSIS: Vomiting (w/nausea)

Discharge instructions: give pedialyte instead of regular feedings for the next 2 feedings and then begin to substitute back in formula for pedialyte 1oz each feeding until pt tolerating pure formula. Return to the ER immediately for inability to tolerate the pedialyte, fever, increased fussiness, or other problems. Follow-up in the ER tomorrow afternoon or night for her to be rechecked unless she is completely asymptomatic.

III. The Errors—Risk Management/Patient Safety Issues

Risk management/patient safety issue #1:

Error: Failure to consider an underlying serious etiology in a vomiting infant.

Discussion: Vomiting is a very common complaint in the ED and, truth be told, the majority of vomiting children have a self-resolving viral infection. Consideration of the differential diagnosis of serious underlying etiologies must occur with every case. If the diagnosis isn't considered, the diagnosis won't be made. Two questions must be asked in the vomiting child:

1. Is this child dehydrated (and require intervention)?
2. Does this child have an underlying emergency causing the vomiting?

Answer to first question: This child looked and acted well according to the documentation. She did not appear clinically dehydrated and intravenous resuscitation was not indicated.

Answer to second question: Is there an underlying emergency causing her to vomit? Some red flags exist in the history. First, the complex social situation deserves mention. The child was in foster care, but was often with her biological mother for unsupervised visits. The child was documented to be alert, smiling and interactive (suggesting that intracranial injury from non-accidental trauma was less likely to be the etiology of her vomiting). Explicit mention that signs of abuse were absent (*i.e.*, no bruising, no focal tenderness, torn frenulum, etc.) would have made this chart more complete.

The child was "vomiting 4-5x today, always after feedings … almost all is coming back up … and pt crying a lot today." Persistent, large volume emesis consistently after each feeding is concerning for obstruction. In young infants, obstruction is most commonly caused by intussusception followed by incarcerated hernia. A benign exam and increased crying/fussiness increase the concern for intussusception. This evaluation does not supply us with the data on which to make our decision; a complete examination of the diaper area/genital area is required to rule out incarcerated hernia or testicular torsion with males. Persistent vomiting and excessive crying in in an infant should raise suspicion of intracranial pathology such as meningitis (even in the absence of fever) or bleeding (intentional or accidental), but the fact that the infant was smiling and interactive makes these etiologies unlikely.

✔ **Teaching point:** Address the underlying cause of the vomiting and if ensuing dehydration needs to be managed.

Risk management/patient safety issue #2:

Error: Incomplete Medical Decision Making (MDM) note.

Discussion: An MDM addressing probable etiology of vomiting should have been documented. The diagnosis of early gastroenteritis was inferred, but not explicitly stated. The process of writing the MDM may prompt the physician to consider other possible diagnoses. Potential maltreatment was also not mentioned in the decision making portion and should have been addressed in a high risk patient.

✔ **Teaching point:** Writing a medical decision making note may aid in consideration of important differential diagnoses.

Risk management/patient safety issue #3:

Error: Failure to ensure appropriate follow up instructions.

Discussion: It is important to recommend timing of return and ensure the ability of the patient's care provider to return. This child should have been asked to come to the ED the following morning for a reassessment and ultrasound if the vomiting persisted. In a young infant, 24 hours is too long to wait to evaluate for dehydration and reassess symptoms.

Ensuring that the patient could return for a follow up would have revealed this child's complex social situation. The foster mother had brought the child in that evening for evaluation but the child was possibly going to be returned to the biological mother during the following day. This information was not known to the providers and may have impacted her disposition decision.

✔ **Teaching point:** Young infants who may become dehydrated and children with potential surgical emergencies should be reassessed in 6–12 hours. If timely follow-up seems unlikely due to social reasons, consider admission.

Risk management/patient safety issue #4:

Error: Sign-out inertia.

Discussion: This patient was seen by a resident who staffed the case with one attending and then discharged the infant with a second attending. The verbal sign-out to the oncoming attending was that this vomiting infant is now tolerating feeds and ready to be discharged after the urine dip resulted. A catheterized urine specimen had been unsuccessfully attempted resulting in spilled urine so a urine bag was now in place. The second attending did not question the prior management plan or read the documentation. An alternate diagnosis was not entertained due to sign-out inertia.

✔ **Teaching point:** Sign-outs are inherently high risk for error. Trust no one. Re-think the case and consider an alternate diagnosis and plan.

IV. The Bounceback

FOLLOW UP WITH THE PCP:

Date: 5/26/13 5:09pm (following day after initial ED presentation)

- HPI: persistent vomiting x 2 days. Pt seen in ER yesterday and told to return if persistent vomiting with decreased amount with increased feedings. per foster mom, pt takes 1 oz q30 min, vomiting liquids, nonbloody, nonbilious, q2-4 hours. not wetting diapers appropriately, changed 1x since yesterday. crying without tears. last BM 2 days ago, no diarrhea.
- PE: General appearance is alert and in no acute distress. Interactive. Abd. soft and nontender. No palpable mass

EMERGENCY DEPARTMENT BOUNCEBACK:

16:43: Vitals: BP: 132/71 P:140 RR: 38 sp02: 99%RA T: 99.1 (rectal)

19:26: Pt is lethargy and not responding to painful stimuli, arousable. possible sepsis vs intussusception. will order PICU labs, KUB, abdominal U/S and start ceftriaxone, IVF resuscitation. will admit to PICU

KUB ABDOMEN

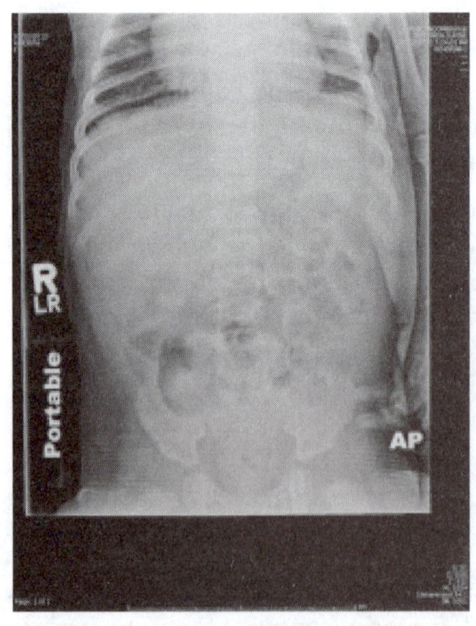

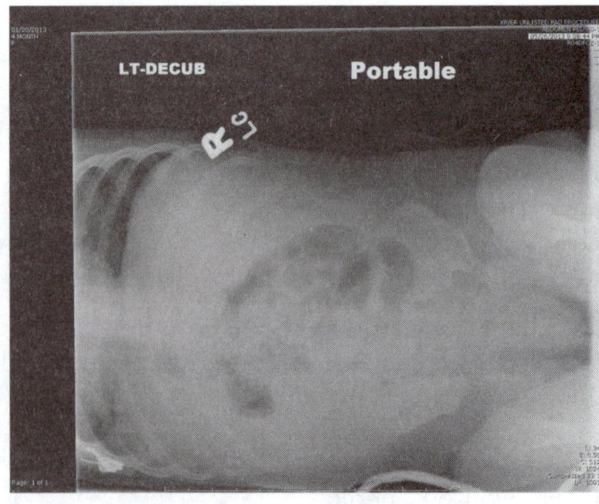

INDICATION: 4-month-old female, evaluate for obstruction.

FINDINGS/IMPRESSION: The KUB demonstrates a nonobstructive bowel gas pattern. The left lateral decubitus view demonstrates a density in the mid-abdomen, which is most consistent with intussusception. There is no radiographic evidence of pneumatosis or free intraperitoneal air.

19:36: Still attempting venous access on pt, difficult likely due to dehydration. Multiple attempts at IV start are unsuccessful. Lab sent. IM ceftriaxone. PICU team at bedside. KUB done with air throughout bowel to rectum. Will get CT head. Foster mom gives history of baby being with biological mom in an unsupervised visit yesterday.

20:20 Attending note: Patient with intussusception on US (Note: see image on page 278). Will consult peds surgery.

20:41: spoke with peds surg: order barium enema and admit.

21:16pm: NICU team at bedside for IV. Surgery resident in ER to see patient. Awaiting BE for intussusception reduction.

RADIOLOGY NOTES: 22:15 – barium enema procedure started. [multiple]attempts were done by Radiologist to resolve intussusception. Second bolus of 100ml Normal Saline was started at **22:39pm** – 2nd bolus 100cc NS infused for 20 mins. Patient during procedure started to shiver and attempts were done to re-warm her. Prn oral suctioning was done for emesis/ secretions. Procedure was not successful; solution kept leaking out of her anus. Patient was also tachycardic with heart rates 180-199 when she was shivering. Oxygen Saturation was 97-98% on room air.

DIAGNOSIS:

1. Intussusception
2. Dehydration
3. Vomiting (with nausea)
4. Lethargy

HOSPITAL COURSE:

In the PICU, the decision was made by the Pediatric surgery team to transfer for higher of care to a facility for surgical reduction by a pediatric surgeon vs repeat barium enema (as the intussusception was nearly reduced).

V. Final Outcome

Faith was transferred to the local Children's Hospital and found to have a spontaneously reduced intussusception. She was discharged the following day. Faith has been brought back to the ED since this event twice for CC: "abdominal pain" by the foster mother and each time was discharged home.

Chapter author comments: I was the attending that discharged this baby. In retrospect, there were some things missed, but I do not think that the care was egregious. The baby looked great, was well hydrated and had a benign exam. I would consider sending this child home again if the child would have been in the care of the foster mother and could have returned the following morning for a re-evaluation. Ideally, I would have clearly articulated to the care-giver that bowel obstruction such as intussusception was on my differential diagnosis. Most serious diagnoses in children have significant overlap with the symptoms of a benign viral infection, particularly on initial presentation. The challenge in caring for children is to find the balance of reassuring anxious parents yet also providing informative return instructions.

VII. Greg Henry Comments

"The number of these children who have a serious cause is small"

The workup of children is examination based, not laboratory based. A four month old vomiting is about as common a complaint as you can get. The number of these children who have a serious cause is small, however, examination is the key. Does the child ~~the~~ look well—yes or no? Children who do not look well get admitted at four months, independent of any particular finding. The hydration status of the child is paramount; a well hydrated child can be handled with reasonable follow up.

I would not suggest that all vomiting four month olds need an ultrasound; this would depend on the entire clinical picture. At the age of four months most serious causes of obstruction should manifest themselves during their acute phase with distention and tenderness. Distended abdomens in this age group do require more aggressive evaluation. The plain film, although of historical interest, is probably not as useful as the ultrasound.

PART 2—THE ANALYSIS

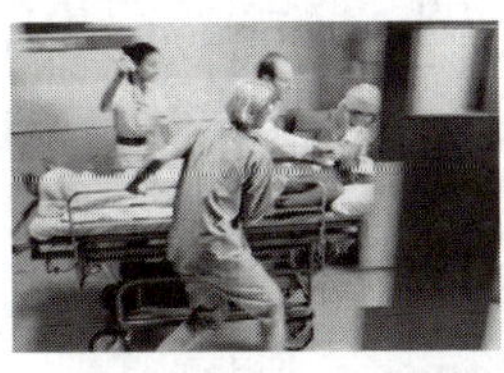

EVALUATION OF THE VOMITING INFANT, MANAGEMENT OF DEHYDRATION, AND INTUSSUSCEPTION

Emily Rose, MD, FAAEM, FAAP, FACEP

Director, Pediatric Emergency Medicine MSIV Clerkship
Assistant Professor of Clinical Emergency Medicine
Keck School of Medicine of the University of Southern California
LA County + USC Medical Center

Evelyn Lee, MS, MD

Emergency Medicine PGY-2 resident
LA County + USC Medical Center, Los Angeles, CA

Evaluation of Vomiting

This infant returned with persistent vomiting. She was alert and interactive initially and then became lethargic and not responsive to painful stimuli fairly abruptly. This is common in intussusception; lethargy may be the only presenting symptom of intussusception. Children may also initially look well, have a normal exam and be asymptomatic between painful episodes. As mentioned before , there are two major concerns when dealing with the child whose chief complaint is vomiting.

1. Is this child dehydrated (and require intervention)?
2. Does this child have an underlying emergency as the cause of vomiting?

Dehydration

The goal of rehydration is to replace the fluid deficit to return to a euvolemic state. Oral rehydration is an option even if a child is severely dehydrated, but it requires significant caregiver investment. Oral therapy should be given to the child in frequent, small amounts. A spoon or syringe may be used to place the liquid in the child's mouth if he is not spontaneously drinking. Five mLs of fluid given every 1–2 min allows 150–300 mL/hour to be given. A good rule of thumb is to give 10 mL/kg of body weight of oral rehydration solution for each watery or loose stool and 2 mL/kg of body weight for each episode of emesis. Breastfeeding should continue during the rehydration process in infants.

Intravenous access may be required for resuscitation of the dehydrated child. Venous access can be a challenge in the young infant. Trans-illuminating lights, infra-red devices and ultrasound may be utilized to enhance ability to obtain peripheral access. Scalp veins are an option in infants. If peripheral access is not easily obtained and the child requires resuscitation, an intraosseous line is a safe, quick and effective option.

An alternative to oral and IV hydration is the subcutaneous route. The recombinant enzyme hyaluronidase (Hylenex) may be injected subcutaneously to facilitate fluid absorption in the child with mild/moderate dehydration.[1,2] A butterfly needle is placed in the subcutaneous tissue (the subcutaneous tissue between the shoulder blades most commonly described). A single dose of 150 U (same dose for all ages, repeated every 24 hours of infusion) is injected subcutaneously followed by fluid infusion. A bolus and maintenance fluid may be administered via this route.

Emergent etiologies of vomiting

The differential diagnosis of vomiting in an infant is broad. Serious etiologies include:

1. Gastrointestinal (obstruction: intussusception, incarcerated hernia, volvulus in a neonate with bilious vomiting, pyloric stenosis)
2. Infectious (sepsis, meningitis, UTI, pneumonia. Note that lower lobe pneumonia associated with ileus can present with vomiting. This is why obstructive radiographs include a chest x-ray)
3. Metabolic (diabetic ketoacidosis, less commonly, inborn errors of metabolism)
4. Ingestion (toxic or foreign body)
5. CNS (increased ICP, tumor, trauma, non-accidental trauma)

Most etiologies can be excluded with a good history and physical examination.

Intussusception

Intussusception is the most common surgical cause of abdominal pain in young children. A majority of cases (80–90%) occur in children <2 years and 60% occur in <1 year.[3] The intussusceptum (proximal bowel segment) telescopes into the intussuscipiens (distal bowel segment) and drags associated mesentery with it. Venous and lymphatic congestion develops along with intestinal edema and the potential for ischemia, perforation, peritonitis and death.

Intussusception most commonly occurs at the ielocecal junction but may occur throughout the small or large bowel. Intussusception in infants is typically idiopathic but associated viral infection is common. Infections may stimulate intestinal lymphatic tissue, causing hypertrophy of Peyer patches in the lymphoid-rich terminal ileum, which may act as a lead point for ileocolic intussusception. Pathologic lead points (i.e., Meckel's diverticulum, polyp, tumor, hematoma, vascular malformation) are more common with intussusception in children >5 years. Intussusception is the most common gastrointestinal complication of Henoch Schoenlein purpura.

Less than 15% of patients with intussusception present with the classic triad of:

- Abdominal pain
- Red currant jelly stool
- Palpable abdominal mass.

Pain is most commonly paroxysms of severe, cramping abdominal pain that progresses in severity. The child may cry and draw up his legs toward the abdomen during the painful episode. Between episodes, the child may appear well, behave normally and have a benign abdominal exam. Vomiting may follow episodes. In two-thirds of patients, a sausage-shaped abdominal mass may be felt, usually in the right side of the abdomen. Up to 70% of patients with intussusception may have gross or occult blood in the stool.[4] As symptoms progress, lethargy is commonly described and is often mistaken for meningoencephalitis. Lethargy or altered mental status may be the only presenting symptom, particularly in infants.

KUB: A KUB may be performed as a screening test if the diagnosis of intussusception is considered, but don't be fooled by relying on this test to "rule-out" the diagnosis. The KUB is not sensitive for intussusception and is only helpful if positive findings are seen. Suspicious findings on a KUB include the "target sign" seen superimposed over the right kidney, a "crescent sign" projecting into the gas of the large bowel, an obscured liver margin, or lack of air in the cecum that prevents visualization from the intussusception itself.

US: Ultrasound is the diagnostic modality of choice for intussusception in many institutions. The diagnostic accuracy of ultrasound approaches 100% sensitivity in the hands of an experienced ultrasonographer.[5] Ultrasound involves minimal risk to the patient and has no radiation exposure. The characteristic sonographic findings are the "target sign" or "bull's eye" or "coiled spring" demonstrating invagination of intestinal layers.

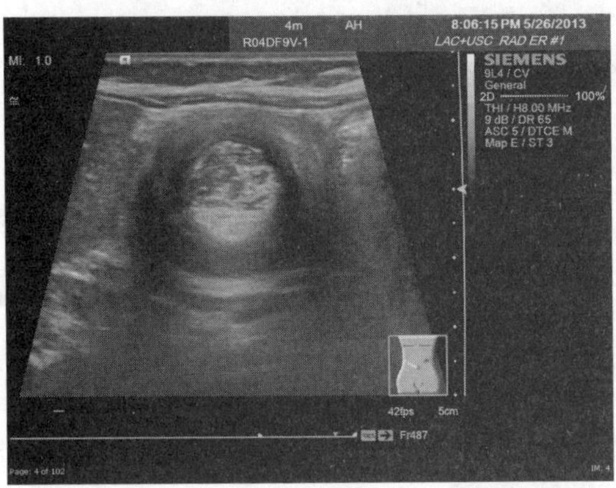

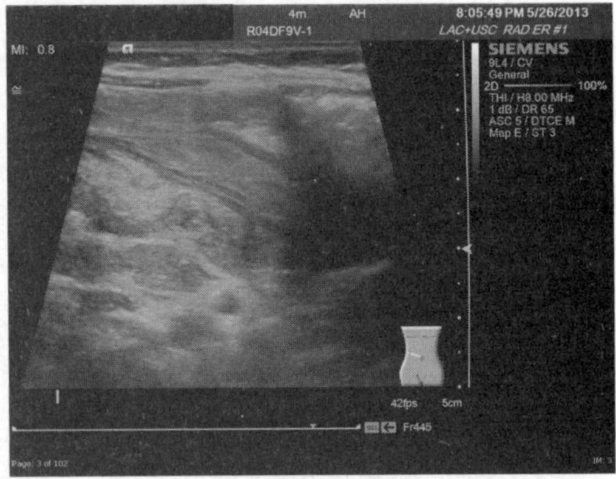

IMPRESSION: 2.9 cm mass in the right abdomen with a targetoid appearance, most consistent with intussusception

- **Imaging:** The ultrasound shows the classic findings of "target sign" with circumferential layers of intestine.

Treatment is non-operative with a hydrostatic (contrast or saline) or pneumatic enema under fluoroscopic or ultrasound guidance. Non-operative management is successful in >90% of cases. Perforation occurs in <1% of enema procedures. Antibiotics are administered prophylactically prior to the procedure in many institutions but have no proven benefit.[6] Approximately 10% of intussusceptions recur; many centers admit for 12–24 hours after reduction. Each recurrence should be treated as if it was the first presentation, provided it was previously successfully reduced non-operatively. Surgical reduction is indicated with evidence of bowel perforation, evidence of a pathological lead point, or when non-operative reduction is incomplete. A delayed (30 min–3 hours) repeat enema may be performed in a child whose intussusception is only partially reduced (as occurred in this case) and may obviate the need for surgery.[7] Small bowel intussusception is less likely to respond to non-operative reduction and more likely to spontaneously reduce.[8]

INTUSSUSCEPTION REDUCTION PROCEDURE:

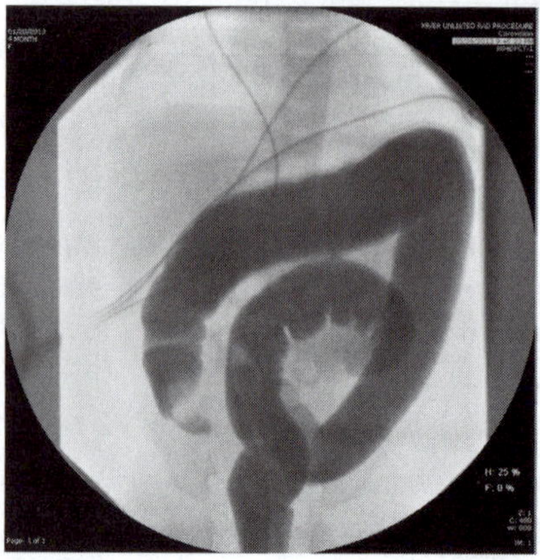

IMPRESSION: Attempted intussusception reduction, unsuccessful after three attempts as described above. Intussusception noted at ileocecal junction.

Clinical Pearls

- Maintain an expanded differential in cases of vomiting
- The triad of abdominal pain, currant jelly stool, and an palpable abdominal mass is present <15% of the time
- KUB has a poor sensitivity for diagnosis whereas US approaches 100%
- Therapy consists of a hydrostatic or pneumatic enema

References

1. Allen CH, Etzwiler LS, Miller MK, et al. Recombinant human hyaluronidase-enabled subcutaneous pediatric rehydration. Pediatrics. 2009;124(5):e858–67.
2. Spandorfer PR, Mace SE, Okada PJ, et al. A randomized clinical trial of recombinant human hyaluronidase-facilitated subcutaneous versus intravenous rehydration in mild to moderately dehydrated children in the emergency department. Clin Ther. 2012;34(11):2232–45.
3. Mandeville K, Chien M, Willyerd FA, et al. Intussusception: clinical presentations and imaging characteristics. Pediatr Emerg Care. 2012;28(9):842–4.
4. Losek JD, Fiete RL. Intussusception and the diagnostic value of testing stool for occult blood. Am J Emerg Med. 1991;9(1):1–3.
5. Hryhorczuk AL, Strouse PJ. Validation of US as a first-line diagnostic test for assessment of pediatric ileocolic intussusception. Pediatr Radiol. 2009;39(10):1075–9.

6. Al-Tokhais T, Hsieh H, Pemberton J, et al. Antibiotics administration before enema reduction of intussusception: is it necessary? J Pediatr Surg. 2012;47(5):928–30.
7. Pazo A, Hill J, Losek JD. Delayed repeat enema in the management of intussusception. Pediatr Emerg Care. 2010;26(9):640–5.
8. Ko YM, Lee SH, Huh J, et al. A fatal case of acute pulmonary embolism caused by right ventricular masses of acute lymphoblastic lymphoma-leukemia in a 13 year old girl. Korean J Pediatr. 2012;55(7):249–53.

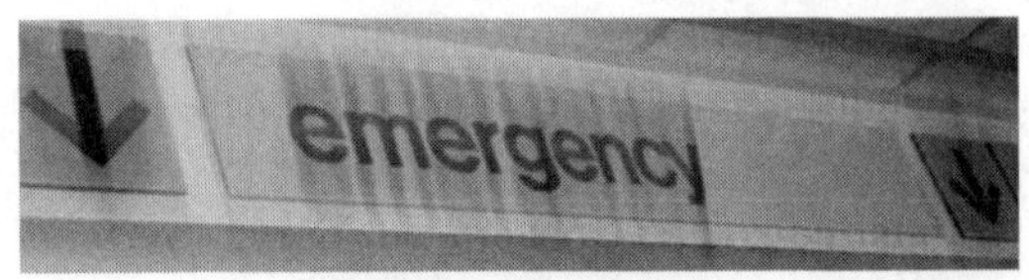

CASE 19

11-YEAR-OLD GIRL WITH MULTIPLE COMPLAINTS

Timothy Horeczko, MD, MSCR, FACEP, FAAP
Assistant Professor of Medicine
David Geffen School of Medicine at UCLA
Department of Emergency Medicine
Harbor-UCLA Medical Center
Torrance, CA

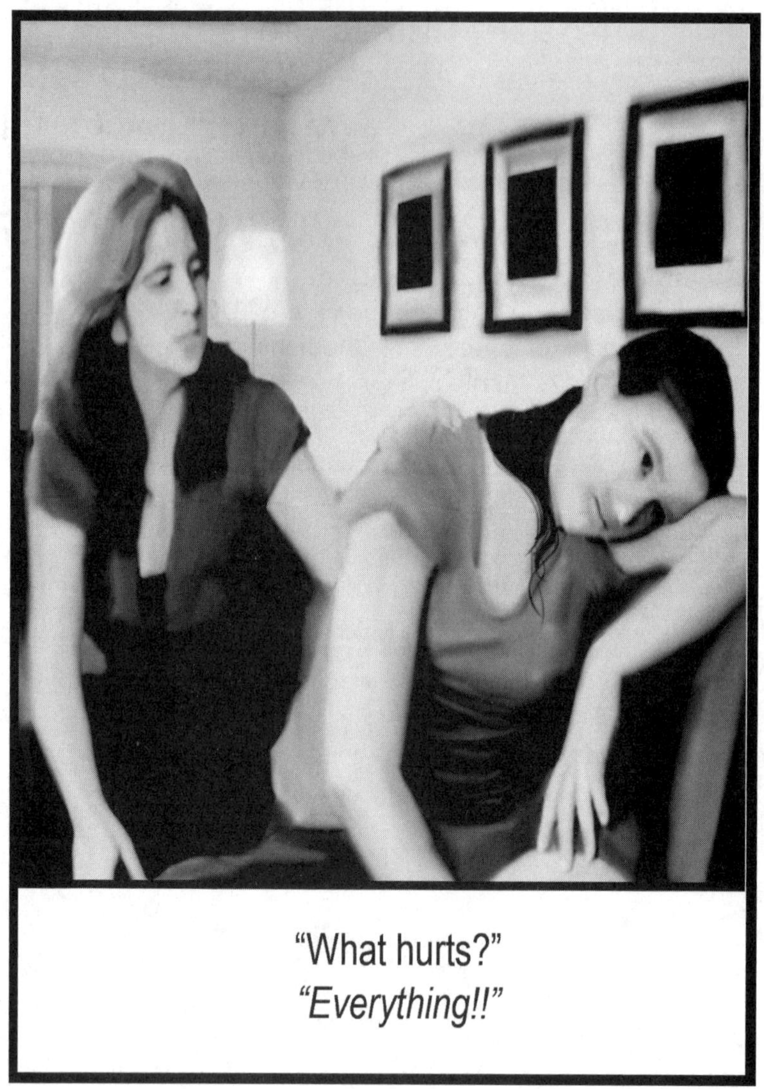

"What hurts?"
"Everything!!"

CASE 19

11-YEAR-OLD GIRL WITH MULTIPLE COMPLAINTS

PART 1—MEDICAL

I. The Patient's Story

Maribel is an 11-year-old girl who lives in a cramped two-bedroom apartment with her mother, father, two older sisters, and her younger brother. She is mildly overweight, and struggles with her school performance. Though both parents work, the family has experienced increased financial hardship of late, and there have been subsequent arguments. Maribel helps out around the home.

Over the last few weeks, she had been complaining of non-specific weakness, fatigue, and that "everything hurts." In anticipation of the start of school, she has been running around the block every day for the past week "to get skinnier," as she has been teased about her weight at school. Her mother describes her as "dramatic." After dinner, Maribel complains again of her body hurting her and begins to cry; her frustrated mother brings her in to the ED.

II.The Doctor's Version (the following is the actual documentation of the provider)

Date: Sunday, August 16th, 2009 at 19:35

Chief Complaint: Body aches

Nurse note: Pt c/o fever, body aches, sore throat x today. Runny nose, mild cough. Pain 7/10.

VITAL SIGNS

Time	Temp(C)	Pulse	Syst	Diast	Sat (RA)
19:40	37.8	126	22	110	99%

HISTORY OF PRESENT ILLNESS (at 20:01): 11 yo girl w/ no PMHx who c/o total body pain, sore throat at home since this afternoon. Mother states that she had tactile fever at home, no thermometer – gave Tylenol prior to arrival. Eating/drinking well. Possible sick contacts at home. Mother states that pt has been feeling this way "off and on" for the past couple weeks – patients states "I feel weak", and today states cannot walk due to weakness—mother thinks due to school starting again tomorrow. No rash, no abdominal pain, no headache. No SOB. Similar sx over past few weeks. On ROS, no neuro sx; complains of dysuria "sometimes". No red flags for abuse or school bullying.

PAST MEDICAL HISTORY:

Allergies: NKDA
Medications: Tylenol prn, Robitussin prn
PMHx: premature at 35 weeks, no sequelae
PSurgHx: None

EXAM (at 20:01):

General: tired, well appearing
HEENT: moist mucous membranes, OP with mild erythema, no exudate, no LAN. Mild rhinorrhea.
Chest: Nl TV/effort; CTAB, no wheeze; no murmur
Abdomen: soft, nt/nd
Extremities: 2+ pulses throughout, full ROM; TTP throughout, R LE > L LE; MAEW.
Neuro: Motor/sensation nl B UE/LE. Ambulates "hunched over", states needs mother to help her walk. Slow, steady gait, ambulates independently with coaching.
Skin: no rash, no petechiae

REPEAT VITAL SIGNS					
Time	Temp(C)	Pulse	BP	RR	SpO2
20:32	38.0	134	108/76	24	100% RA

Orders (20:40): Motrin 10 mg/kg suspension, UA, Gram stain and culture

Results (reviewed at 21:52) - **UA**: WBC 7, LE +, nitrite neg, few bacteria, multiple squamous cells, otherwise nl

Orders (21:59): Keflex 25 mg/kg PO x 1

Repeat exam (22:20): Pt states "I feel better"; ambulatory, taking PO. Walks to bathroom unassisted, steady gait. Leg pain improved.

Discharge vitals (22:25 at discharge) **T** 37.6 **HR** 112 **BP** 112/78

Medical decision making: 11 yo girl w/ influenza-like illness, appears well. No e/o pneumonia by H&P. Given some urinary sx and suggestive UA will treat for UTI. RTED precautions and f/u PMD this week.

Impression:

1. UTI
2. Influenza-like illness

Disposition: Home with mother

III. The Errors—Risk Management/Patient Safety Issues

Risk management/patient safety issue #1:

Error: Relegating all signs and symptoms to the grab bag of "viral syndrome."

Discussion: Viral illness is very common; children present to the ED in overwhelming numbers with mild illness in disproportion to its severity. In this forest of URIs, we need to seek out and identify the "sapling of sepsis" early to improve outcomes. Typically a thorough history and physical will be all that is needed to decide when to ramp up the diagnostic machinery. The acute-on-chronic nature of her complaints does not readily fit a viral illness, or even serial viral illnesses. Occam's razor needs some sharpening here.

✔ **Teaching point:** Do not assume a child with vague symptoms has viral syndrome until proven otherwise.

Risk management/patient safety issue #2:

Error: Relegating all signs and symptoms to a positive laboratory result.

Discussion: Urinary tract infection (UTI) is common in girls. However, as in any diagnostic testing, pretest probability must inform ordering and interpretation of the result. This girl had an unconvincing history of intermittent urinary symptoms. When directly asked, she passively and vaguely endorses them; "complains of dysuria sometimes." When a technically poor urinalysis is suggestive of an infection, the clinician experiences premature closure and anchoring biases. This may be a case of "true-true and unrelated," but at best we have only half of the picture.

✔ **Teaching point:** Order and interpret tests using pre-test probability; make decisions based on post-test probability.

Risk management/patient safety issue #3:

Error: Cobbling together unrelated findings to construct a "Frankendiagnosis."

Discussion: Admittedly, the patient with multiple complaints presents a potentially challenging case. However, it can be unwise to "pick and choose" various complaints and findings from a menu of possible multiple diagnoses to fit a composite impression. For example:

- body aches?—*ah, must be the flu*
- fever?—*flu again*
- possible dysuria—*suggestive urinalysis result*
- not feeling well?—*must be a urinary tract infection*
- Unable to walk previously due to pain?—*must be all of the above and her dramatic personality*

The thought process is disjointed. If anything, systemic symptoms in a girl with a UTI (although probably not in this case) would be unified in a diagnosis of pyelonephritis, not influenza-like illness plus lower tract infection.

✔ **Teaching point:** Instead of pushing a square peg in a round hole, try taking a step back to check that you have the right pieces to the puzzle.

IV. The Bounceback

Date: Wednesday, August 19th, 12:50 (3 days after initial ED visit)
Chief Complaint: Leg pain

Nurse note: Seen here on Sunday for flu and UTI. Pt states she cannot walk, brought in by ambulance. Pain 10/10.

VITAL SIGNS					
Time	Temp(C)	Pulse	Syst	Diast	Sat (RA)
12:50	39.6	168	32	108	98%

HISTORY OF PRESENT ILLNESS (at 13:00): Pt at school, states cannot walk from class to class, feels weak, not enough time. No paresthesias, no bowel or bladder complaints, no trauma, no falls. No dizziness, headache, or vision changes. States legs hurt the most, R more than L. Fevers at home. Pt does not remember the last time she was well. No rash. No dysuria. Not taking medication Rx in ED 3 days ago. No Tylenol or Motrin at home. Spoke w/mother on phone (consent), no other illnesses – mother concerned about bullying at school.

EXAM

General: tearful, uncomfortable, lying in gurney
HEENT: moist mucous membranes, TM/NP/OP clear, neck supple
Heart: tachycardic, regular, no murmur
Lungs: no wheeze, rales, or rhonchi
Abdomen: soft, nt, nd
Back: No CVA TTP
Extremities: R LE with full ROM, nl hip, knee, ankle, foot. Pt has marked TTP R thigh – no edema, erythema, crepitus, or skin changes. 2+ pulses DP/PT B LE.
Neuro: does not ambulate due to right thigh pain. 5/5 strength and normal sensation B UE and LE. 5/5 strength hip/knee/ankle flexion and extension. Normal L4/L5/S1 sensation B LE. Full ROM/no TTP C/T/L/S spine.
Skin: no rash, 1 sec CR, flushed

ORDERS (13:32)
CBC, CHEM 10, ESR [erythrocyte sedimentation rate], CRP [C-reactive protein], CK, R hip XR series, R knee XR series, R tib-fib XR series, blood culture, nasopharyngeal swab, 20 mL/kg NS bolus, ibuprofen 10 mg/kg PO x 1.

PROGRESS NOTE (14:20): Persistently tachycardic in 140s – repeat NS bolus – remains febrile now to 39 C. DDx includes bacteremia, myositis, osteomyelitis. Less likely necrotizing fasciitis given no crepitus, bullae, skin changes, skip lesions. Less likely septic joint given full ROM, no TTP hip/knee/ankle – no erythema, edema, or increased warmth.

RESULTS (14:45)

- WBC: 23.4 with 22% bands
- Chemistry: Na 136 K 3.4 Cl 108 HCO3 14 BUN 22 Cr 1.2 Gluc 128 AG 14
- ESR 42 mm/hr CRP 5 mg/dL CK 88 U/L
- UA: neg
- XR hip/knee/tib-fib series: no evidence of fracture or periosteal elevation, nl alignment

PROGRESS NOTE (14:50): **T** 37.8 **HR** 126 **BP** 114/80

Pt continues w/ discomfort after Motrin, will add morphine. Improves w/ NS bolus x 3, will continue to volume replete. Pt with compensated shock, sepsis syndrome, and concern for osteomyelitis. Repeat exam shows no signs or sx of necrotizing fasciitis or myositis. However, given marked systemic signs, will perform CT non-con RLE, consult Surgery. Pt with sepsis, not a candidate to withhold abx for OR biopsy. If osteo—will give ceftriaxone and clindamycin. Discussed plan with mother who is now here.

RESULTS (16:05): CT non-con RLE shows no evidence of stranding, abscess, gas formation. Surgery concurs.

PROGRESS NOTE: (16:20): Admit to Pediatric ICU. Pt improved hemodynamically, now more comfortable. Compensated shock resolving, now urinating. Discussed case with resident; admit to monitored bed. MRI from inpatient, ID consult, Orthopedics consult.

IMPRESSION:

1. Septic shock, fluid-responsive
2. Fever
3. Likely osteomyelitis, R femur

HOSPITAL COURSE: :

- **Blood culture:** *Staphylococcus aureus* sp
- **Urine culture** (9/16/11): negative (final)
- **MRI of the pelvis and lower extremities** (August 20th, 2009): "the shaft of the right femur shows evidence of osteolysis with a sclerotic border with septated periosteal reaction and soft-tissue swelling"…. "consistent with osteomyelitis"

FINAL DIAGNOSIS: Acute osteomyelitis, bacteremia due to Methicillin-resistant *Staphylococcus Aureus*

IV. Greg Henry Comments

"It is not necessarily negligent to misdiagnose such a case on the first visit"

Anyone who says that this would be an easy diagnosis is either deranged or an out and out liar. The vast majority of children we see do have viral conditions and this mixed bag of symptoms is difficult at best. There are general rules that apply to a child this age.

The first rule of emergency medicine is all families are dysfunctional albeit in their own way. Family problems are the rule not the exception. The ability to put family situation, mother, daughter problems or onset of adolescence, into some type of perspective is difficult at best. But objective findings don't lie. The child has a pulse rate of 126. Could it be from a virus? Of course, but it is something to consider.

Secondly, examination is just that, examination. My main criticism with the initial examination is that there is no notation as to actual pain with manipulation of the joints and extremities; no one asked her to simply point to the location of maximal pain and direct an exam to this area. The fact that the patient says she feels better is also a difficulty. Does this support the diagnosis of hysteria? Does this mean that a mild amount of Motrin has cured a viral disease? It is difficult to know. This is one of those cases where the only decent test is time.

In all honesty, any emergency physician who has practiced for a reasonable length of time has had such cases. It is easy to say this patient would have been admitted, given blood cultures, and diagnosed on the first visit, but in most places, she would have been sent home, possibly with a prescription for Cephalexin.

It is interesting to note that the bounce back takes place three days later. The reasonable question that might be asked is what were the patient and parents doing in the interim? With an initial discharge pulse rate of 134 it would seem prudent that the patient be examined the next day to see if she was improving. It is not necessarily negligent to misdiagnose such a case on the first visit, but with diagnostic uncertainty, setting up short term interval follow up is the most reasonable thing to do; three days is problematic.

On the return visit the retrospectoscope is 20/20. The patient is a totally different person; febrile, heart rate of 168, and clearly focal problems. The real questions now are bone v. soft tissue infection, medical v. surgical?

The main area of potential medical legal jeopardy stems from the actual wording on the initial discharge instructions; were they instructed to "return as needed" or was there a specific follow up plan?

PART 2—THE ANALYSIS

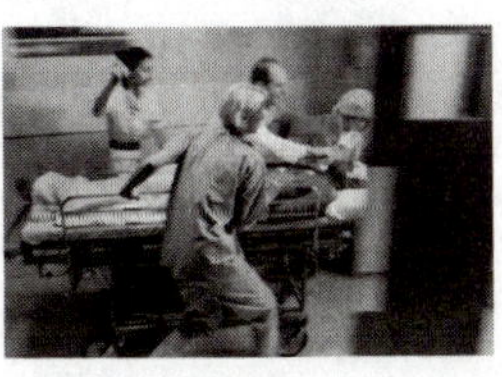

EVALUATION OF PEDIATRIC MYALGIAS, INABILITY TO AMBULATE, AND OSTEOMYELITIS OF APPENDICITIS AND THE ROLE OF ULTRASOUND

Timothy Horeczko, MD, MSCR, FACEP, FAAP

Assistant Professor of Medicine
David Geffen School of Medicine at UCLA
Department of Emergency Medicine
Harbor-UCLA Medical Center
Torrance, CA

Maribel is an 11-year-old girl with multiple psychosocial stressors, including her family's financial situation, being overweight, underperformance in school, and a difficult relationship with her mother. This is an illustrative case of the multi-factorial nature of pain: it has a physical, emotional, experiential, cultural, and contextual basis, all of which inform the patient's presentation. In the ED, of course, we assume an organic etiology until proven otherwise. The difficulty here is discerning what ratio of the above factors may explain the severity of her symptoms—is this a minor illness with a major personality component? Is this a significant illness and the patient is amplifying it, prompting those around her (including the provider) to downplay her symptoms?

The focal tenderness to palpation of her right femur is not directly addressed in the initial visit. Specific objective findings need to be accounted for or investigated further. Perhaps a more concerted follow up plan (and potentially the diagnosis itself) could have been made with some persistence in the initial evaluation. With some reflection and reframing, the etiology of her presentation may be more readily accessible; subacute symptoms of pain in a pre-adolescent with fever and focal tenderness to palpation. This may have prompted earlier investigation. On the second visit, she presents with worsening of her symptoms and systemic features. The differential diagnosis was appropriately kept open and dangerous diagnoses were considered.

When she returns, the critical action is the identification and rapid treatment of her compensated septic shock. Recall that children compensate for shock very well, as evidenced by a marked tachycardia, until they precipitously fall off the cliff into decompensated shock (i.e., hypotension, which in children is often rapidly followed by cardiac arrest). This case demonstrates the multi-faceted nature of septic shock: hypovolemic (volume depletion due to fever, insensible losses) and distributive (flushed skin and flash capillary refill as a sign of pathologic vasodilation). She received immediate and repeated isotonic boluses and responded well. She was "pulled off the cliff" just in time.

Refusal to walk and inability to ambulate in children

The etiology of acute limb pain, the refusal to walk, or inability to ambulate in children is dependent on age (e.g., toddler's fracture in children and slipped capital femoral epiphysis seen more commonly in adolescents). We'll focus here on the differential diagnosis that applies across age ranges. The four main categories for the emergency physician to consider are:

- Trauma
- Infection
- Hematologic-oncologic
- Non-traumatic orthopedic

Note: Refusal to walk or limp without leg or hip pain should prompt consideration of an expanded differential diagnoses including abdomen (appendicitis), genitalia (testicular torsion, inguinal hernia), and neuro systems (epidural abscess). Other etiologies such as inflammatory, neurologic, developmental, and psychiatric will likely either be evident by other means (e.g., limp in a child with Henoch-Schönlein purpura hopefully is diagnosed in the context of purpura), or are not essential to diagnose in the ED (e.g., growing pains, conversion disorder, or reflex sympathetic dystrophy).

1. **Traumatic conditions** should always be considered for two main reasons: a) abuse can present with vague and potential "non-acute" symptoms particularly in the preverbal children; b) children have the following mentality, "play or die." They are not interested in slowing down after acute injury and the exam may be misleading, especially when the all-too-important growth plate may be involved.
2. **Infectious etiologies** are the sneakiest of the four. Fevers abound in children, and it can be difficult to flesh out if the new symptom of pain or gait disturbance is related. In the ED, it's best to assume so until proven otherwise. Septic arthritis presents as a febrile, irritable child with resistance to bear weight or allow movement of the affected joint (note that the joint may not show signs of edema and/or erythema, particularly in the hip joint). In less straightforward cases, a thorough history and physical exam in conjunction with WBC, erythrocyte sedimentation rate (ESR), C-reactive protein (CRP), plain films, and/or joint ultrasound may help to distinguish septic arthritis from its benign distant cousin, transient (toxic) synovitis. When in doubt, tap that joint!

    - Osteomyelitis, discitis (vertebral osteomyelitis), and myositis are the trickiest of these sneaky infectious causes of gait disturbance in children, due to their sometimes-vague complaints and indolent nature.
    - Inflammation of an intervertebral disc may present with back pain, abdominal pain, vomiting, or simply refusal to walk. These children are often deceptively well appearing, but the majority will harbor a low-grade Staphylococcus aureus infection.
    - Myositis presents with features that heavily overlap with osteomyelitis. If bacterial in origin, myositis presents as a systemically ill child with focal tenderness to palpation; if viral in origin (i.e., benign acute childhood myositis), the child will present typically in the context of an influenza epidemic, with tenderness in his calves and a mildly elevated creatinine kinase. With suggestive symptoms, range every joint and percuss each vertebra.

- When considering an infectious etiology of limp or leg pain, some less common but important infectious causes may be missed: retroperitoneal abscess, epidural abscess, psoas abscess, adenitis, meningitis, and meningococcemia (bilateral leg pain is a very early presentation for meningococcemia).

3. **Hematologic-oncologic**—Bone tumors, both benign and malignant, may present with vague symptoms over a prolonged period of time. Consider with prolonged systemic symptoms, pain at night, and pain after rest. Prolonged pain or swelling after a relatively minor injury may be a harbinger for a bony tumor of childhood. Leukemia may present with bone and joint pain. A thorough skin exam may uncover easy bruising or petechiae. When in doubt, risk stratify with a WBC, and ensure close follow-up as the diagnosis may present itself in a delayed manner. Bone and joint pain in children with hematologic disorders such as sickle cell disease or hemophilia will vary in their presentation (e.g., infarction versus hemorrhage) and pathophysiology of gait disturbance.
4. **Non-traumatic orthopedic causes**—Avascular necrosis of the hip (Legg-Calvé-Perthes disease: LCP). Children typically present with slow-onset worsening pain and a trendelenburg gait (if they will walk at all) caused by weakness of the abductor muscles of the lower limb, gluteus medius and gluteus minimus. They often have limited range of the hip (especially internal rotation and abduction). Plain films may be diagnostic (see below), but MRI may be needed with high clinical suspicion. Non-concerning non-traumatic orthopedic causes include apophysitis, tendonitis, and growing pains.

Radiographic Findings of LCP

Initial findings:

Ossific nucleus fails to grow and looks smaller;
Surrounding bone may become osteopenic, causing nucleus to look more dense;
Cartilage of femoral head continues to grow and therefore medial joint space looks widened;
Crescent sign (Caffey's sign) may be seen; represents pathologic fx of resorbing femoral head and is best seen on a frog leg view of the pelvis;

Avascular stage: ossific nucleus is small, dense, and uniform;

Fragmentation stage:

Epiphysis is seen to fragment;
The dense avascular bone is replaced by radiolucent granulation tissue;

Re-ossification stage:

Radiopaque areas replace radiolucent areas;
Normal bone density returns

Overview of Osteomyelitis

Osteomyelitis in children is most often due to hematogenous spread. The primary infection may have been local, transient, trivial, and may be resolved. However, once the bone is seeded with bacteria, the course of illness is often indolent. Children may present with the refusal or inability to walk, fever, and focal tenderness to palpation, with or without outward signs of swelling. Children of all ages are at risk, especially those with recent trauma or strenuous activity. In our case, the patient was running around the block. The most common pathogens include methicillin-sensitive staphylococcus aureus (MSSA), methicillin-resistant staphylococcus aureus (MRSA) (presenting with considerably more pain, tachycardia, and fever), and Kingella kingae (difficult to culture and the most common cause in children under 4 years of age). In addition, salmonella should be considered as a causative organism in patients with sickle cell disease.

Diagnosis of Osteomyelitis

The most important step in diagnosing osteomyelitis in children is the first one: to consider it. In a child with symptoms and suggestive of osteomyelitis (focal pain and otherwise unexplained fever), obtain a CBC with differential, serum CRP and ESR, plain films, and a blood culture. If all negative (and blood culture pending) in a child with low suspicion for osteomyelitis, the patient may be discharged with close follow-up; ideally repeat CRP or ESR with serial examinations are performed until the cause of the patient's symptoms is clear.

If any of the above are suggestive (ESR, CRP, or plain films), the child should be admitted and an MRI with gadolinium, radionuclide bone scan, or CT should be used to evaluate further. The child with a high clinical suspicion of osteomyelitis—regardless of the benignity of emergency department testing—should be treated the same: admission and advanced imaging. It is perfectly rational and reasonable to admit the child with a strong suspicion of osteomyelitis and a negative initial work-up in the ED for observation and to complete the full work up in-house.

Treatment of osteomyelitis

Source control is important to address early; culprit cutaneous and intraosseous abscesses should be drained as soon as possible. The initial medical treatment of osteomyelitis is intravenous. Specific agents used will depend on the presentation and institutional practice, but considerations include: clindamycin if MRSA suspected; vancomycin for areas with high clindamycin resistance; a beta-lactam for patients younger than 4 years of age at risk for Kingella kingae; a third-generation cephalosporin for children with sickle cell disease at risk for Salmonella infection.

A reasonable initial choice for children in general is clindamycin and ceftriaxone or cefotaxime (especially if younger). Blood culture results and infectious disease specialist input later may inform the final antibiotic regimen. If the child is not systemically ill, antibiotics may be held until a deep bone biopsy can be performed. Any sign of systemic illness should prompt immediate antibiotic administration in parallel with volume resuscitation (bone biopsy may be done even after antibiotics are started, albeit with diminished yield).

Children are typically treated with parenteral antibiotics in the hospital for a few days; serial examinations, WBC, and CRP are helpful to monitor effect of therapy. Traditionally treatment is continued via a peripherally inserted central catheter (PICC) until a planned transition to oral therapy is possible. A new treatment trend in select patients with proven MSSA infection involves a week of IV antibiotics, followed by oral therapy. For all, total treatment time (regardless of setting and route) is 4–6 weeks.

Bringing it all home

In retrospect, initially Maribel had many features suggestive of osteomyelitis: vague prolonged symptoms, pain with ambulation, fever, and focal tenderness to palpation, all out of proportion to the proposed umbrella diagnosis of viral illness. Her increased strenuous physical activity just prior to her presentation may have caused some microtrauma and put her at increased risk. Not every child with flu-like symptoms should get a work-up, but the above unexplained features, even in a relatively well appearing child, warrant close follow-up. With diagnostic uncertainty, a good fail-safe for emergency physicians is a frank discussion with the family that a definitive diagnosis has not been established—only with time and another look may the diagnosis emerge. Sometimes our good habits are the only things that save us from occult illness.

References

1. Arnold JC, Cannavino CR, Ross MK, et al. Acute bacterial osteoarticular Infections: eight-Year analysis of C-reactive protein for oral step-down therapy. Pediatrics. 2012;130(4): e821–e8.
2. Dartnell J, Ramachandran M, Katchburian M. Haematogenous acute and subacute paediatric osteomyelitis: a systematic review of the literature. J Bone Joint Surg Br. 2012;94-B:584–95.
3. Frank AL, Marcinak JF, Mangat D, et al. Clindamycin treatment of methicillin-resistant Staphylococcus aureus infections in children. Pediatr Infect Dis J. 2002;21:530–4.
4. Harik NS, Smeltzer MS. Management of acute hematogenous osteomyelitis in children. Expert Rev Infect Ther. 2010; 8(2):175–81.
5. Lazzarini L, Lipsky BA, Mader JT. Antibiotic treatment of osteomyelitis: what have we learned from 30 years if clinical trials? Int J Infect Dis. 2005;9:127–38.
6. Liu C, Bayer A, Cosgrove SE, et al. Clinical practice guidelines by the infectious diseases society of America for the treatment of methicillin-resistant Staphylococcus aureus infections in adults and children. Clin Infect Dis. 2011; 52:e18–e54.
7. Pääkkönen M, Kallio MJT, Kallio PE, et al. Significance of negative cultures in the treatment of acute hematogenous bone and joint infections in children. J Pediatric Infect Dis Soc. 2013; 2:119. DOI:10.1093/jpids/pis108.
8. Pääkkönen M, Kallio MJT, Kallio PE, et al. Sensitivity of erythrocyte sedimentation rate and c-reactive protein in childhood bone and joint infections. Clin Orthop Relat Res. 2010; 468:861–6.
9. Peltola H, Pääkkönen M. Acute osteomyelitis in children. N Engl J Med. 2014;370:352–60.
10. Peltola H, Pääkkönen M, Kallio PE, et al. Clindamycin vs. first-generation cephalosporins for acute osteoarticular infections of childhood—a prospective quasi-randomized controlled trial. Clin Microbiol Infect. 2012;18:582–9.
11. Riise Ø, Kirkhus E, Handeland K, et al. Childhood osteomyelitis-incidence and differentiation from other acute onset musculoskeletal features in a population-based study. BMC Pediatrics. 2008;8:45. DOI:10.1186/1471–2431-8–45.
12. Tse SML, Laxer RM. Approach to acute limb pain in childhood. Pediatr Rev. 2006; 27(5):170–80.
13. Yagupsky P, Porsch E, St Geme JW. Kingella Kingae: an emerging pathogen in young children. Pediatrics. 2011;127(3):557–65.

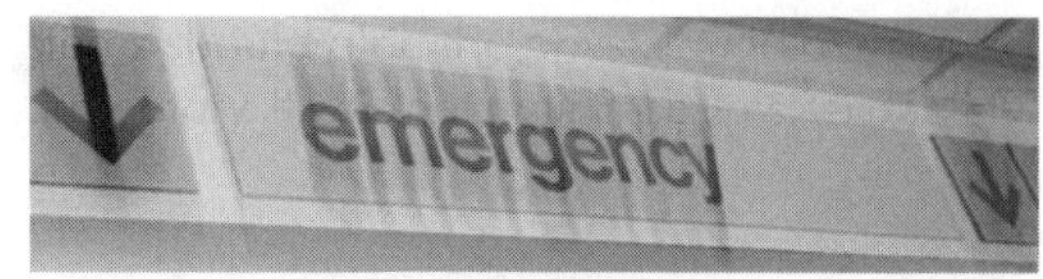

CASE 20

A 15-YEAR-OLD GIRL WITH SHORTNESS OF BREATH

J. Matthew Blickendorf, MD
Chief Resident, Department of Emergency Medicine
Wexner Medical Center at The Ohio State University

Jonathan Stevens, MD, FAAEM
Attending Emergency Physician, Immediate Health Associates
Mt. Carmel St. Ann's Hospital, Columbus, OH

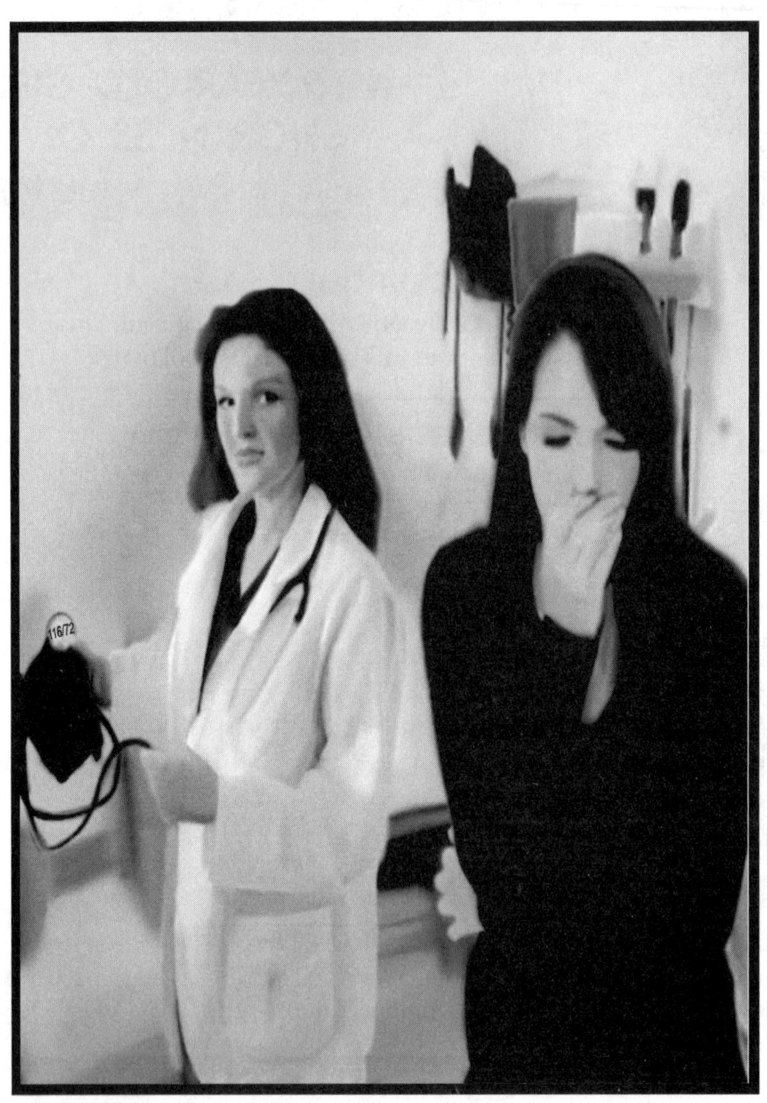
116/72

CASE 20

A 15-YEAR-OLD GIRL WITH SHORTNESS OF BREATH

PART 1—MEDICAL

I. The Doctor's Version (the following is the actual documentation of the provider)

Date: February 24, 2008 at 12:51
Chief Complaint: Shortness of breath
Nurse's Note: Sore throat, difficulty breathing, cough-barky. c/o hoarse voice for 2 days and sore throat and SOB? Patient noted to be hoarse. O2 sat 100% in RA. Pain scale 5/10.

HISTORY OF PRESENT ILLNESS (Per resident physician, Dr. Stephen Lewis):
15 y/o F h/o migraines p/w sore throat and cough. Symptoms started 3 days ago. Cough described as productive, deep with occasional throat tightening and SOB. Now has hoarse voice, bilateral ear pain, shoulder pain, myalgias. No rash, vomiting, diarrhea, dysuria. UOP ok. Decrease in PO intake but still w/ adequate fluids. Possibly had sick contact w/ friend last week.

REVIEW OF SYSTEMS: keep consistent

Constitutional: Negative for fever
ENMT: Positive for nasal congestion.
Respiratory: Positive for cough, difficulty breathing and shortness of breath
Gastrointestinal: Negative for vomiting and diarrhea.
Musculoskeletal: Positive for myalgias.
Skin: Negative for rash.
Neuro: Positive for headache.

PAST MEDICAL HISTORY:
Allergies: Sulfacetamide
Medications: Topamax
PMH: None
Social history: Exposed to tobacco smoke, attends school
Immunizations: current

EXAM:

VITAL SIGNS							
Time	Temp(C)	Rt	Pulse	Syst	Diast	Resp	Sat
12:49	37.4	oral	104	116	72	22	100%on RA

Constitutional: alert, calm, cooperative, ill appearing, non toxic state
Head and face: atraumatic, normocephalic
Eyes: conjunctivae and lid normal, EOMI, PERRL
Pharynx: oral mucosa moist
Nose: nasal mucosa normal
Ears: tympanic membrane normal
Throat: uvula midline, pharynx erythematous
Neck: supple, non-tender, ROM-full, no meningeal signs. submandibular lymphadenopathy
Respiratory: breath sounds equal bilaterally, no rales, rhonchi or wheezes, normal respiratory effort/excursion
Cardiovascular: NSR – no murmur, no friction rub, distal pulses present, strong, cap refill <2 seconds, NL S1/S2
Gastrointestinal: abdomen soft, non-tender, non-distended, no hepatosplenomegaly
Skin: skin pink, warm, and dry
Neuro: A&Ox3

ED COURSE:
12:52 – Acetaminophen 650mg PO for pain 5/10
13:42 – Rapid Strep test: negative
14:27 – XR soft tissue neck. Indication: dyspnea. Result: normal airway

MDM (15:14) - Per resident physician Dr. Stephen Lewis:
DDx includes bronchitis, strep, pneumonia, laryngitis. Croup is less likely given her age. Likely viral syndrome. Will need to treat symptomatically w OTC meds and humidified air. VS stable. No problems with breathing during ED stay

DIAGNOSIS: Laryngotracheitis

DISPOSITION (15:17): Patient was discharged home with prescriptions for acetaminophen and ibuprofen with instructions to call pediatrician or clinic, or return to ED if struggling to breathe or symptoms worsen.

MDM ADDENDUM (17:04) Per attending physician Dr. Larry Prescott:
15 y/o with hoarse voice and cough. On my exam alert, no distress, well hydrated, dry cough, no wheezing, heart murmur. Probable viral syndrome. Discussed mother and indications for return and follow up

Stephen Lewis, MD (resident)
Larry Prescott, MD (attending)

➢**Author's note (MW):** Surely there aren't any risk management or patient safety issues on this case, right? The initial visit was a slam-dunk benign flu or viral URI case. While we certainly don't advocate for a million dollar workup for URI cases, there are subtleties to the case documentation that can leave one wondering if there was more to this girl's presentation.

II.The Errors—Risk Management/Patient Safety Issues

Risk management/patient safety issue #1:

Error: Triage chief complaint does not match physician chief complaint.

Discussion: It doesn't take an emergency physician, or any physician for that matter, to know that shortness of breath or difficulty breathing is often greater cause for concern than a sore throat or cough. Despite recording the chief complaint as SOB, the triage nurse assigns this patient as low acuity and even appears to question the complaint of difficulty breathing in the note: "c/o hoarse voice for 2 days and sore throat and SOB?" The physician note minimally explores the patient's shortness of breath, the documented reason for visiting the ED. The workup and documentation aren't bad if the patient presented for sore throat and cough—but the triage note tells a different story.

✔ **Teaching point:** Chief complaints included in nursing notes should be addressed in the physician's note.

Risk management/patient safety issue #2:

Error: Triage Cueing.

Discussion: : Interestingly, this patient was triaged with a chief complaint of "SOB" but was assigned an acuity level 4 (the second to lowest level of acuity). In a busy ED, it is OK for the physician to check with nurses about the degree of SOB to verify the accuracy of the acuity level. This is one of the advantages of electronic medical record and track board. But note that the triage-assigned acuity level or location can lead to anchoring bias or diagnosis momentum. As emergency physicians, we can't let our guard down when a patient is triaged as low acuity or downplayed by other emergency department staff.[1]

✔ **Teaching point:** The provider should not be falsely assured just because a patient is assigned a low triage category.

Risk management/patient safety issue #3:

Error: Abnormal vital signs not addressed.

Discussion: The advent of the electronic medical record (EMR) and pre-populated historical components, vital signs, or physical exam findings can result in pertinent information "flying under the radar." The patient is described as "ill appearing, nontoxic." An ill appearing patient with borderline abnormal vital signs heightens the attention more than a nontoxic appearing patient with normal vital signs. This patient technically meets SIRS criteria given her mildly elevated heat rate and respiratory rates. While many patients with viral syndromes meets SIRS criteria and have self-limiting illnesses, the girl's abnormal vitals could indicate a poor trajectory and should be addressed in the note.

✔ **Teaching point:** Abnormal vital signs should be acknowledged in the note.

Risk management/patient safety issue #4:

Error: No repeat vital signs documented.

Discussion: From time of presentation to time of disposition, this patient was in the department for 2.5 hours without documentation of repeated vital signs. If this patient still had an elevated heart and respiratory rates after treatment of her pain and hours of observation, a reassessment may reveal progression of illness and an underlying diagnosis.

✔ **Teaching point:** Repeat abnormal vital signs even if they are borderline.

Risk management/patient safety issue #5:

Error: Incomplete diagnostic workup for differential diagnosis.

Discussion: The physician appropriately records a differential diagnosis and an associated diagnostic plan. Bronchitis, pneumonia, strep throat, and laryngitis are included with a plan for a rapid strep test and soft tissue neck x-rays. Soft tissue neck x-rays are often completed to aid in the diagnosis of croup, epiglottitis, retropharyngeal abscess, or enlarged tonsils and adenoids. Only one of these is included in the differential while no diagnostic test is ordered to evaluate the lower airways for bronchitis, pneumonia, or another etiology of the patient's dyspnea.

✔ **Teaching point:** Diagnoses considered in the differential should have an appropriate associated diagnostic test or an explanation of why no further workup was pursued.

Risk management/patient safety issue #6:

Error: Differential diagnosis too narrow.

Discussion: Just because it's cold and flu season doesn't mean it's always cold or flu. Since laryngotracheitis was listed as the final diagnosis, a bacterial etiology could have been entertained. In addition, was there any consideration of noninfectious causes? The patient could be tachypneic because of metabolic acidosis caused by DKA from undiagnosed diabetes. She could be tachycardic because of a pulmonary embolism or hoarse because of compression of the recurrent laryngeal nerve.

✔ **Teaching point:** Consider bacterial infections and noninfectious causes for symptoms usually attributed to viral infections.

Risk management/patient safety issue #7:

Error: Inadequate discharge instructions.

Discussion: The attending documents discussing "indications for return and follow-up." What were these specific indications? Were they geared towards upper respiratory complications such as stridor or inability to handle secretions, or lower respiratory complications such as chest pain, tachypnea or retractions? Some or all of these may have been discussed, but since it wasn't documented, the reader, and if it becomes a legal issue… the jury is left to speculate. There is also no mention of how soon the follow-up should be.

✔ **Teaching point:** Give specific indications for return and specific timeframes for follow-up. Ensure a patient has the ability and reliability to follow-up.

III. Greg Henry Comments

"There is no question that patients coming to the fast track can be just as sick as people in the main emergency department"

It is difficult to make much out of the first emergency department visit. The vast majority of 15-year-olds with these presenting complaints have viral disease. The fact that she is essentially afebrile, has normal blood pressure and a sat of 100%, tends to mitigate against severe illness. The fact that the patient's lungs are clear, heart sounds and mentation are normal also argue against severe disease. I'm in agreement that we should always keep a "high index of suspicion" for disease, but believe me, in most emergency departments this patient would not be a high priority case.

I will agree with the fact that the triage complaint and the physician chief complaint are somewhat different. This patient is here for shortness of breath. That is not the usual complaint of a 15-year-old. There is no question that patients coming to the fast track can be just as sick as people in the main emergency department. Anchoring bias affects us all.

The real risk management take home point is that a short term interval should follow such cases. Repeating abnormal vital signs is important, but even if they had been back into the normal range, if the patient is not substantially improving in the next 12 hours, she needs to be seen. Calling to get an examination date within three weeks at a primary care office is not acceptable. The discharge instructions need to be time and action specific.

✔ **Madeline Matar Joseph teaching point:**
Though many of these patients will improve with symptomatic treatment, including antipyretics, a patient described as "ill appearing" should not be placed directly into the urgent care setting. Some children with 104 temperature look ill, but after getting the fever down, they are bouncing off the walls and the parents are asking to go home!

IV. The Bounceback

February 26, 2008 at 9:37am (2 days after ED visit) – Phone call to ED. Patient now complaining of pain in side of chest. Wants to know if she should return to ED. RN recommends calling PCP office to arrange follow-up appointment.

February 26, 2008 at 10:21am – Phone call to PCP. Patient with entire chest hurting, very difficult to breathe, feels short of breath. Patient difficult to understand due to raspy voice. Referred to ED.

ED RETURN – Feb 27th (3 days after initial ED visit)

VITAL SIGNS							
Time	Temp(C)	Rt	Pulse	Syst	Diast	Resp	Sat
12:19	38.2	oral	162	125	64	62	78% on RA

- Physician notes previous visit. Chest exam with decreased aeration in bilateral bases with right-sided crackles. CXR shows pneumonia and patient is admitted.
- 15:52 – Pt decompensates and is placed on BiPAP in PICU. Viral swab positive for Influenza A. Blood culture is gram stain positive for MRSA.
- Patient continues to decompensate overnight and is intubated.
- Remains on high frequency ventilation. Cool extremities but stable blood pressures.
- February 28th ECMO is initiated.
- Bronchoscopy is performed: There are copious brown secretions indicative of ongoing bleeding and obstructive clots. There are specimens of material with appearance suspicious for lung parenchyma.
- Patient's mental status decompensates and she has brain CT which shows large frontal and parietal intracranial hemorrhage (ICH) and right intraocular hemorrhage.
- ECMO is discontinued. Morphine is administered.
- Family agrees with comfort care and patient is pronounced in the early evening.

AUTOPSY – March 11, 2008

Final anatomic diagnoses (abbreviated):

- Bilateral necrotizing pneumonia, MRSA, s/p influenza A infection
- Multiple pulmonary abscesses
- Bilateral pulmonary congestion and hemorrhage
- Subarachnoid hemorrhage involving both frontal lobes, temporoparietal lobes, and left occipital lobe
- Right frontal lobe hematoma (3.5cm x 3.0cm)

In summary, this patient died as a result of respiratory failure secondary to a severe necrotizing pneumonia caused by *Staphylococcus aureus* (MRSA) complicating an influenza A virus infection leading to sepsis with DIC accounting for bleeding in the lungs and brain.

IV. Greg Henry Comments—Continued

"All I can say is, I'm glad I wasn't the physician on the first visit"

The tragedy in this case is the patient may have had a treatable illness. Not all cases such as this will survive, but at least they should be seen back in a time frame within which action can be taken. Parenthetically, the patient's visit three days later presents a totally different disease and a totally different level of illness. A pulse rate of 162 and a pulse of 104 have nothing to do with each other. All I can say is, I'm glad I wasn't the physician on the first visit.

PART 2—THE ANALYSIS

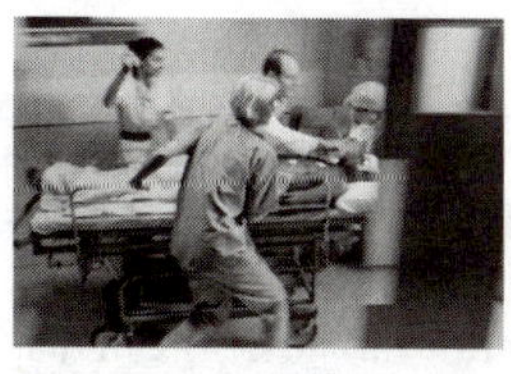

UPPER RESPIRATORY TRACT INFECTIONS AND METHICILLIN-RESISTANT STAPHYLOCOCCUS (MRSA) PNEUMONIA APPENDICITIS AND THE ROLE OF ULTRASOUND

J. Matthew Blickendorf, MD
Chief Resident, Department of Emergency Medicine
Wexner Medical Center at The Ohio State University

Jonathan Stevens, MD, FAAEM
Attending Emergency Physician, Immediate Health Associates
Mt. Carmel St. Ann's Hospital, Columbus, OH

Differentiating URI histories

This otherwise healthy 15-year-old girl presented with chief complaints among the most common to emergency medicine. Most of us saw this girl or someone similar during our last shift in the ED—and depending on the season, we may have seen 10–15 such patients during the same shift! Keeping the mantra of emergency medicine, "think worst first," is difficult in the peak of flu and cold season.

The approach to this patient should be no different than any other emergency department patient: Construction of a differential diagnosis and diagnostic workup based on the history and physical examination. Reviewing the triage notes, vital signs, and nursing assessment prior to evaluating the patient helps direct the history and physical.

In this case, the attending's understanding of this girl's presentation was framed first by the resident—potentially leading to anchoring bias, diagnosis momentum, or premature closure. As discussed in Risk Management/Patient Safety Issue #1, the resident records the chief complaint as "sore throat and cough" while the patient's "shortness of breath and difficulty breathing" are barely mentioned in the note. A resident presentation focused on a chief complaint of dyspnea may have elicited an alternative differential and workup from the attending physician, perhaps a chest x-ray. Those working with resident physicians or MLPs must be cognizant of the high potential for overlooked historical elements or exam findings. Reconfirming the chief complaint with the patient upon the reexamination by the attending is very important to avoid such bias. (It also helps with the patient satisfaction scores.)

This girl's symptoms do not uniquely fit into one illness script. Influenza causes fever, chills, myalgias, headache, cough, and rhinitis. The common cold causes nasal congestion, rhinorrhea, sneezing, sore throat, and dry cough.[2] These viral syndromes explain all her symptoms except… the shortness of breath (which was her chief complaint!)

Shortness of breath is a symptom of *lower* respiratory illness. The physician note identifies bronchitis and pneumonia as potential diagnoses. Patients with bronchitis experience cough, fever, myalgias, sore throat, nasal congestion, and even dyspnea or chest discomfort. The physical examination may be normal or demonstrate tachypnea, tachycardia, fever, wheezing, rhonchi or rales.

Critical to the diagnosis of bronchitis, however, is the *lack* of pneumonia, asthma or an alternative explanation of symptoms. Tintinalli states, "The primary objective in patient evaluation is carefully excluding pneumonia, either clinically or radiographically."[2] In the case of a young girl who bounces back with severe necrotizing pneumonia after presenting with flu or bronchitis symptoms initially, the question is whether an early pneumonia was missed at the first visit. With a second presentation 3 days later, pneumonia (as a complication of flu) seems to have developed. Hence, in pediatrics we prefer 24 hour follow up in case something early is "brewing."

Workup of URI symptoms...to image or not to image, that is the question

One could argue that this presentation may not have required any further workup past a simple H&P. Regarding the sore throat, this patient had a Centor Criteria score of one, recommending no further testing or antibiotics.[3, 4] Regarding the neck x-rays, the patient was tolerating PO without stridor, dysphagia, neck stiffness, or drooling. The physician properly stated that croup was unlikely due to age. Based on her symptoms, a decision was made to image the upper airway instead of the lower airway. Was the pretest probability high enough to warrant a soft tissue neck x-ray?

In reviewing the medical record of this case, it's interesting to note that the repeat ED visit note, the admitting H&P, and even the autopsy report mention that the patient had a negative chest x-ray during the initial ED visit, a study that was not actually done. The admission notes almost imply that *of course* a chest x-ray was ordered during the initial visit. Does a patient's complaint of shortness of breath warrant a chest x-ray? Was the physician's clinical gestalt enough to rule out pneumonia?

Based solely on the history and physical exam, physicians are poor at distinguishing pneumonia from other respiratory illnesses in adults[5-8] and children.[9] Adults who lack abnormal vital signs or physical exam findings can be identified as low risk for pneumonia,[7, 8, 10] and studies of children have demonstrated similar findings.[11-13]

While she had no positive findings on chest auscultation, this young girl did have abnormal vital signs. Her only recorded vital signs were from triage with a respiratory rate of 22 and heart rate of 104 beats per minute. Especially in light of presenting with a chief complaint of shortness of breath and difficulty breathing and ill appearing, an early pneumonia may have been picked up on a screening chest x-ray. But would the diagnosis and treatment of a typical community-acquired pneumonia have altered this girl's prognosis?

MRSA pneumonia

Staphylococcus aureus has been well recognized for decades as a cause of community-acquired pneumonia (CAP). An infrequent cause of CAP, *S. aureus* pneumonia is more common in patients with chronic lung disease, patients with laryngeal cancer, immunosuppressed patients, nursing home patients, intravenous drug users, or others at risk for aspiration pneumonia.[14, 15] In healthy patients, *S. aureus* pneumonias have been well described after viral illnesses like influenza. Despite a typically insidious onset of disease with low-grade fever, sputum production, and dyspnea, chest x-rays demonstrate extensive disease with empyema, pleural effusions, cavitation, and multiple areas of infiltrate. These patients often require ICU admission.[14, 15]

Until recently, methicillin-resistant *S. aureus* (MRSA) pneumonia has been almost exclusively confined to the health-care setting. The first fatal community-acquired MRSA (CA-MRSA) pneumonia and bacteremia in the U.S. was reported in children in 1999[16] and in adults in 2005.[17] Since then, descriptions of this severe form of CAP have been limited mostly to case reports and series.

The prevalence and incidence of invasive CA-MRSA infections likely varies geographically. In the United States, 2% of CA-MRSA infections cause invasive pneumonia, and 14% of all invasive MRSA infections are CA-MRSA pneumonia.[18] Albeit uncommon, CA-MRSA pneumonia generally affects young and previously healthy patients, especially in the post-influenza setting.[15, 18] In a case series of 10 patients during the 2003–2004 influenza season, the median age was 17.5 years and all had preceding or concurrent influenza-like illness.[21]

Community-associated strains of MRSA are more likely to cause severe disease. The severity of disease in CA-MRSA has been linked to the presence of a staphylococcal toxin known to be associated with tissue necrosis called Panton-Valentine leucocidin, a toxin that is found in less than 5% of health-care associated strains of MRSA (HA-MRSA).[18]

Clinical presentation is typically a severe pneumonia with high fever, hypotension, and hemoptysis progressing rapidly to septic shock requiring ventilator support.[18] The rapid progression of this disease distinguishes it from HA-MRSA and other severe pneumonias. In two case series the median time from symptom onset to death was 4 days (range 1 to 33 days)[19] and 3.5 days (range 2 to 25 days).[21] In contrast to other bacterial pneumonias, leukopenia is prominent feature and indicates a poor prognosis. Like other non-MRSA staphylococcal pneumonias, more than a quarter of patients with CA-MRSA pneumonia have multi-lobar infiltrates and/or cavitation on imaging studies.[18] Among 46 cases noted during the 2006–2007 influenza season, initial chest x-rays were abnormal in 91% of patients.[19] Many reports from the U.S. and Europe note mortalities greater than 50%.[18]

Despite the many publications describing CA-MRSA pneumonia, our understanding is limited to case reports. We have limited data to predict who is at higher risk of CA-MRSA pneumonia.[20] No clinical, radiographic, or laboratory findings clearly identify patients with *S. aureus* pneumonia.[19]

It is recommended that patients presenting to the ED with severe, life threatening, community-acquired pneumonia warranting admission to step-down or the ICU be empirically treated for MRSA with vancomycin or linezolid.[15, 18, 20, 21] Empiric treatment for CA-MRSA would also be appropriate with suspicion of recent or concurrent influenza, a rapid progression of symptoms, necrotizing appearance on chest imaging, or history of MRSA infection.[20, 21]

Back to our case

Regarding the case of this unfortunate young girl, it's difficult to know if a radiographic pneumonia would have been present on a chest x-ray during the initial visit. It's even more difficult to assume that her ED disposition or subsequent clinical course would have been altered by the diagnosis and appropriate treatment of a community-acquired pneumonia—antibiotics with inadequate coverage of MRSA pneumonia—at the initial visit. However, explicit return precautions emphasized prior to discharge may have resulted in a sooner return to the ED.

The choices of empiric antibiotics given during the second ED visit are unknown, but earlier empiric treatment with vancomycin or linezolid based upon her bounceback vital signs and physical exam may have lead to a better outcome. While not every ED patient with URI symptoms should have a screening chest x-ray and not every discharged CAP should be treated with MRSA coverage, we must keep CA-MRSA pneumonia on our radars, especially during influenza season in otherwise healthy adolescents and young adults.

Chapter Summary

This is a tragic case of an otherwise healthy 15-year-old girl with a relatively benign physical exam who reported symptoms that are a dime-a-dozen in any emergency department. It is hard to accuse the initial physicians of missing an obvious or even occult pneumonia, let alone necrotizing MRSA pneumonia. However, the cases in this book are not designed to help the physician reach the standard of care, but to prompt consideration of subtle clues, enhance the differential diagnosis, and provide tips on documentation to reach *excellence* in care.

✔ Teaching points about case

- Differential diagnosis and workup needs to reflect the chief complaint.
- Be vigilant for red flags in patients triaged to lower acuities.
- Have an explanation for unexplained abnormal vital signs and repeat prior to discharge.
- "Ill-appearing" patients require more attention to borderline abnormal vital signs and repeat vitals after intervention. If the patient is sent home, arranging for a closer follow up time is important.
- Give specific discharge instructions with appropriate follow-up timeframes and inquire regarding any obstacles to such follow up.
- Community-acquired MRSA pneumonia is a complication which can be seen in young and healthy patients with preceding influenza infection.

References

1. Croskerry P. Achieving quality in clinical decision making: cognitive strategies and detection of bias. Acad Emerg Med. 2002; 9(11):1184–204.
2. Lefebvre CW. Acute Bronchitis and Upper Respiratory Infections. In: Tintinalli JE, Stapczynski JS, Ma OJ, et al (eds). Tintinalli's Emergency Medicine. 8th Ed. New York, NY: McGraw Hill; 2014. http://accessemergencymedicine.mhmedical.com.proxy.lib.ohio-state.edu/content.aspx?bookid= 693&Sectionid=49251512. Accessed May 03, 2014.
3. Centor RM, Witherspoon JM, Dalton HP, et al. The diagnosis of strep throat in adults in the emergency room. Med Decis Making. 1981; 1(3):239–46.

4. Bisno AL, Gerber MA, Gwaltney JM, et al. Infectious Diseases Society of America: Practice guidelines for the diagnosis and management of group A streptococcal pharyngitis. Clin Infect Dis. 2002; 35(2): 113–25.
5. Emerman CL, Dawson N, Speroff T, et al. Comparison of physician judgment and decision aids for ordering chest radiographs for pneumonia in outpatients. Ann Emerg Med. 1991; 20(11):1215–19.
6. Graffelman AW, le Cessie S, Knuistingh Neven A, et al. Can history and exam alone reliably predict pneumonia? J Fam Pract. 2007; 56(6):465–70.
7. Metlay JP, Kapoor WN, Fine MJ. Does this patient have community-acquired pneumonia? Diagnosing pneumonia by history and physical examination. JAMA. 1997; 278:1440–45.
8. O'Brien WT Sr, Rohweder DA, Lattin GE Jr, et al. Clinical indicators of radiographic findings in patients with suspected community-acquired pneumonia: who needs a chest x-ray? J Am Coll Radiol. 2006; 3:703–6.
9. Ayalon I, Glatstein MM, Zaidenberg-Israeli G, et al. The role of physical examination in establishing pneumonia. Pediatric Emerg Care. 2013; 29(8):893–6.
10. Nolt BR, Gonzales R, Maselli J, et al. Vital-sign abnormalities as predictors of pneumonia in adults with acute cough illness. Am J Emerg Med. 2007; 25(6):631–6.
11. Lynch T, Platt R, Gouin S, et al. Can we predict which children with clinically suspected pneumonia will have the presence of focal infiltrates on chest radiographs? Pediatrics. 2004; 113(3 Pt 1):e186–9.
12. Bilkis MD, Gorgal N, Carbone M, et al. Validation and development of a clinical prediction rule in clinically suspected community-acquired pneumonia. Pediatric Emerg Care. 2010; 26(6):399–405.
13. Neuman MI, Monuteaux MC, Scully KJ, et al. Prediction of pneumonia in a pediatric emergency department. Pediatrics. 2011; 128(2):246–53.
14. Tintinalli JE, et al, eds. Community-acquired pneumonia. In Tintinalli's Emergency Medicine: A Comprehensive Study Guide, 7th ed. (2010 McGraw-Hill).
15. Moran GJ, Talan DA. Pneumonia. In: Marx JA, Hockberger RS, Walls RM (eds). Rosen's Emergency Medicine. 8th Ed. Philadelphia, PA: Elsevier Saunders; 2014:978–87.
16. Centers for Disease Control and Prevention. Four pediatric deaths from community-acquired methicillin-resistant Staphylococcus aureus: Minnesota and North Dakota, 1997–1999. JAMA. 1999; 282:1123–5.
17. Francis JS, Doherty MC, Lopatin U, et al. Severe community-onset pneumonia in healthy adults caused by methicillin-resistant Staphylococcus aureus carrying the Panton-Valentine leukocidin genes. Clin Infect Dis. 2005; 40:100–7.
18. Hidron AI, Low CE, Honig EG, et al. Emergence of community-acquired methicillin-resistant Staphylococcus aureus strain USA300 as a cause of necrotizing community-onset pneumonia. Lancet Infect Dis. 2009; 9:384–92.
19. Kallen AJ, Brunkard J, Moore Z, et al. Staphylococcus aureus community-acquired pneumonia during the 2006 to 2007 influenza season. Ann Emerg Med. 2009; 53(3):358–65.
20. Moran GJ, Talan DA. MRSA community-acquired pneumonia: should we be worried? Ann Emerg Med. 2009; 53(3):366–68.

21. Talan DA, Moran GJ, Pinner R. Update on emerging infections: news from the Centers for Disease Control and Prevention. Ann Emerg Med. 2007; 50(5):612–4.

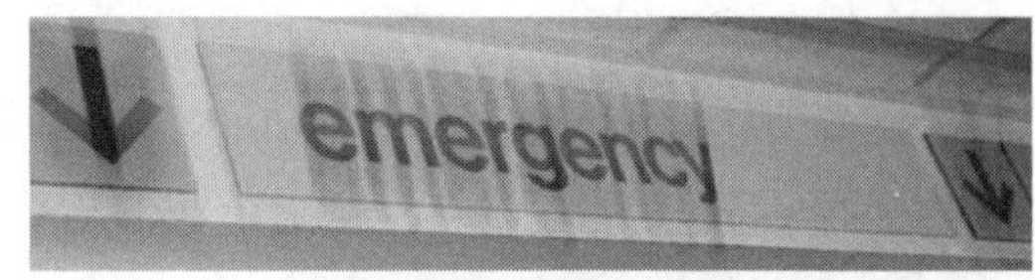

CASE 21

9-YEAR-OLD WITH FEVER AND HEADACHE

Madhu Hardasmalani, MD, FACEP, FAAP
Pediatric Emergency Medicine
Keck school of medicine
LAC+USC Medical Center

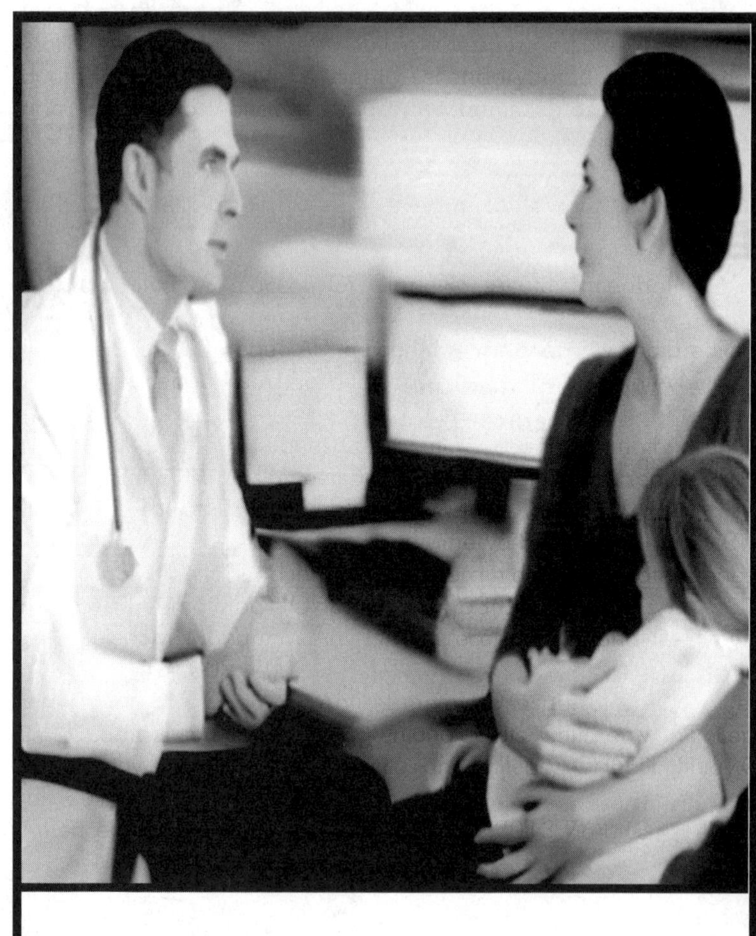

"She has a headache, fix her!"

CASE 21

9-YEAR-OLD WITH FEVER AND HEADACHE

PART 1—MEDICAL

I. The Doctor's Version (the following is the actual documentation of the provider)

Date : 11/30/2013 at 21:37.

Chief Complaint: Headache, nausea, vomiting and dizziness.

Nurse note: Headache 10/10, fever 5hrs ago, +nausea, +vomiting, + dizziness, no nuchal rigidity, no photosensitivity, no trauma. Alert, attentive, no acute distress, Cap refill <2secs, no rash.

HISTORY OF PRESENT ILLNESS (Per resident): 9yr, presents with fever x 1 day and headache, no cough, ear pain, sore throat, + congestion, vomiting x 1.
No abdominal pain, diarrhea, dysuria, no change in mental status, no rash. Fever to 104°F resolved with Tylenol. No photophobia.

REVIEW OF SYSTEMS : Positive for chills, nausea.

PAST MEDICAL HISTORY : H/O Septic arthritis (ankle) 1 year ago, H/O Urinary tract infection.
Allergies – NKDA.
Social History: Lives with mom and 2 siblings, attends school.

VITAL SIGNS

Time	Temp	Heart Rate	Resp	Syst	Diast
21:37	98	143	20	107	71

General: Well nourished, alert, attentive, A&O x 3. Uncomfortable but nontoxic. Smiling. No acute distress.
Head : Pain to palpation over frontal head.
Eyes: PERL. —PERRL.
Ent: oropharynx clear, neck supple, + congestion on exam.
Lungs: CTA bilaterally.
Heart: normal rate, rhythm.
Abdomen: soft, nontender.
Neuro: responds appropriately, motor-grossly intact, normal gait.

Extremities: no deformities/edema.
Skin: no rash.

DECISION MAKING: 9yr F with headache and fever x 1 day. Patient well appearing, neck supple, uncomfortable but nontoxic and congested on exam. Will treat with Motrin, check urine, if negative will dc home as this is likely Viral URI. Very low suspicion for meningitis given the well appearance of patient and supple neck.

ED COURSE: PO Motrin 400 mg administered.
Urine dipstick +large hemolyzed blood. Negative ketones, glucose, leucocytes and nitrites. Headache improved.

DIAGNOSIS (22:43): Viral URI.

DISPOSITION: Return if symptoms get worse or any concerns.

➢Authors' Note (MW):
For this case, we will let the reader draw their own conclusions ... were there red flags not addressed? Were there positive test results not explored further? Was the bounceback avoidable? Following is the return visit, then an in-depth exploration of the initial visit by Dr. Hardasmalani, followed by some personal comments, and as always, Greg Henry's wit and wisdom!

II.The Bounceback

ED visit # 2:12/01/2013 17:01 (Almost 17hours after initial ED visit).

Chief Complaint: Headache and vomiting worsening. Not acting right. Patient ambulated to the room.

VITAL SIGNS

Temp	Pulse	Resp	Syst	Diast	O2 sats
97.4	163	22	87	49	100%

O/E: A&O x 3. Patient appeared confused, she called her father her brother. In obvious distress. Patient complained of headache and abdominal pain. Also bloody emesis about 10 times.
HEENT: WNL. Neck – supple.
Lungs: Clear bilaterally.
Heart: S1S2- normal.
Abdomen: distended, epigastric tenderness, absent bowel sounds.
Neuro: Deferred complete neuro exam. Nonfocal and grossly intact.
Skin: warm , cap refill <2 secs. No rash.

ED COURSE :

- Blood was sent for full sepsis evaluation. IV fluid bolus initiated. As the fluid bolus was administered patient stated she felt better. She asked for water. Her vital signs improved. Heart rate decreased to 130/min.

- Her lab results started pouring in : Bicarb of 9, Platelets- 19000, WBC- 3500, PT/PTT-43.1/131.2 , Creat-2.5, AST- 250, ALT- 220, lactate- 16, fibrinogen <3, d-dimer>10000.
- Chest X-ray – no infiltrate.
- As the second fluid bolus and IV Ceftriaxone were started she appeared edematous and developed ecchymosis on the thighs.
- She was transferred to PICU at 19:50. Vitals at time of transfer: Pulse 133, Resp 29, BP 93/56, sat 100%

ED DIAGNOSIS: Septic Shock with DIC.

HOSPITAL COURSE:

- Despite fluid resuscitation in the PICU, her clinical condition continues to deteriorate and she becomes hypotensive
- Pt is started on vasopressors. IV Vancomycin, Zosyn, Amikacin were administered. Blood pressure remains low
- She is intubated
- Condition worsens with increased ecchymosis, bleeding, low cardiac output.
- Pt suddenly goes into pulseless electrical activity (PEA). CPR is started.
- Despite 20 minutes of CPR, spontaneous circulation could not be attained. She is pronounced dead at 0040.
- Microbiology department calls PICU – blood culture positive for Group A streptococcus

AUTOPSY:

- Lungs – With areas of atelectasis and bronchopneumonia. Heart – normal. Brain and meninges- normal.
- Appendix- hyperemic with pus in the lumen.
- Tissues with evidence of significant capillary leak.

CAUSE OF DEATH (per autopsy): Septicemia due to appendicitis.

PART 2—THE ANALYSIS

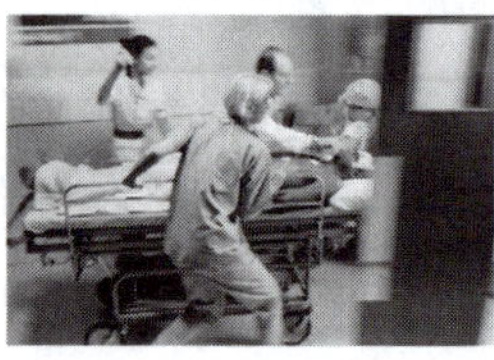

EVALUATION OF HEADACHE AND DIZZINESS, PEDIATRIC SEPSIS + THE STORY BEHIND THE STORY/ A PERSONAL NOTE

Madhu Hardasmalani, MD, FACEP, FAAP
Pediatric Emergency Medicine
Keck school of medicine
LAC+USC Medical Center

A personal note

I was the attending when the patient bounced back. It was scary!!

She was tachycardic, tachypneic denied neck pain or headache but kept saying that her belly hurts. She had epigastric tenderness, slightly distended abdomen and the overlying skin looked a bit erythematous. No rash. There were no bowel sounds. Her extremities were warm, flash capillary refill. As the first bolus was half way through, she stated "she felt better," she asked if she could have some water to drink. Her heart rate dropped from 163 to 130/min.

Blood pressure measurement was an issue. We were using adult pressure cuff, because with the pediatric cuff her reading was abnormally high, like 150/110, which we knew was not accurate. Our differential was sepsis but to evaluate for specific etiologies, such as pneumonia, pancreatitis, appendicitis, volvulus, initial presentation of DKA (which was ruled out soon by accucheck of 65mg/dl), meningitis and encephalitis.

As soon as she got IV Ceftriaxone she went downhill. She became edematous. Her thighs now had purpura; it was bad. She was slowly slipping away. I had to sit down. I knew her chances of surviving were very slim. She was pronounced at midnight in the PICU exactly one day after initially presenting with headache, dizziness and fever.

Debriefing

I discussed the case with the physicians who were involved in the initial visit. At that visit the mother seemed concerned about the patient mainly because she had lost her other daughter to meningitis! The patient's symptoms of headache, fever and vomiting worried mom and so she brought her to the ED.

"But the patient looked so good!!," the physicians said. Both the attending and the resident had sat down in the room with mom and reassured her that there is no signs of meningitis, no neck stiffness, no photophobia, normal mentation, she probably has a virus and would be better in 2–3 days.

We get this frequently; patients do come to get a breast lump checked out "because my aunt was recently diagnosed with breast cancer" or "My child has headaches, I'm worried because my cousin's son was recently diagnosed with brain tumor. He too had headaches." Do we evaluate them for breast cancer or do a brain CT of the child who looks like a peach?? Certainly not.

In this case a sibling died of "meningitis." Also the patient had 2 significant past histories of significant infections —pyelonephritis requiring inpatient management and septic arthritis. Were these be clues to an underlying immunodeficiency?

Greg Henry Comments

"I hate this case! Reading it sends chills up and down my spine"

I hate this case! Reading it sends chills up and down my spine. How many children like this have you seen in your career? It seems that the examination clearly ruled out meningitis, and indeed that was not the cause of her demise. It is interesting to note that with appendicitis from streptococcus this child had no abdominal pain, and no abdominal tenderness.

The term sepsis is thrown around too much these days. Under the new guidelines the average strep throat could be considered sepsis. This is done to show "how effective" our sepsis protocols are. I think the first visit in the child, except for the non-repeat of the pulse, was reasonable. Even with an elevated heart rate, exactly what would have caused you to work this child up for appendicitis? This is a one in a million case. I'm glad I was not the initial physician.

Continuation of Dr. Harasmalani's Discussion

Dissecting the case—the initial visit

For now, let's dissect this case: Presenting complaint—headache, fever, vomiting, dizziness and final diagnosis—Sepsis.

First of all pediatric sepsis is the buzz word now in the medical community. Early recognition is being emphasized very vigorously by ACEP and Pediatric Critical care physicians.[1,2]

There is a certain baggage that is associated with using the term septic shock. Shock for most of us is a child who is obtunded, hypotensive, mottled who needs the ICU. But that is too late in the game. The catch is to identify patients very early in the sepsis continuum.[3] A child who is febrile, tachycardic, tachypneic, with cap refill of 3 seconds and cool extremities is in septic shock even with normal blood pressure and normal urine output. Early recognition requires identifying those patients before any major organ dysfunction, patients with subtle changes in signs and symptoms that need to be explored, evaluated and managed expeditiously.[4,5]

Some can argue that the panel's broad definition of sepsis—systemic inflammatory response syndrome (SIRS) plus infection—would encompass a disproportionate number of infants and children in the emergency department.[6] This is probably true because we encounter febrile children all the time that are tachycardic and tachypneic. Considering sepsis in every child who comes to the ED for fever and is tachycardic is ridiculous, because Viral illness is the most common diagnosis. We should not be inserting IV's, fluid resuscitating and giving antibiotics to these patients!!

Clues which could have altered the outcome

Let's analyze this case and look for clues that may have altered the outcome.

The patient, 9-year-old female, with past medical history significant for urinary tract infection and septic arthritis presented to the emergency department with acute onset of headache, fever, vomiting and dizziness. She was well appearing, ambulatory and without any focality. She had no runny nose or sore throat nor did she have ear pain. She had no symptoms of upper respiratory tract infection!! So how can we diagnose her condition as a URI?? Her symptoms of headache, vomiting and dizziness point to central nervous system or a systemic condition.

In the ED she was afebrile but yet her headache was 10/10 which seems odd. Most headaches that are due to fever (secondary to vasodilation) resolve when the fever resolves. But in our patient it persisted.

Headache is a common complaint in the pediatric emergency department and most of them are due to URI.[7] Our patient had tenderness over frontal sinuses so what does this mean? I don't know. Frontal sinuses do not fully develop until adolescence; sinusitis is unlikely in that age group. Could her headache be due to be meningitis? She had a normal neurologic examination and a supple neck, but in many cases of meningitis, neck stiffness may not develop for 12–24 hrs. Neck pain, neck stiffness, positive kerning's and positive brudzinski's are useful if present but useless to rule out the disease if absent.[8]

Her initial complaint in triage was also dizziness. There is no mention of this in the physician H&P. This could mean one of two things: either the physician did not specifically ask for this or asked but the patient denied. If patient denied it needs to be discussed in the note. If there is a discrepancy with the nursing triage complain this should be corrected by the physician.[9]

Dizziness could mean either she was vertiginous or felt lightheaded. My guess is that she was light headed. However, a better description of this symptom in the physician's H&P would have been valuable.

The most important clue—tachycardia and sepsis

But the most important clue in this case is the tachycardia. A resting heart rate of 143/min is significantly high in a 9-year-old patient; a normal heart rate in a patient this age is 60–100/min. This is a huge red flag. To me it suggests that at this visit she was compensating to the decreased peripheral vascular tone by increasing her heart rate and maintaining a normal blood pressure. She was in the SIRS stage. The decreased peripheral vascular could also explain her dizziness/light headedness.

There is no explanation for her tachycardia. She wasn't febrile. She could be anxious or was in pain—had headache 10/10 when she first came into the hospital so tachycardia could be because of that. But it should have been repeated. Not doing so is an error. If heart rate was repeated and still elevated then the most prudent thing to do would be continued observation and reassessments. If she had sustained tachycardia, then sepsis work up and treatment was warranted.

Heart rate abnormalities will be present early in the course of sepsis.[10] Tachycardia is the hallmark of compensated shock. This simple vital sign measurement will help in diagnosing patients early on before sepsis or septic shock develops. Aggressive treatment at this stage has shown to significantly improve outcomes.[10]

In the busy emergency department, there are many barriers to shock recognition in the early compensated stage. These include variation in health care worker experience, high background rates of pediatric tachycardia leading to blunted recognition, tachycardia attributed to other causes or tachycardia unrecognized as a sign of compensated shock.[11]

Febrile children will typically be tachycardic; usually 10 beats for every 2° F elevation in temperature.[12] Anything outside that range needs explanation, such as pain, anxiety, crying, febrile, dehydrated!!

Also, was there an unrecognized immunodeficiency condition in the family? The sister died of meningitis and the patient herself had two significant infections in the past.

That being said, she had Group A Streptococcal sepsis, which is extremely aggressive with high morbidity and mortality. Most patients are seen early in the course of the disease by primary care physicians or emergency physicians only to return in the next 12–24 hrs in full blown sepsis. Initially the signs and symptoms are mild and nonspecific. Eighty percent of patients develop clinical signs of soft tissue infection that progress to necrotizing fasciitis or myositis. Of the 20% of cases without soft tissue findings, a variety of clinical presentations have been observed, such as myositis, perihepatitis, peritonitis, myocarditis, and overwhelming sepsis.[13]

My take on this case (Madhu)

My two cents, yes the standard of care was violated; heart rate should have been repeated to make sure there was no sustained tachycardia. If the elevated heart rate persisted then work up and treatment of sepsis should have been initiated.

Madeline Matar Joseph Comments: Reading this case hurts my stomach!

The last assessment before being discharged home indicated that the patient was "uncomfortable but nontoxic." What does that mean? Where was the source of her *discomfort*? It seems that the concentration by the physician was on one system only: CNS/meningitis. One of the most common serious bacterial infections in females with high fever is UTI/pyelonephritis, but there was not a good history of urinary symptoms or exam (CVA tenderness) which explored for this. She had + large blood on the urine point of care testing (POCT), so this is one possibility. Most of children with UTI initially look good even in the presence of bacteremia.

Chapter Summary (Madhu)

To avoid death in less than 24hrs from overwhelming sepsis in a seemingly well child during the winter season when most emergency departments are teeming with flu and viral illness cases consider the following:

1. Be cautious while diagnosing Viral URI. Patients should have symptoms of upper respiratory tract infection, such as nasal discharge, sore throat or otitis media.
2. Read the triage note carefully and document any discrepancies in history or physical exam findings.
3. Pay attention to less sought after histories such as past medical and family history and look for any connection to the presenting complaint.
4. Most importantly—repeat abnormal vital signs!! Recording, analyzing and treating abnormal vital signs is the standard of care.

References

1. Surviving Sepsis Campaign Committee. Surviving Sepsis Campaign: International Guidelines for Management of Severe Sepsis and Septic Shock: 2012, Critical Care Med. 2013;41(2):580–637.
2. Brierly J, et al. Clinical practice parameters for hemodynamic support of pediatric and neonatal septic shock: 2007 update from the American College of Critical Care Medicine. Critical Care Med. 2009;37(2):666–88.
3. Goldstein B, Giroir B. International pediatric sepsis consensus conference: definitions for sepsis and organ dysfunction in pediatrics. Pediatr Crit Care Med. 2005;6 (1):2–8.
4. Han YY, Carcillo JA, Dragotta MA., et al. Early reversal of pediatric-neonatal septic shock by community physicians is associated with improved outcome. Pediatr. 2003;112(4):793–9.
5. Launay E, Gras-Le Guen C, Martinot A, et al. Suboptimal care in the initial management of children who died from severe bacterial infection: a population-based confidential inquiry. Pediatr Crit Care Med. 2010;11(4):469–74.
6. Kissoon N. Sepsis Guideline Implementation: benefits, pitfalls and possible solutions. Crit Care. 2014;18(2):207.
7. Lewis DW, Qureshi F Acute headache in children and adolescents presenting to the emergency department. Headache. 2000;40 (3):200–3.
8. Amarilyo G, et al, Diagnostic accuracy of clinical symptoms and signs in children with meningitis. Pediatr Emer Care. 2011;27:196–9.
9. Anderson RE. Medical malpractice: a physician's sourcebook. 1st ed. 2005:104–5.
10. Graves GR, et al ,Tachycardia as predictor of sepsis. Ped Infect Dis J.1984;3:404–6.
11. Cruz AT, et al.Test characteristics of an automated age and temperature adjusted tachycardia alert in pediatric septic shock. Ped Emerg Care. 2012;28 (9):889–94.
12. Hanna CM, Greenes DS. How much tachycardia in infants can be attributed to fever? Ann Emerg Med. 2004;43(6):699–705.
13. Stevens DL. Group A streptococcal sepsis. Curr Infect Dis Rep. 2003;5(5):379–86.

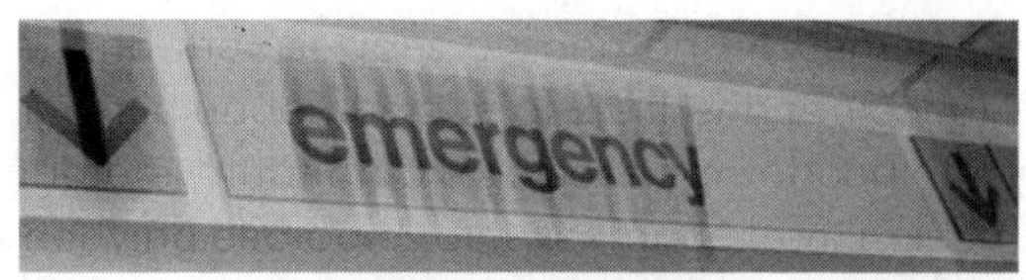

CASE 22

9-YEAR-OLD GIRL WITH ANKLE PAIN

Emilie Cobert MD, MPH
Attending Physician
MedStar Franklin Square Medical Center
Baltimore, MD

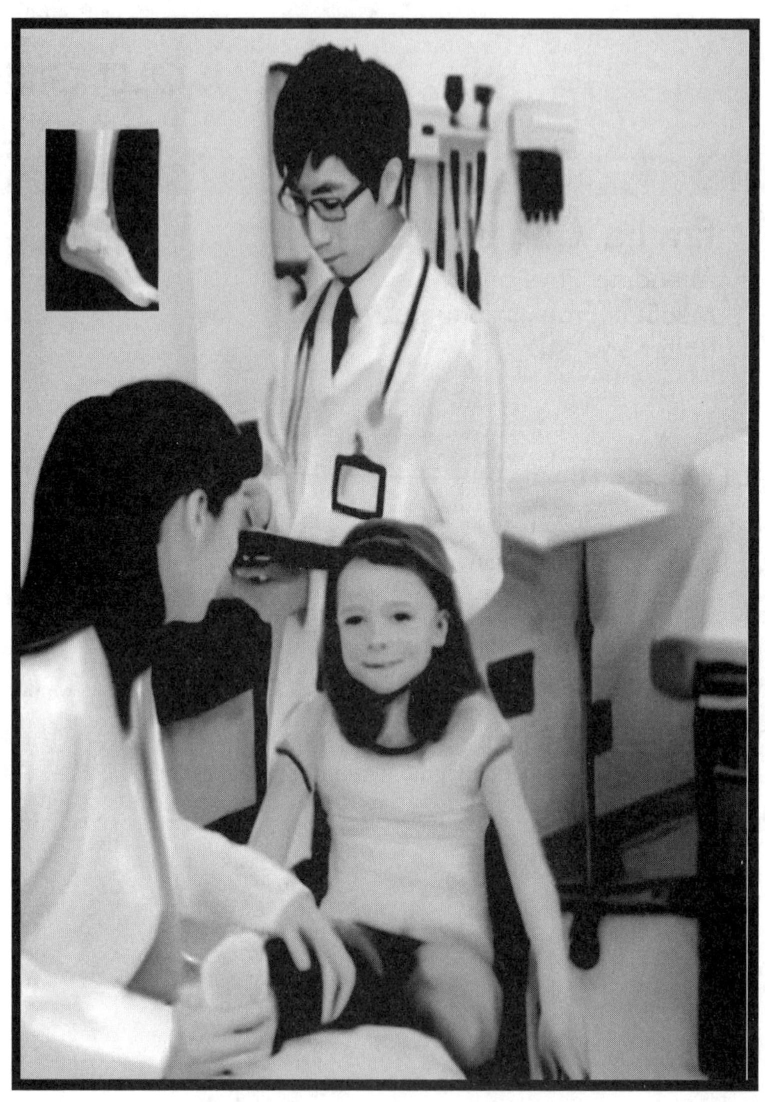

CASE 22

9-YEAR-OLD GIRL WITH ANKLE PAIN

PART 1—MEDICAL

I. The Patient's Story

Priscilla is like any other 9-year old girl in 3rd grade; active, "hyper" (per her parents) and chatty, particularly at school. Priscilla enjoys playing with her friends, dancing, and arts & crafts. She doesn't have much interest in sports, but never shies away from running around during school recess.

Priscilla is lucky enough to have a younger brother and close-knit family with grandparents, aunts, uncles and cousins. Her family is of very modest means; mom waits tables and dad is a laborer. Her family has recently fallen on hard times as local construction jobs are sparse and dad has been out of work for extended periods. While her parents never went to college, they encourage Priscilla's schoolwork and education. Priscilla's uncle has had a life-long struggle with drug addiction and, when not in rehab, he lives with Priscilla's family.

Pediatrician visits have been uneventful, yearly events for Priscilla. She has a diagnosis of mild asthma, and after an evaluation for difficulty focusing and 'picking' when nervous, a child psychiatrist diagnoses depression, OCD and ADHD, starting her on medications. She has responded well and has been stable for the last several years.

One morning, Priscilla wakes up with a painful right ankle. Her mother brings her to a local urgent care. There is no specific trauma, but Priscilla had been running around during recess the previous day, and after a negative ankle x-ray, Priscilla is diagnosed with an ankle sprain and put in an air cast.

The next day, Priscilla awakes with a fever of 102°F, wheezing, and worse ankle pain. Mom brings her to a local ED, where a second ankle x-ray is normal. The ED treats Priscilla with an albuterol nebulizer and diagnoses her with an upper respiratory infection-induced asthma exacerbation and ankle sprain.

On day 3 from her initial symptoms, Priscilla's fever rises to 104°F, she vomits twice, and her ankle pain is worse. She refuses to ambulate. Mom brings her to a different ED. This "bounceback" is detailed below.

II. The Doctor's Version and Bounceback (the following is the actual documentation of the provider)

Date: November 1, 2012

TRIAGE (13:01)

RN: Right ankle swelling, fever x 4 days, n/v

VITAL SIGNS						
Time	Temp(F)	Pulse	Resp	Syst	Diast	Pain
13:04	102.9	154	26	130	72	6/10

Weight: 119 lbs

Triage Intervention (advanced protocol in place): Tylenol given. IV established, IVF started, urinalysis and rapid strep sent.

HISTORY OF PRESENT ILLNESS – recorded by physician (15:29): 9-year old AAF c/o 4 days of right ankle pain. Woke up with pain. No injury. Went to [urgent care] 3 days ago, neg. XR. DX: sprain. Next day pt with inc. pain, unable to bear weight, inc. swelling and also wheezing. No redness or warmth. Went to another ED, another neg. XR, no IV or labwork or CXR, given splint. Rec'd albuterol aerosol for wheezing and d/c'ed. Fever x 3 days (Tm 104), N/V last night (NBNB x 1). No emesis today. No diarrhea. Last BM 2 days ago. Dec. po today. No runny nose, sore throat, cough, SOB. Ankle still hurts posterior calcaneus, "better" but still painful to WB [weight bear]. Abdominal pain today, diffuse, constant. No vision changes or rash. Flushed since 8 AM. No other joint involvement. No dysuria. No other pain. **Meds:** Adderall, bupropion, hydroxyzine, Advil, acetaminophen.

REVIEW OF SYSTEMS:
Physician circled: constitutional, GI, MS, Skin

PAST MEDICAL HISTORY:

Allergies: NKDA

Meds: see above

PMH/PSH: asthma, depression, ADHD, OCD, tonsils/adenoids. IUTD [immunizations up to date]

FamHx: mom – h/o abscess. No MRSA.

SH: Lives with parents/brother/extended family. 3rd grader.

PHYSICAL EXAM:

Constitutional: febrile 39.4, 130/73, RR26, HR 154 (sinus tach w/ fever), 97% RA, well-developed, well-nourished AAF, mildly ill-appearing, NAD

HEENT: NL TMs, PERRL, EOMI, dry MM, throat: posterior erythema, no exudates

Neck: supple, shotty LAD, no meningismus

Lungs: CTA B/L, RR tachy

Card: tachy, no m/r/g

Abd: soft, diffuse tenderness w/ voluntary guarding, no rigidity, no focality, NABS diffusely, no mass

Ext: no lower leg edema, right ankle tenderness over Achilles insertion point on calcaneus w/o erythema/swelling, ROM limited 2° pain

Skin: flushed facial cheeks, diffuse old scars 2° bug bites, no other rash

ED COURSE:

15:27: Patient had received a weight-based fluid bolus and acetaminophen in triage.
CBC: WBC 7, H/H 12.4/35.7, plt 101
CMP: Abnormalities: Na 132/ Cr 0.5/ Alb 3.4/ Alk Phos 256/ AST 116/ ALT 64
CRP: 120
Lyme: negative
Rapid strep test: negative

15:56: MD ordered additional labs including: CRP, Lyme titer, Strep antibodies, blood and urine cultures

ED MD PROGRESS NOTE:

20:58: Pt defervesced, flushing resolved, less ill-appearing, tol. PO. Labs show nrl. WBC, Rapid strep test No UTI. Pt with pain out of proportion to exam. No trauma. No skin findings. Exam not consistent with joint infection but suspect this is source of fever. No empiric antibiotics indicated at this time. Will observe to follow clinical course. Possible bone scan/ MRI to r/o osteo; ortho consult. Mom aware of plan.

ED DIAGNOSIS: Fever, calcaneal pain

DISPOSITION: Observation

III. Greg Henry Comments

"Non-traumatic bone and joint pain in children is infective until proven otherwise"

It's not very often that these words pass my lips, but I honestly believe that the emergency department visit fell below the standard of care; non-traumatic bone and joint pain in children is infection until proven otherwise. Bugs get there by direct injection into the bone or joint or by traveling somewhere in the blood stream. While this approach may be perfectly acceptable in most kids at most times, if an infectious process is not included in the differential, you will eventually get burned.

I applaud them for thinking broadly about Lyme disease, but a search for osteomyelitis was needed also. The only real place where such infections come from is the heart. An evaluation which lacks aggressiveness early on is fraught with difficulty. Obtaining cultures, administration of antibiotics, and an echo cardiogram seem reasonable. Such cases are rare; but would you be comfortable with this workup if it was *your* child?

IV. Madeline Matar Joseph Comments

Ankle sprain is unlikely to occur in children before the age of 11–13 years since the distal tibia starts ossifying at that age and the growth plate (physis) is still open. Since the growth plate is weaker than the ligaments, a fracture through the physis will occur before or associated with a ligamentous injury. In addition, minor trauma can portend infection of the bones or the joints. I agree with Dr. Henry; do not play with fire. If you are concerned about an infection of a joint or bone, observation alone is not sufficient.

OBSERVATION COURSE:

Nov. 1 22:00 [from admitting MD note]:

MSK: Right ankle tender to touch, dec. ROM, but complete exam w/o pain while distracting. No erythema/warmth.

SKIN: multiple 1 mm open lesions on forearms consistent with skin picking. Remainder physical exam negative.

Nov. 2 17:09 [RN note]: BP taken is 88/50 while patient lying in bed. Patient flushed, but not itching. No complaints of difficulty breathing, no other signs of flushing or rash. Patient almost finished 1st dose of vancomycin. MD aware of BP and is in room to see patient. Will continue to monitor.

Nov. 2 21:30 [RN note]: D/w MD because on assessment all joints appear to be slightly inflamed and painful. Patient denies right ankle injury prior to symptom onset. Pain on palpation to area on left outer aspect of knee appears slightly red and tender. Pt also c/o general neck/ shoulder/elbow pains. Per MD, will reassess.

Nov. 3 01:11 [RN note]: Patient noted to have increased RR and appears SOB. O2 sats 86-91% on RA. Placed on continuous monitoring and 1.5L NC O2 with sats up to 96-98%. MD aware and at bedside for reevaluation of hypoxia and change in respiratory status. MD ordered CXR. Orders pip-tazo and ceftriaxone. MD at bedside to discuss findings w/ family and discuss plan of care to transfer to Peds ICU.

Nov. 3 08:30: Additional labs ordered: CBC, coagulation panel, d-dimer, reticulocyte count, ANA. Repeat CBC: WBC 5.7, H/H: 10.6/31.2, Plt: 39. INR 1.3. PT 15.8, PTT 40.4. DD>5000. Lactate 1.9. BMP normal. ANA+.

Nov. 3 09:44: Lab called with preliminary positive blood cultures showing Staphylococcus aureus.

Nov. 3 11:05: CXR shows bilateral pulmonary infiltrates

Nov. 3 12:21: Patient transferred to ICU for SIRS.

INPATIENT COURSE:

The patient transferred to the ICU for sepsis with gram-positive cocci in clusters from blood culture. The patient's respiratory and cardiovascular status has decompensated with hypoxia, respiratory distress, tachycardia, and hypotension.

The intensivist noted on his history that the patient had been camping two weeks prior in Pennsylvania, but had no subsequent rash or signs of tick bites. :

ICU Labs repeated on admission:

CBC: 5.2>10.8/31.5<37
CMP: Na 145/ K 3.5/ Cl 108/ BUN 8/ Cr. 0.45/ Glc 96/ Ca 8.3/ Mg 1.9/ Phos 3.4
TPr 5.1/ Alb 2.6/ AST 73/ ALT 58/ Alk Phos 211/ TB 0.7
Fibrinogen: 349/ PT 15.5/ INR 1.2/ PTT 40
ESR: 12
CRP: 22.1

ICU Imaging:

CXR: patchy bilateral pulmonary opacities which may reflect pneumonia. Small bilateral pleural effusions, left greater than right.

ECHO: Two mobile echogenic structures attached to the anterior leaflet of the mitral valve measuring 1.6 to 1.9 cm and 0.9 to 1.1 cm in length consistent with vegetation. Findings consistent with infective endocarditis.

CXR #2: Stable bilateral air space opacities, which may reflect infection and/or edema. Small bilateral pleural effusions.

R ankle/foot XR: No radiographic findings of osteomyelitis. Soft tissue edema.

CT head: Multiple, small wedge-shaped areas of edema involving the posterior circulation of bilateral occipital lobes and the right cerebellum, suspicious for embolic infarcts.

Abdominal US: Geographic area of decreased echogenicity and vascularity in the superior left kidney suspicious for area of renal infarction. Small amount of ascites.

CT Chest and CT Angio Abd/Pelvis: Moderate bilateral pleural effusions with diffuse bilateral airspace opacities and cardiomegaly, concerning for pulmonary edema. Superimposed infectious process cannot be excluded. Ill-defined wedge-shaped region of hypoattenuation within the spleen.

MRI/MRA Head/Neck: Central septic emboli with multiple small intraparenchymal abscesses in occipital lobes and cerebellum. Associated hemorrhage within abscessed areas. Mild edema without shift or herniation. No aneurysm.

V. Hospital Course and Follow up

On ICU Day 2, the patient has increasing respiratory distress despite placement of 30L high-pressure nasal cannula and requires intubation. She develops mitral regurgitation.

1. Cardiothoracic Surgery: The patient was taken to the OR on ICU Day 3 for mitral valve repair, requiring midline sternotomy and intra-operative aorta cross-clamp and bypass.
2. Infectious Disease →MSSA sepsis by blood culture
3. Ophthalmology: to evaluate for retinal infarct → not present
4. Orthopedics: to evaluate for osteomyelitis → negative on MRI
5. Neurosurgery: no surgical intervention
6. Urology: to evaluate renal infarct → small affected area; non-surgical

The patient is discharged home after two weeks in the hospital. She requires a PICC line for home IV antibiotics. Three-month follow-up reveals improvement in her mitral valve function, improvement in her neurologic status without sequelae, resolution of the ankle pain, and normal renal function.

Discharge diagnoses:

1. Infective endocarditis with mitral valve vegetations
2. Mitral valve regurgitation
3. MSSA sepsis
4. Cerebral/cerebellar septic emboli
5. Renal infarct
6. Bilateral pleural effusions with respiratory failure
7. Coagulopathy

PART 2—THE ANALYSIS

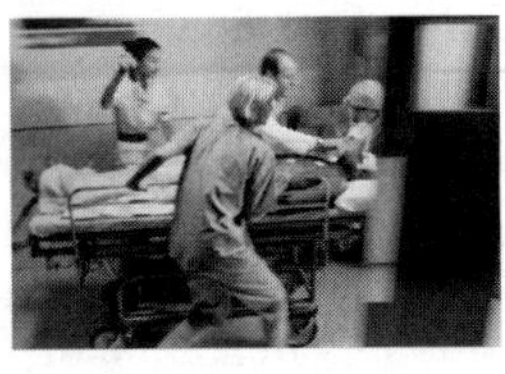

SEPTIC ARTHRITIS, SYSTEMIC INFLAMMATORY RESPONSE SYNDROME (SIRS), AND INFECTIVE ENDOCARDITIS

Emilie Cobert MD, MPH
Attending Physician
MedStar Franklin Square Medical Center
Baltimore, MD

Overview

This case is a bit of a head-scratcher because of its unusual chief complaint. It is rare, but not unheard of, for endocarditis to present with arthralgias, particularly polyarthralgias.[13] Arthralgias indicate dissemination of infective emboli that result in diffuse inflammatory symptoms.[9] But that is our endpoint and easily explained by the retrospectoscope.

Initial evaluation

Priscilla's first work-up at the urgent care was reasonable considering her chief complaint of ankle pain without other systemic symptoms. She first complained of fever at the following ED visit; that is where the problems begin.

At the very least, fever plus ankle pain equals septic arthritis until proven otherwise. Priscilla's symptom of ankle pain with fever should prompt the ED physician to look further. Presumably the ED physician stopped the diagnostic work-up at viral URI-induced asthma exacerbation and ankle sprain because, after all, common things are common. A patient may inadvertently guide the provider to a diagnosis if the patient is convinced of a certain diagnosis. Alternatively, a physician may piggyback off of a previous diagnosis if she does not approach a patient anew. Either way, diagnostic momentum limits the differential and risks diagnosis. *However*, the crux of emergency medicine is ... well ... ruling out emergencies.

Occam's razor states that among competing theories, the simplest hypothesis should be chosen. While elegant in its succinctness, this is not how the emergency physician should view the world. Is it more likely that Priscilla had two distinct pathologies: ankle pain and a viral URI causing a fever and an asthma exacerbation? Even if the ED physician doesn't stick a needle in every febrile ankle pain or do an x-ray of every wheeze with fever, the physician should justify on the chart why those actions were not taken.

Systemic symptoms involving multiple organ systems should alert the physician to a systemic process, e.g., infectious, hematologic, and inflammatory. It was not until Priscilla's second ED visit that the astute ED physician went that route.

Bounce back visit

The second ED physician suspected a systemic infectious process with the ankle as the source; however, she noted that Priscilla's ankle was underwhelming on the physical exam. Admitting Priscilla for an observation period to see how her signs, symptoms, exam, and diagnostic data evolved was an entirely reasonable and prudent clinical step.

Septic arthritis in children

Acute septic arthritis is uncommon with an incidence in the developed world of approximately 6/100,000,[9] a high morbidity that can lead to permanent joint dysfunction and pain. Septic arthritis is uncommon in the pediatric population, but when it occurs, 50% of cases are under the age of 3 years.[9] Causative organisms vary by age group and risk factors. *Staphylococcus aureus* is overall the most common bacteria to affect children over age 2.[9] If there are physical examination signs of joint infection (effusion, erythema, warmth), then aspiration is warranted.

Osteomyelitis in children

Pediatric osteomyelitis is uncommon in the developed world, with an incidence of 8/100,000 and with boys being affected twice as often as girls.[12] *Staphylococcus aureus* is the most common bacteria followed by *Streptococcus pyogenes and S. pneumoniae.*[12] Bacteria reach the bone via direct inoculation (e.g., trauma), spread from adjacent tissue (i.e., cellulitis or septic arthritis), or hematogenous spread. The latter is the most common cause of osteomyelitis in children.[12] Classic clinical manifestations include limping or the inability or refusal to walk, fever, focal tenderness, and sometimes focal redness or swelling.[12] Initial evaluation in suspected pediatric osteomyelitis includes obtaining CRP, blood cultures, and radiographs.[12]

While Priscilla did have joint pain and fever, she ultimately did not have septic arthritis or osteomyelitis. Her polyarthralgias were manifest of the systemic infectious process caused by the endocarditis she was brewing.

Systemic inflammatory response syndrome (SIRS)

Priscilla also met SIRS criteria on her 3rd presentation. To meet SIRS criteria, a child must have two of four criteria (one of which *must* be abnormal temperature or leukocytosis): Core temperature >38.5°C or <36°C, tachycardia (varies by age group), tachypnea (varies by age group), leukocytosis.[4]

Priscilla's joint was not alarming enough to all three physicians to aspirate; however, by her third presentation, she appeared constitutionally unwell enough to require observation. She met SIRS criteria by her core temperature, tachycardia, and tachypnea. Current pediatric sepsis guidelines recommend prompt antibiotic initiation after drawing blood cultures.[4] Vancomycin, a good choice agent for *S. aureus*, was given before the blood cultures were positively reported, but it was nearly 20 hours before they were started.

Patient Safety Point: Do not rely on the admitting team to start antibiotics. If you are concerned enough about a septic joint or osteomyelitis to admit the patient, start the 1st dose of antibiotics in the ED.

Infective endocarditis

Infective endocarditis (IE) peaks in infancy and late adolescence.[1] *Staphylococcus aureus* is the most common organism to cause IE.[1] Nearly half of all children with IE have an underlying preexisting heart disease (congenital, prosthetic, or rheumatic).[1] Fever with multiple symptoms or signs of infection suggest a systemic process and should alert to an infective embolic phenomenon or hematologic spread.

The Duke criteria[3] is a clinical diagnostic tool for infective endocarditis. A patient meets criteria if she has 2 major criteria OR 1 major criterion plus 3 minor criteria OR 5 minor criteria. Before Priscilla received an echocardiogram, she did have 1 major criterion (+ blood cultures) and 1 minor criterion (fever). However, it is possible that an earlier chest x-ray may have prompted consideration that the infiltrates were in fact pulmonary infarcts from emboli (a vascular phenomenon satisfying a minor criterion). Additionally, the +ANA may have prompted obtaining a rheumatoid factor test, which is also a minor criterion.

Duke Criteria for Diagnosis of Infective Endocarditis

Definite Infective Endocarditis
- Pathologic criteria
  - Microorganisms: demonstrated by culture or histology in a vegetation, *or* in a vegetation that has embolized, *or* in an intracardiac abscess, *or*
  - Pathologic lesions: vegetation or intracardiac abscess present, confirmed by histology showing active endocarditis
- Clinical criteria, using specific definitions listed in Table III
  - 2 major criteria, *or*
  - 1 major and 3 minor criteria, *or*
  - 5 minor criteria

Possible Infective Endocarditis
- Findings consistent with infective endocarditis that fall short of "Definite," but not "rejected."

Rejected
- Firm alternate diagnosis for manifestations of endocarditis, *or*
- Resolution of manifestations of endocarditis, with antibiotic therapy for 4 days or less, *or*
- No pathologic evidence of infective endocarditis at surgery or autopsy, after antibiotic therapy for 4 days or less

Source: Durack DT, Lukes AS, Bright DK. New criteria for diagnosis of infective endocarditis: utilization of specific echocardiographic findings. Duke Endocarditis Service. Am J Med. 1994;96(3):200–9. Table II.

Priscilla's inpatient management prior to her upgrade to the ICU was choppy; while the physician did evaluate her promptly at the bedside when her respiratory status was decompensating, there was a marked 10-hour delay in obtaining a chest x-ray, a 7-hour delay in obtaining any additional laboratory diagnostics, and a nearly 12-hour delay in upgrading her level of care. The physician recalls thinking that a rheumatologic process was at the forefront of the differential, especially in light of the +ANA, lack of leukocytosis, lack of recurrent fever, and polyarthralgias. He later related that the expansion of ATB coverage after his bedside evaluation was evidence that he was covering for sepsis.

Patient outcome and summary

Priscilla's remarkable recovery left her with few sequelae. While she underwent a rocky clinical course and received a new mitral valve, she was left with no neurologic, renal, pulmonary or musculoskeletal deficits.

The take-away lesson from this case is to consider a diagnosis that ties together all signs and symptoms. Do not fall victim to the diagnoses of least resistance. Signs and symptoms that involve multiple organs warrant a search for a hematologic, infectious, systemic inflammatory, or embolic process.

References

1. Calza L, Manfredi R, Chiodo F. Antibiotic therapy for infective endocarditis in childhood. J Pediatr Pharmacol Ther. 2006;11:64–91.
2. Day MD, Gauvreau K, Shulman S, Newburger JW. Characteristics of children hospitalized with infective endocarditis. Circulation. 2009;119:865–70.
3. Durack DT, Lukes AS, Bright DK. New criteria for diagnosis of infective endocarditis: utilization of specific echocardiographic findings. Duke Endocarditis Service. Am J Med. 1994;96(3):200–9.
4. El-Wiher N, Cornell TT, Kissoon N, Shanley TP. Management and treatment guidelines for sepsis in pediatric patients. Open Inflamm J. 2011;4(Suppl 1-M11):101–9.
5. Goldstein B, Giroir B, Randolph A. International pediatric sepsis consensus conference: definitions for sepsis and organ dysfunction in pediatrics. Pediatr Crit Care Med. 2005;6:2–8.
6. Horowitz DL, Katzap E, Horowitz S, et al. Approach to septic arthritis. Am Fam Physician. 2011;84(6):653–60.
7. Johnson JA, Boyce TG, Cetta F, et al. Infective endocarditis in the pediatric patient: a 60-year single-institution review. Mayo Clin Proc. 2012;87:629–35.
8. Nade S. Acute septic arthritis in infancy and childhood. J Bone Joint Surg Br. 1983;65:234–41.
9. Nade S. Septic arthritis. Best Pract Res Clin Rheumatol. 2003;17:183–200.
10. Netzer RO, Zollinger E, Seiler C, et al. Infective endocarditis: clinical spectrum, presentation and outcome. An analysis of 212 cases 1980–1995. Heart. 2000;84:25–30.
11. Paul R, Neuman MI, Monuteaux MC, et al. Adherence to PALS Sepsis Guidelines and Hospital Length of Stay. Pediatrics. 2012;130:e273–e280. (doi: 10.1542/peds.2012-0094)
12. Peltola H, Paakkonen M. Acute osteomyelitis in children. N Engl J Med. 2014;370:352–60.
13. Vincent P, Davis R, Roy D. Group B streptococcus tricuspid endocarditis presenting with arthralgia in a postpartum woman: a case report. J Med Case Rep. 2012;6:242.

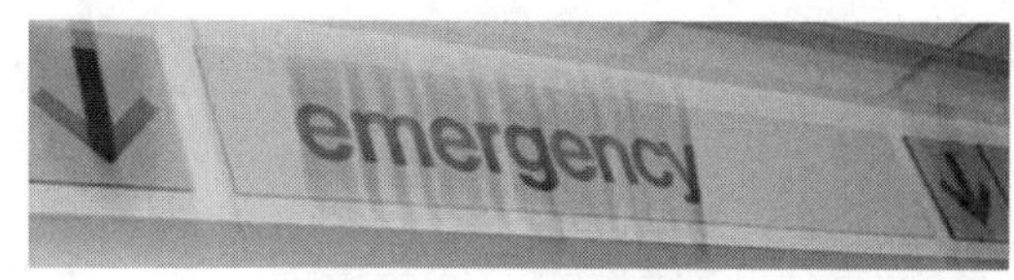

CASE 23

14-YEAR-OLD GIRL WITH TACTILE FEVER AND BACK PAIN

Jon Juhasz, MD
Emergency Medicine Physician
Wright Patterson Air Force Base, OH
OIF and OEF War Veteran

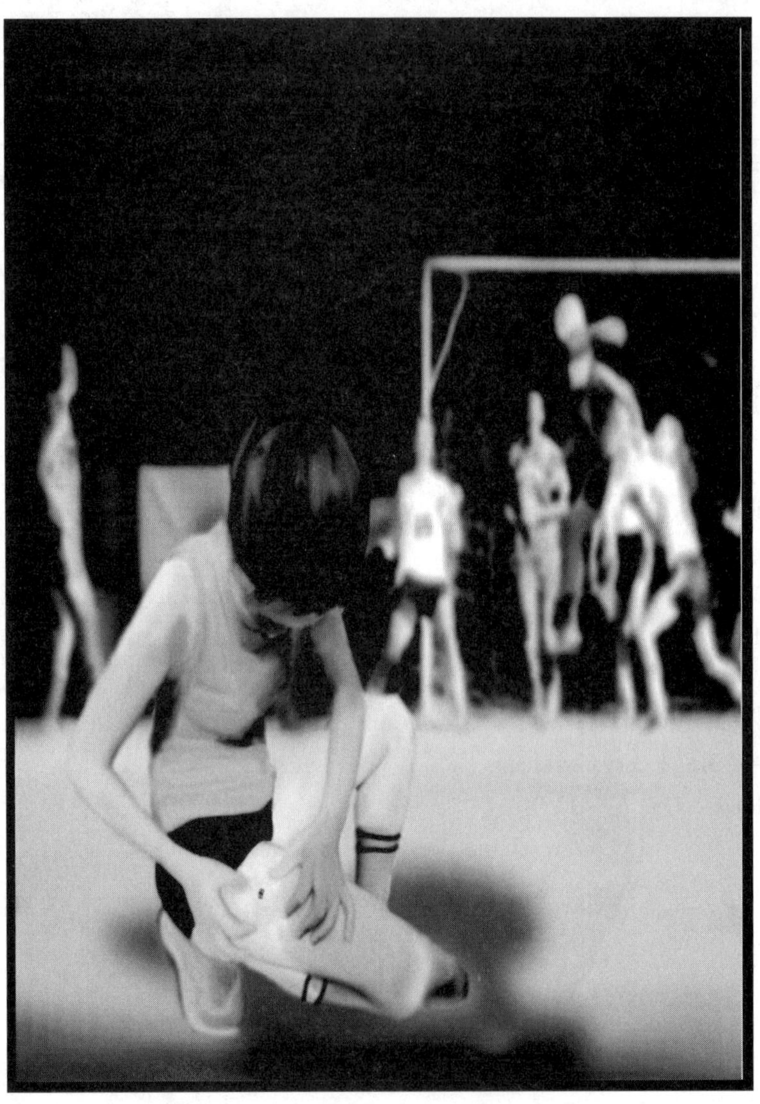

CASE 23

14-YEAR-OLD GIRL WITH TACTILE FEVER AND BACK PAIN

PART 1—MEDICAL

I. The Patient's Story

Jacqueline is an athletic 14-year-old straight-A high school student, excited about the fall soccer season on the junior varsity team. She is an only child, pushed by her mother to excel on the field and in the classroom. She doesn't smoke or drink, and is actively involved in her church youth group.

During a 4 mile training run, she feels like she is bitten on her right leg by a "weird bug." Over the next few days, she develops some redness around the bite, subsequently developing back pain, nausea and low grade fevers. Her mother takes her to the family physician, who places her on a 2 week course of Bactrim for cellulitis but her fevers and nausea continue. She attributes the back pain to her rigorous exercise routines.

II.The Doctor's Version (the following is the actual documentation of the provider)

Date: August 20, 2012 at 20:53
Chief complaint: Back Pain, Nausea, Fever
Nurse note: c/o back pain, +n, -v, -d, and fevers but mom states hasn't taken temperature. Pain scale 6/10

HISTORY OF PRESENT ILLNESS – (Per R2 ER Resident, Dr. Adrian Kelly): Patient had onset of tactile fever and pains in the lower back while out and about this afternoon. Mom treated with ibuprofen and got some relief. She identifies the pain in the lumbar region without lateralization. LMP 8/15, last sexual activity Dec 2011. No urinary symptoms. No hematuria. Nausea present no vomiting.

REVIEW OF SYSTEMS: All other systems reviewed and are negative.

PAST MEDICAL HISTORY:
Allergies: NKDA
Medications: Ibuprofen, Bactrim, Multivitamin
Pmh: none
Social History: Nonsmoker

EXAM

VITAL SIGNS						
Time	Temp(F)	RT	Pulse	Resp	Syst	Diast
21:08	99.5	TM	74	16	115	74

Constitutional: Alert and oriented x3, well-developed, well-nourished, no distress
Head: Normocephalic and atraumatic
Eyes: PERRL, EOMI, no discharge bilaterally, conjunctiva normal.
Ears: bilateral external ears normal
Throat: oropharynx is clear and moist, no oropharyngeal exudate
Neck: Normal Range of motion, No JVD. No tracheal deviation. No thyromegaly.
Lungs: Effort normal. No Stridor. No respiratory distress. Breath sounds normal. No wheezes. No rales.
Heart: Normal rate, normal heart sounds, no gallop, no friction rub, no murmur, intact distal pulses
Abdomen: Soft. Bowel sounds normal. No distension, no tenderness, no rebound, no guarding
Musculoskeletal: Normal range of motion. No edema and no tenderness
Neurological: Normal reflexes. Normal muscle tone. Coordination normal.
Skin: Warm and dry. No rash noted. Not diaphoretic. No erythema. No pallor.

ED COURSE:
Labs – Urinalysis normal; Urine pregnancy negative
21:50 – Ibuprofen 600mg PO
22:20 – Repeat Vitals: T 98.6, HR 78, BP 119/78, RR 18.
22:35 – Doctor's Progress Note: There is no focal evidence for infection. The urinalysis showed no infection, bacteria or blood to suggest UTI or ureteral stone. Patient is afebrile. Felt better during her stay in the ED. This is likely myalgias associated with a virus or possibly related to her activity playing soccer. No evidence of emergent medical condition.

DIAGNOSIS: Back pain and Nausea

DISPOSITION (22:40): Patient was discharged home and is to follow-up with her PCP in 1- 2 days. Condition upon discharge stable. Rx for ibuprofen 600mg TID. Return to the ED if symptoms worsen.

Adrian Kelly, MD, R2
Kenneth Johansen, DO

III. Patient Safety Points per Madeline Matar Joseph

Patient Safety Point #1: Back pain is not a very common complaint in children. Therefore, a thorough history and physical examination should be done to rule any serious underlying disease. Most young adolescents will be embarrassed to talk about loss of bladder or bowel control unless asked directly. Physical examination should include a good neurological examination.

Patient Safety Point #2: The "weird bug bite." The art of listening to our patients can be challenging in the busy ED. How many times a day do you see patients checking in with the chief complaint of "spider bite" to end up being a MRSA infection? But hearing the word "weird bug" prior to the presentation of systemic symptoms should prompt an examination of the skin to look for ticks.

IV. The Patient's Story (continued)

August 22, 2012 – Jacqueline's symptoms have worsened. Her nausea has now lead to multiple episodes of vomiting. Her back pain and headache are worse. She returns to the same ED.

V. The Bounceback (2 days after initial visit)

ED visit #2 – August 22, 2012

- 9:05 PM – **Triage vitals**: Temp 101.8, pulse 85, resp 20, BP 115/51.
- 9:20 PM - **HPI/PE:** Jacqueline is evaluated by Dr. Jimmer Whohaski (ED resident) and Peds ED attending Dr. Mohamed Tezlardifer (colleague of initial ED attending): "Ill-appearing and much worse than 2 days ago, +n/v, decreased po intake, +flank pain that is new, + ongoing back pain, fevers to 102, reports 14 days of Bactrim completed for resolved RLE/thigh cellulitis from a bug bite; +mucus membranes dry, +R flank ttp, has bilat lower lumbar tightness/ttp, no saddle anesthesia, 5/5 strength in bilat LE, no incontinence, nml gait"
- 9:35 PM- iv, Zofran, 1 L NS, morphine for pain, and motrin for fever/pain.
- 10:10 PM - Blood cultures taken. Rocephin.
- **Labs:** CBC: WBC= 2.4; 60% Segmented Neutrophils, Platelets 78. BMP is nml. Urine preg negative, UA shows 8-10 wbcs, 1+bacteria
- **Assessment:** "Leukocytopenia, thrombocytopenia perhaps represents serious side effect of Bactrim (?agranulocytosis), meets SIRS criteria, could have pyelo with her UA wbc 8-10, this would explain her flank pain but usually UA is more impressive. Will admit for further treatment and workup."
- **ED diagnosis:**
  1. Fevers
  2. Nausea and vomiting
  3. R flank pain, likely pyelonephritis
  4. Leukocytopenia
  5. Thrombocytopenia

HOSPITAL COURSE

- Pt admitted to the floor and improves with fluids. Given unclear source of infection, rocephin is discontinued
- **Hospital day #1 (8/23/12):** Approximately 24 hours after admission, patient develops confusion and altered mental status.
- Lumbar puncture was performed, and patient started empirically on Vancomycin 15mg/kg iv, Rocephin 2 Gm iv, Acyclovir 15mg/kg iv; Patient was transferred to the ICU with consults to: Pulm/critical care, Infectious Disease, General Surgery, Neurology, Ophthalmology, and Neurosurgery.
- CT Head w/o contrast, 8/23/2012 (hospital day 1): Initial night hawk preliminary reading: "negative for any acute abnormalities." Morning official read: "Findings with minimal diffuse cerebral edema, such as in the setting of encephalitis. At some point when the patient is stable, MRI without and with contrast would be more sensitive."
    - Lumbar puncture results, CSF protein, ++++ 544+++ (15-45 mg/dL), Glucose 98 ++ (40-80 mg/dL), WBC 6++ (0-5), RBC 2++ (0), Neutrophils 5% (<10%), Lymphocytes 76 % (65-75%), Monocyte 14 (24-35%), appearance/color: clear and colorless; Opening Pressure +++29 cm/H2O
- Concern for cerebral edema and increased intracranial pressures: Mannitol 25 Gm iv and 3% Saline 4ml/kg
- **Hospital day #2 (8/24/12):** Pt begins to seize resulting in intubation. She later is noted to have decorticate posturing
- MRI Brain and Spine w/ and w/o contrast: The cord is normal in morphology and signal intensity. There is no syrinx. There is no area of cord edema to suggest myelitis. Marrow signal is normal. There is a minimal ill-defined edema in the lower lumbar paraspinal muscles.
- EEG: Mildly abnormal EEG by the presence of a slow and poorly regulated background
- ICU notes: "Mother voiced her feeling that the workup and treatment were delayed (prior to ICU) and symptoms minimized (in previous ER and PCP visits)."
- **Hospital day #3 (8/25/12):** CT HEAD w/o Contrast "There is loss of extra-axial fluid in the region of the perimesencephalic cistern and in the posterior fossa which would be consistent with the clinical suspicion of increased intracranial pressure. The ventricles remain small. The fourth ventricle is smaller in comparison with the prior study"
- Infectious disease workup:
    - Blood Culture – Negative from 2 separate days
    - Urine Cultures - Negative x2
    - Leukins Culture - Negative x2
    - CSF Culture – Negative
    - Resp infectious disease panel –negative
    - EBV – Negative
    - Mycoplasma PCR of throat swab and serum – Negative
    - Malaria Screen – Negative
    - VDRL – NonReactive
    - ParvoB19 -+++ 7.13 IgG (<0.89 negative, >1.11 positive), 0.25 IgM (>1.11), this may possibly represent previous immunity
    - HHV6 – Negative
    - HSV CSF – Negative

- o Anti-DSDNA - None Detected
- o Myeloperoxidase Ab, IgG - None
- o (ANCA), Serine Protease3 IgG - 1 (RR 0-19) (ANCA)
- o Procalcitonin - 0.12 (Normal)

- Nuclear Cerebral Flow Study, 8/25/2012, No intracranial blood flow is demonstrated
- **Hospital day #4 (8/26/12):** ICU progress note "EMU (Epilepsy Monitoring Unit) abnormal, with progressive worsening and in the end a period of flat lining. Exam consistent with brain death. Cerebral blood flow study supporting diagnosis of brain death. Repeat clinical exam consistent with brain death.
- After extensive discussions with family, care is withdrawn at 1251 with Asystole at 1315, declaration of death at 1317... the patient had progressive worsening of mental status, with eventual herniation likely secondary to intracellular swelling due to viral encephalitis, though etiology at time of death unknown."
- Pending Studies at time of death all turned out to be negative: Ehrlichia Abs and PCR, HIV1 DNA PCR, RPR, Arbovirus battery, Eastern Equine and St. Louis encephalopathy Abs, CSF Ig's, Lymphocytic Choriomeningitis (LCM), ANA, Anti-Neutrophil Cytoplasmic Ab, Mycoplasma IgG/M, Throat viral culture, West nile Ab panel serum, Borrelia Ab's, CMV titers

FINAL DIAGNOSIS: Encephalitis, Cerebral Edema, Brain Death

Carbon County News Journal—Posted: 4 p.m. Thursday, Sept. 6, 2012

Girl's death remains mystery; West Nile ruled out

14-year-old Jacqueline, a sophomore and varsity soccer player at Carbon County High School died of encephalitis, or inflammation of the brain and spinal cord, at Regional Children's Medical Center.

What she and county health officials don't know—and are trying to find out what triggered the encephalitis, which is most often caused by a viral infection. Bacterial and fungal infections can also cause encephalitis. Carbon County Health officials confirmed it was not West Nile virus, now a public health threat in 48 states.

Losing a child is heartbreaking enough, the patient's mother said, but adding to her pain are online posts on social media sites and speculation about what caused her daughter's death. She said some of the posts mention West Nile virus, others say her daughter suffered a stroke.

"I'm sick of Facebook and all the lies people are posting," she said. "To this day, I still can't tell you what happened to my daughter."

The patient had just started her sophomore year, and it was going great, her mother said. She was on the varsity soccer team and had a boyfriend who was a member of the football team. "She liked going to football games and wearing his jersey. She only got to wear it once, but I'm glad she got to experience that," Mother said. "This was going to be the year. I couldn't wait to see what was going to happen for her."

Mother said she cannot go back to work yet as an office manager.

"If I'm home, I'm with her," she said.

FINAL AUTOPSY (report completed October 6, 2012):

- The autopsy macroscopic findings included marked brain edema, marked left ventricle myocardial thickening, moderate splenomegaly, thymic atrophy, and two paratubal cysts on the right fallopian tube. The microscopic study shows brain edema without inflammatory exudate or viral inclusions. Sections of heart reveal lymphocytic exudate and focal necrosis more marked on the left ventricle. The spleen presents diffuse hemorrhage and marked decrease of lymphoid tissue.
- Additional review by a Forensic Neuropathologist, October 13, 2012, "My perspective on the case is that it certainly appeared that this young woman probably had an encephalitis of some sort from clinical findings. It did not appear that her heart was particularly involved in whatever was going on. In any case the photo of the brain clearly shows some injection and congestion and swelling but not much else that is obvious."

IV. Greg Henry Comments

"Good luck is as important as a good doctor when it comes to viral encephalitis."

And so it goes, another disease for which we have essentially no therapy. Even with herpes simplex virus, the use of acyclovir or ganciclovir is only minimally effective. It follows the chicken soup theory that it probably can't hurt, but to think that there is literature which shows a clear trend is to delude ourselves. Virtually all the other viral illnesses are a crap shoot at best.

Lowering intracranial pressure with Mannitol *seems* like a nice idea, but there is not much literature to support this . A surgically placed drain in the ventricles theoretically may help, but good luck in finding that literature base. In medicine there are many things that "seem like a good idea at the time" only to be destroyed by the fact that almost nothing works. Good luck is as important as a good doctor when it comes to viral encephalitis.

The physicians all seemed to care and did all they could in search for treatable illness. At some point in time there is a limit to our capabilities. Criticizing a physician for refraining to perform tests unsupported by the evidence is a criminal act that destroys the treating doctor and undermines confidence in the healthcare system.

PART 2—THE ANALYSIS

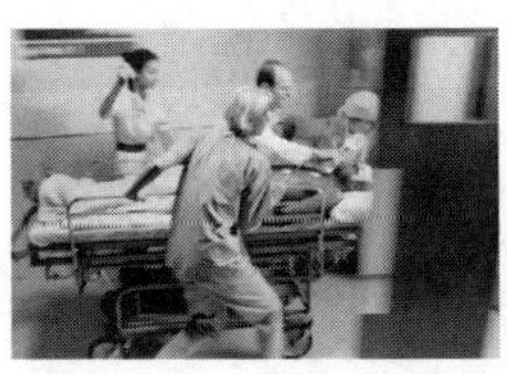

MEDICAL DISCUSSION: EVALUATION AND TREATMENT OF ENCEPHALITIS

Jon Juhasz, MD
Emergency Medicine Physician
Wright Patterson Air Force Base, OH
OIF and OEF War Veteran

Diagnoses that elude us:

This case demonstrates that even with the best available medical care, sadly, an etiologic diagnosis may elude us. In less than 50% of cases of encephalitis are we able to identify a definite source.[1] We deceive ourselves by thinking that we are smart enough to save these patients. This can be frustrating for the treatment team but even more devastating for the patient's family

Many unanswered questions:

This patient sought care from her primary care provider and the emergency department, but neither impacted the final outcome. Did the bug bite have anything to do with her final diagnosis and why wasn't it addressed in the first ED visit? A bite in the late summer months should prompt consideration of encephalitis.[2-4]

Another possibility considered was that the Bactrim prescribed for her bug bite/cellulitis caused her symptoms and abnormal labs. The fact that the fever and headache began prior to initiation of Bactrim makes this doubtful. Maybe it was a combination of effects? Was her spleen enlarged because it was sequestering platelets and leukocytes? Could this have been an autoimmune encephalitis, better understood since the 2007 finding of Anti-N-methyl-D-Aspartate (NMDA) receptor encephalitis?[5-8]

Her headache did not seem to coincide with classic meningeal signs. In hindsight, it is easier to see her encephalitis progression; the altered mental status and seizures represented the fulminant state of her cerebral edema.

The devastated mother of this patient was very upset regarding her perceived "delay in care," but even if her West Nile virus testing had come back positive, what could have been done differently? Every parent would be expected to analyze all aspects of their child's care. Communication and realistic expectations are important.

Evaluation of possible encephalitis?

On her first day of admission, Jacqueline exhibited a significant neurologic decline. A lumbar puncture was not done until after she had altered mental status. The LP was suggestive of a viral infectious process: an elevated opening pressure, a high protein level and minimally elevated white blood cells with a lymphocytic predominance.[8,9] Her brain CT showed cerebral swelling that was consistent with encephalitis. Should these tests have been done earlier? Many ED physicians would argue they were not indicated until more concerning symptoms developed.[1] Some neurologists would argue they should have been accomplished with the headache to rule out other pathology (SAH, neoplasms, abscess).[10,11] In the end, the care remained supportive. An infectious source was likely the cause of her symptoms, but this was not shown definitively.

The patient's encephalitis was worked up with numerous inpatient viral tests. Late summer viral encephalitis, as in this case, should be considered to come from some type of arthropod. The diagnosis of West Nile virus and other arboviruses (*arthropod borne* viruses) was entertained given her history of mosquito bites. This was appropriate to have high on the differential.[12-15] Good thought ... but testing was negative. There are newly emerging vector-borne viruses in the U.S., such as Chikungunya virus that cause encephalitis.[16] Another possibility is an autoimmune process.[5]

Encephalitis pathophysiology

Encephalitis is an infection of the brain parenchyma causing a variety of neurologic abnormalities.[2-4, 17] The typical and most common offenders in the U.S. are viruses that include:

- Herpes simplex virus (HSV)
- Varicella zoster virus (VZV)
- Epstein Barr Virus (EBV)
- Cytomegalovirus (CMV)
- West Nile virus
- La Crosse virus
- Western Equine virus
- Eastern Equine virus
- St. Louis Equine virus
- Rabies virus [10]

On autopsy, this patient was also found to inflammation of her myocardium. Viruses that are reported to cause both encephalitis and myocarditis include: Encephalo-myocarditis Virus (EMCV),[18] some enteroviruses[19] (specifically Coxsackievirus strains), West Nile virus,[20] Parvovirus B19[21] (which this patient had +titers), Ljungan Virus,[22] and the Swine Flu [23] (H1N1).

Bacteria represent a less commonly encountered cause of encephalitis. Bartonella, the cause of cat scratch disease, has been described to cause a variety of neurologic manifestations including encephalitis. Mycoplasma can cause a direct (invasive) or indirect (immune-mediated or post-infectious) neurologic abnormalities. Additionally, tick-borne encephalitis should be suspected in the correct epidemiologic setting. Vector borne agents such as Rickettsia and Borrelia may need to be included in the differential diagnoses. Amebic meningoencephalitis which may be caused by Naegleria, may present in a similar fashion and should be suspected in the right epidemiologic setting (e.g., exposure to or immersion in a body of warm water). A wet mount study of fresh cerebrospinal fluid may detect the amebic organism.

In viral encephalitis, the gray matter of the brain is usually affected to greater degrees. This leads to impairment in the patient's cognitive abilities and may present with psychiatric signs. Lethargy and seizures are also commonly described in severe cases. New psychiatric symptoms are more associated with HSV.[10] HHV-6 can be quite devastating in the immunocompromised.[24] The impairment in cognition leads to aphasia, amnesia and confusion, followed by seizures. The arboviruses (West Nile and St. Louis Equine) have been associated with movement disorders.[12] Fever is almost always present and meningeal signs and symptoms are common.

The diagnosis can be supported by CT Head showing cerebral edema. Contrast enhancement may be helpful in distinguishing inflammatory processes from other etiologies. In cases of HSV encephalitis, cranial imaging shows medial, temporal, and inferior frontal gray matter changes.[25] Lumbar puncture often shows increased intracranial pressures and HSV meningoencephalitis is usually hemorrhagic and often has cerebrospinal fluid with increased red blood cells. The differential diagnosis includes subarachnoid hemorrhage, Lyme Disease, meningitis, brain abscess, bacterial endocarditis, and toxic/metabolic encephalopathies.[2,3]

Encephalitis Treatment, What more could have been done?

This patient was given excellent supportive care, and in cases of encephalitis where no definitive treatment of an etiologic agent is available, this is all that is indicated.[2] The patient was given broad spectrum coverage with parenteral acyclovir, ceftriaxone and vancomycin but this obviously was not life-saving. It is hard to say that anything more could have been done.

Treatment for HSV (beyond the neonatal period) and VZV encephalitis is with acyclovir 10 mg/kg iv q8 hours. Ganciclovir 5mg/kg iv q 12 hours is recommended for CMV encephalitis.[1,2] Ribavirin, interferon-alpha, and West Nile virus specific immunoglobulin remain controversial for the treatment of West Nile Virus as outcomes seem to vary.[14,15]

Encephalitis causes severe swelling of the brain. This cerebral edema can result in tonsillar herniation leading to brain death. This process can be slowed by osmotic agents reducing the amount of brain swelling. Typical agents include Mannitol 0.5–1 gm/kg iv and 3% saline (range from 1.5–10 mL/Kg with 2 mL/Kg being the most commonly used).[2,26]

Encephalitis Disposition

Patients suspected to have encephalitis should be admitted to the hospital, preferably the ICU.[2] This patient went to the pediatric medicine floor because she did not yet have the definitive diagnosis.

Chapter Summary

What is the take home message if you encounter a 14-year-old soccer player deteriorating in your ED?

- Fevers with headache, photophobia, vomiting, or unusual back or neck pain can be representative of encephalitis, specifically meningeal inflammation from the encephalitis. Though it did not identify the exact source, a lumbar puncture to define the diagnosis is the test of choice. Be sure to include an opening pressure.
- Encephalitis symptoms in their most fulminant state include altered mental status, new onset psychiatric symptoms, ataxia, cognitive defects, seizures and motor deficits.

- MRI is more sensitive than CT in diagnosing encephalitis. If a CT is done, perform both without and with contrast to look for meningeal contrast enhancement and/or parenchymal brain abscess.
- Treatment for suspected viral encephalitis is with Acyclovir and Ganciclovir (for CMV encephalitis).[1,2] Ribavirin, interferon-alpha, and West Nile virus specific immunoglobulin remain controversial. Potential bacterial infections should be covered with broad spectrum antibiotics (usually vancomycin and ceftriaxone), steroids are usually indicated to reduce inflammation.
- Brain death from encephalitis is usually secondary to cerebral edema and tonsillar herniation. Consider osmotic agents such as Mannitol and/or 3% saline.

References

1. Weingarten L, Enarson P, Klassen T. Encephalitis. Pediatr Emerg Care. 2013;29 (2):235–41.
2. Simon DW, Da Silva YS, Zuccoli G, Clark RS. Acute encephalitis. Crit Care Clin. 2013;29(2):259–77.
3. Dubray K, Anglemyer A, LaBeaud AD. Epidemiology, outcomes and predictors of recovery in childhood encephalitis: a hospital-based study. Pediatr Infect Dis J. 2013;32(8): 839–44.
4. Britton PN, Dale RC, Booy R, Jones CA. Acute encephalitis in children: progress and priorities from an Australasian perspective. J Paediatr Child Health. 2014 Jun 22. doi: 10.1111/jpc.12650. [Epub ahead of print].
5. Erol I. Autoimmune encephalitis in children. Minerva Pediatr. 2013; 65(3):295–305.
6. Twilt M, Benseler SM. Childhood inflammatory brain diseases: pathogenesis, diagnosis, and therapy. Rheumatology (Oxford). 2014;53(8):1359–68.
7. Jones KC, Benseler SM, Moharir M. Anti-NMDA receptor encephalitis. Neuroimaging Clin N Am. 2013;23(2):309–20.
8. Lin JJ, Lin KL, Hsia SH, Chou MI. Anti-N-methyl-D-aspartate receptor encephalitis in Taiwan—a comparison between children and adults. Children with Encephalitis and/or Encephalopathy Related Status Epilepticus and Epilepsy (CHEESE) Study Group. Pediatr Neurol. 2014;50(6);574–80.
9. Kelly D. An encephalitis primer. Adv Exp Med Biol. 2013;764:133–140.

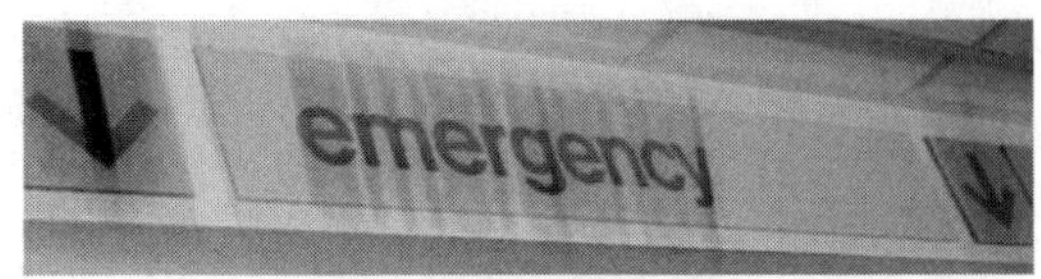

CASE 24

8-WEEK-OLD GIRL WITH COUGH AND "FEVER"

Jessica Mason, MD
Emergency Medicine Resident, 2nd year
Metro Health, Cleveland Ohio
Producer and Co-Host: Resident Call Room Podcast. HippoEM.com

Christopher Wyatt, MD
Assistant Professor
Case Western Reserve University, School of Medicine

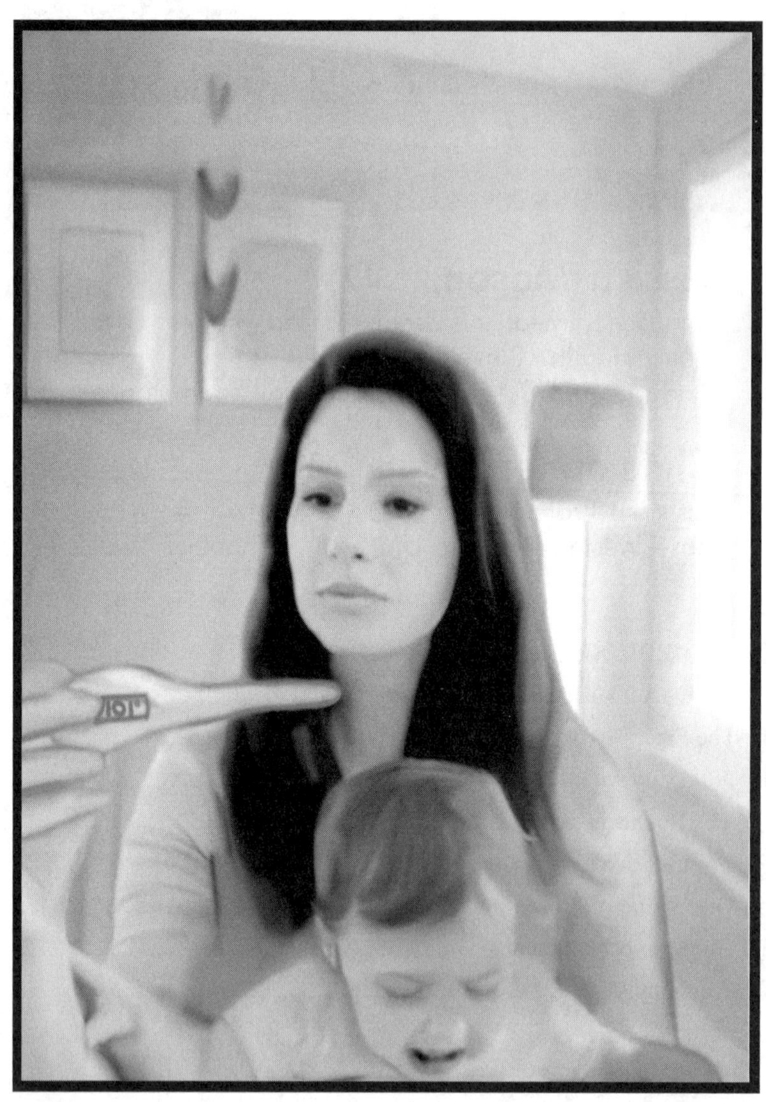

CASE 24

8-WEEK-OLD GIRL WITH COUGH AND "FEVER"

PART 1—MEDICAL

I. The Initial Visit with the PCP (the following is the actual documentation of the provider)

CHIEF COMPLAINT (2/2/14 at 19:53): Fever

VITAL SIGNS				
Time	Temp(F)	Pulse	Resp	O2 Sat
1939	100.0	163	38	100% RA
2130	100.2	144	32	100% RA
2200	100.2	150	32	100% RA

HISTORY OF PRESENT ILLNESS: 8wkF brought in by mom for fever. Starting today, felt warm, Tmax reportedly 101, no anti-pyretics given, dry cough, rhinorrhea. Getting green/yellow mucous when bulb suctions nostrils. Also sleeping more today.
Only 6 oz milk since last night (pumped breast milk so could measure)

6 wet diapers today
Brother is home from hospital yesterday after RSV and bacterial pneumonia.
Born term, vaccination are UTD

ROS
+eyes slightly pink
Denies v/d, signs of abd pain, bloody bm's, new rash, lethargy, bulging from head

EXAM:

Pulse 150 | Temp(Src) 100.2 °F (37.9 °C) (Rectal) | Resp 32 | Wt 4.627 kg | SpO2 100%

Constitutional: active, interactive and appropriate for age. Well hydrated.
Head: Normocephalic, atraumatic. Font soft, flat
Ears: Right TM unremarkable. Left TM unremarkable.
Nose/Throat: MMM. Symmetric palate. Posterior pharynx clear; no exudates. No palatal petechiae. No rhinorrhea
Eyes: Conjunctivae nml. No scleral icterus.
Neck: Neck supple; no evidence of meningismus. No cervical LAD
Cardiovascular: Normal rate. Regular. No m/r/g; Well perfused.
Pulmonary/Chest: CTAB; no retraction, nasal flaring, grunting or accessory muscle use. No respiratory distress.
Abdominal: s/nd/nt; No crying or grimacing with deep palpation

Musculoskeletal: MAEx4. Brisk capillary refill.
Skin: Skin is warm and dry. Neonatal acne on chest
Neurological: Alert and interactive. Moves all extremities. Age appropriate behavior and development.

RESULTS:

Respiratory virus panel – pending
CXR – Low lung volumes, no focal infiltrates

MEDICAL DECISION-MAKING:

8wk F evaluated for fever, cough. Pt well appearing, vitals wnl, afebrile in ED w/o anti-pyretics prior, well hydrated, font soft/flat, lungs clear, no inc wob. Mom is physician. Spoke with child's PCP, had wanted to evaluate for hypoxia and possible bacteremia. Low suspicion for meningitis or UTI, more likely respiratory etiology given URI sxs and sick contact. CXR w/o focal pna, but poor inspiration. Tolerated 2oz pedialyte. Observed in ED, vitals repeated, afebrile, no hypoxia. Low suspicion for bacteremia. RVP pending. Has f/u tmrw.

-Resident, MD

Attending Note:

URI sx, reported fever at home, brother with RSV; temp 100.2 on arrival, well appearing, no hypoxia, tachypnea, g/f/r, well hydrated, no respiratory distress. > 30 days old and clear source of infection (URI) and exposure (brother with RSV). Discussed with mother urine culture/blood culture/CBC, but not felt to be necessary by this MD. CXR and RVP high yield tests; CXR without infiltrate; tolerated po in ED. Low risk for SBI; has f/u at 12 pm tomorrow, stable for d/c home with suction/nasal saline, monitor for respiratory distress (mom is a physician).

I saw and evaluated the patient. I personally obtained the key and critical portions of the history and physical exam. I reviewed the resident's documentation and discussed the patient with the resident. I agree with the resident's medical decision-making as documented in the resident's note.

-Attending, MD

Nursing Notes:

(2055) Baby suctioned with saline drops to nares, no secretions
(2131) Baby drank 2 oz of pedialyte
(2235) Baby drank 3 oz of breast milk from bottle

DIAGNOSIS:

URI, likely RSV

DISPOSITION (2235):

Home in stable condition. Follow-up with PCP tomorrow as scheduled. Prescriptions: Nasal saline

II. The Errors—Risk Management/Patient Safety Issues

Risk management/patient safety issue #1:

Error: Inadequate birth history.

Discussion: The birth history only mentions that the child was born "term." A more detailed history to delineate risk factors for underlying serious bacterial infections should be obtained including: prolonged ruptured membranes prior to delivery, vaginal versus Cesarean birth, maternal infections (i.e., Group B strep, chorioamnionitis, genital herpes and chlamydia).

✔ **Teaching point:** Mother's birth history is an important part of the newborn's history.

Risk management/patient safety issue #2:

Error: Inadequate vaccination history.

Discussion: Immunization status is frequently documented as "up to date" without further description. For children less than 2 months old, "up to date" only includes the initial Hepatitis B vaccination. The risk of serious bacterial infection decreases with the administration of the pneumococcal vaccinations typically administered at 2 months of age.[1] Of note, pertussis can mimic RSV in its clinical presentation due to the lack of classic "whooping cough" in this age group.

✔ **Teaching point:** For children near 2 months of age, it is important to note if the child has received their "2 month" immunizations against pneumococcal, Haemophilis influenzae type B infections and pertussis (DPT).

Risk management/patient safety issue #3:

Error: Documentation of "no evidence of meningismus" in an 8-week-old.

Discussion: Many clinicians feel that documentation of "no meningismus" obviates them from a meningitis work-up. Meningismus in an infant is difficult to assess, is frequently absent and should not be used to exclude meningitis in an ill-appearing infant. Lethargy, irritability, inconsolability, poor feeding, bulging fontanelle, and increased sleeping are more common signs of meningitis than meningismus.

✔ **Teaching point:** Lack of nuchal rigidity does not exclude meningitis in an infant.

Risk management/patient safety issue #4:

Error: Obtain reliable data on temperature prior to arrival.

Discussion: When an afebrile patient has a complaint of "fever" prior to arrival, it is important to learn if a thermometer was used, the route (rectal, oral, tympanic, axillary, forehead), and whether antipyretics were given prior to the ED presentation. Currently, there are numerous thermometers in the market and if the parents "added a degree," this could result in an unnecessarily septic work-up, however, the subjective report of fever (not the extent) is often accurate. Of note, hypothermia is an ominous sign of overwhelming infection in infants.

✔ **Teaching point:** The decision to initiate a febrile work-up should be based upon reliable and complete data.

Risk management/patient safety issue #5:

Error: The diagnosis needs to be supported with appropriate documentation.

Discussion: In the first 2 months of life it is important to differentiate between URI and bronchiolitis based on a thorough respiratory examination, including documentation of nasal flaring, supra-sternal retractions, inter-costal retractions, tachypnea, and wheezing. RSV bronchiolitis can present between 4–12 weeks of age. The gestational age is important to obtain as their post-natal age should be adjusted accordingly. For example a 34 week gestation infant with wheezing who is a 2 months old is truly only 2 weeks post-natal (from a lung maturity point of view) and perhaps, should be admitted due to the high risk of apnea. History should be elicited for chronic lung disease (formerly called broncho-pulmonary dysplasia) in premature babies, particularly if the infant was admitted to the NICU and was intubated or was on high flow oxygen/CPAP or sent home on oxygen.

✔ **Teaching point:** unique problems in occur in premature infants.

Risk management/patient safety issue #6:

Error: Inadequate differential diagnosis

Discussion: Caring for children of physicians is always challenging. Even if the parents are in the medical profession, treat them as "parents." Go over the discharge instructions in detail using appropriate medical terms (to avoid insulting them), but also use layman's terms to ensure understanding. It is difficult for parents to "doctor" their children in an objective fashion and they are looking to you for medical guidance.

✔ **Teaching point:** Even with health care workers or physicians, be sure to discuss in layman's terms discharge instructions and strict warning signs for return.

Summary of risk assessment:

The overall documentation in this case is quite good. There is documentation of a detailed history including term birth, immunization status, tolerance of feeds, number of wet diapers and URI symptoms. The exam includes non-templated descriptions of what seems to be a well-appearing, non-toxic infant without signs or symptoms of dehydration or respiratory distress. There are several sets of repeat vital signs and nursing note updates demonstrating that the child tolerated bottle feeds while in the ED. There is ensured follow-up with the primary care provider the next day.

The work-up seems appropriate, although some physicians may have ordered blood tests and a catheterized urine sample. The child was over 8 weeks of age without prematurity, or immunocompromise, and was afebrile in the emergency department with an apparent URI with known recent exposure to RSV.

Complete blood counts, blood cultures, and urine cultures are commonly obtained in well-appearing infants between 30–60 days of age to determine risk of occult serious bacterial infection. In children who have been immunized against pneumococcal infections, however, the routine use of CBC and blood cultures may not be recommended.[2,3] Children between the ages of 2–24 months presenting with the clinical scenario of bronchiolitis have been found to be at a lower risk of bacteremia and UTI's.[4] The respiratory virus panel seems appropriate. The value of chest x-ray in an afebrile child without hypoxia, respiratory distress or focal lung findings likely treated the expectations of the parent more than the clinical need of the child. In this case, further testing would not have changed the diagnosis or disposition.

III. Follow up with the PCP—1 day later (2/3/14)

- Vitals: 100.2
- Still frequent coughing reported, breathing not labored or rapid. Lungs clear, no GFR, good air entry.
- RVP still pending.
- Fever, cough over last 2 days, likely RSV given brother's recent illness -- clinically just URI at this time, no lower respiratory tract findings
- She is over 60 days old, she is not toxic appearing here, not actually febrile here -- discussed doing more workup such as UA/urine culture and CBC/blood culture but reviewed with parents that the risk of serious bacterial infection is low
- Supportive care
- Follow up in 2 days for recheck, mom knows to continue to monitor for resp distress, wheezing, apnea, dehydration

➢**Authors' note:** Was the patient having a normal "periodic breathing" or episodes of apnea?

Periodic breathing occurs when the breath pauses for up to 10 seconds at a time. There may be several such pauses close together, followed by a series of rapid, shallow breaths, then the breathing returns to normal. This is a common condition in premature babies in the first few weeks of life. Even healthy full-term babies sometimes have spells of periodic breathing.

Apnea on the other hand occurs when breathing stops for at least 20 seconds. The infant may become limp. There may be a change in skin color (such as blue or pale/gray color around the mouth) and a drop in heart rate before the baby starts breathing normally again. Sometimes the baby must be stimulated to restart breathing. None of this happens with periodic breathing.

In light of our patient's presentation with change in breathing patterns, high fever, decreased oral intake and urination and a positive RSV, a close follow up and perhaps same day ED evaluation was warranted.

IV. The Bounceback—2 days later (2/4/14)

- **EMS:** Child brought to ED by EMS after apparent life-threatening event (ALTE).
- **HPI:** This morning the child stopped breathing, turned ashen, received rescue breath by her mother. Upon EMS arrival, the child was hypoxic at 89%.
- **PE:** In the ED, the child was hypoxic at 92% and appeared dehydrated with basilar crackles and tachypnea.

- **MDM:** She was placed on supplemental oxygen, labs obtained with 13% bands and repeat CXR revealed right middle lobe and left retrocardiac infiltrates/atelectasis. Respiratory virus panel from initial visit was positive for RSV.
- **Disposition:** The child was admitted to the Pediatric Intensive Care Unit (PICU).

Diagnosis: RSV bronchiolitis; Possible pneumonia; hypoxia; dehydration; ALTE

HOSPITAL COURSE:

- Admitted to PICU and treated with ceftriaxone pending cultures for 48 hours. Required Vapotherm (high flow oxygen) therapy for 5 days and eventually weaned off supplemental oxygen.
- Transferred to pediatric floor on 2/8/14 after 5 days in PICU
- Discharged home on 2/9/14

PART 2—ANALYSIS

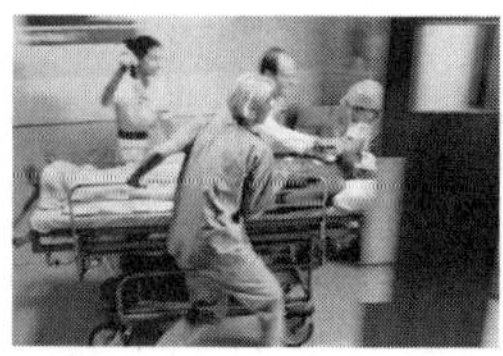

EVALUATION OF PEDIATRIC FEVER, DIFFERENTIATING BRONCHIOLITIS FROM PNEUMONIA, AND APPARENT LIFE-THREATENING EVENTS (ALTEs)

Jessica Mason, MD

Emergency Medicine Resident, 2nd year
Metro Health, Cleveland , Ohio
Producer and Co-Host: Resident Call Room Podcast. HippoEM.com

Christopher Wyatt, MD

Emergency Medicine Resident, 2nd year
Metro Health, Cleveland Ohio
Producer and Co-Host: Resident Call Room Podcast. HippoEM.com

Introduction

For the non-pediatric emergency physician, the chief complaint of pediatric fever often elicits a guttural moan:

Why can't they just see their pediatrician?! Why do I work at a hospital without a separate pediatric emergency department?! If I have to convince another overly concerned parent that their child isn't sick I'm going to ...

Children with fever account for as many as 20% of pediatric emergency department visits. Every pediatric "season" is accompanied by fever: influenza season, RSV season, croup season, rotavirus season, enterovirus season, and the list goes on and on. It seems like pediatric fever never takes a vacation and every child under the age of 2 either has a cough and fever or diarrhea and fever. The appropriate evaluation and disposition of pediatric patients with fever is a common challenge. Underlying etiologies of fever range from mild to severe, from viral infections to the most serious bacterial infections, including meningitis and sepsis.

Clinical guidelines have been published and frequently debated, with no definite algorithmic conclusion that can satisfy every situation. Emergency medicine residents train under teaching physicians with varying risk tolerances who often practice differently. Because pediatric fever is so common, the emergency physician should be knowledgeable about febrile illnesses affecting a variety of age groups, the risk factors associated with more serious infections, and guidelines regarding the approach to care for children with fever.

However, even the most ardent and knowledgeable clinician following the most recent guidelines will eventually have the pediatric fever *bounce back*. Sometimes, the discussion with parents regarding warning signs and indications for return are far more important than the tests ordered during their ED visit. This case lends us many points for discussion.

Was she febrile?

What is a fever? Fever is either present or absent, but temperature is on a continuum. We define fever so we can study it, and then we use this to shape our clinical impression of a patient. The exact temperature cut-off that defines a fever varies based on age of the patient, site, local custom and clinical scenario.[5,6,7] There may also be varying definitions depending on medical specialty (i.e., emergency physicians versus pediatricians).[6] Some studies suggest no single value should define fever since there is such variability among individuals, age, and time of day.[8]

The currently accepted custom for defining acute fevers in infants evaluated in the emergency departments in the U.S. is a rectal temperature of 38.0°C (100.4°F).[9, 10] This cut-off was used to define "fever" in the landmark studies that gave us the Boston Criteria and Rochester Criteria for the work-up of febrile infants.[9, 10] Interestingly or perhaps frustratingly), a third major U.S. study, giving us the Philadelphia Criteria, used 38.2°C (100.76°F) as their definition of fever. The British Thoracic Society uses 38.5°C (101.3°F).[7] The exact temperature defining fever may seem a moot point, but it is often the catalyst in triggering an invasive and thorough work-up looking for a serious bacterial infection.

In this case we have an infant with a temperature of 37.9°C (100.2°F) on initial visit. Using a binary interpretation of fever, she is afebrile. Should 1/10th of a degree change your clinical impression and work-up? At her initial ED visit, she is described as well appearing and afebrile. Chest x-ray was normal and a RSV swab was sent. Had she been "febrile," the work-up would have likely changed to include urinalysis, possibly blood cultures and lumbar puncture.

But again, this child is "well appearing," the physician has low suspicion for serious bacterial illness, there is good follow-up arranged for the next day and a reasonable parent is in agreement with the plan. In this case, would this additional and invasive work-up have changed the outcome? Probably not, though it does raise concern for a purely algorithmic approach as opposed as to a clinical impression which may better serve our patient.

How old is she?

In addition to being on the cusp of a fever, she is also on the cusp of two age categories that are significant in the work-up of an acute pediatric fever, well-appearing infants age 30–59 days versus 60–90 days. Data comparing these two populations is limited, and the approach is based more on recommendations than evidence. Well-appearing infants 30–59 days are studied in the Philadelphia Criteria. Well-appearing infants 60–90 days show no significant difference to those older than 90 days.[11] The primary difference between the work-up of well appearing febrile infants <60 days versus well appearing febrile infants >60 days is that lumbar puncture is generally recommended in the <60 day group.[12]

In this case, the patient's exact age in days is not stated, but we can infer if she is 8 weeks, that she is around 56–63 days. Again, she is right at the cusp of two categories, defined largely for the purpose of research and developing clinical decision making tools. Should this child have gotten a lumbar puncture? Would it have changed anything? I don't think so. It is well documented that she has a reliable caregiver and next-day follow-up.

Should she have gotten blood cultures, urine cultures, and urinalysis? Not if you are strictly interpreting the definition of fever and are calling this a well-appearing afebrile child. Would this have changed her outcome? Even with the benefit of hindsight, I don't think this would have changed her disposition. She bounced back before blood cultures would have been available, they may never have grown bacteria, and the urine also may not have grown bacteria.

Comparison of the Boston, Rochester, and Philadelphia Criteria for Evaluation of Pediatric Fever

In our attempts to approach medicine as scientists we must remember that evidence based medicine has the flaw of human design.

Table 1: Comparison of the Boston, Rochester, and Philadelphia Criteria for Evaluation of Pediatric Fever

Location	**Boston**	**Rochester**	**Philadelphia**
Year published	1992	1994	1999
Age	28-89 days	0-60 days	29-60
Rectal temperature	38.0°C	38.0°C	38.2°C
Work-up	CBC with differential Blood cultures Urinalysis Urine cultures Stool WBCs (if diarrhea) Lumbar puncture, CSF cytology and culture CXR (if respiratory symptoms)	CBC with differential Blood cultures Urinalysis Urine cultures Stool WBCs (if diarrhea) If starting antibiotics → lumbar puncture, CSF cytology and culture	CBC with differential Blood cultures Urinalysis Urine cultures Stool WBCs (if diarrhea) Lumbar puncture, CSF cytology and culture CXR
High risk (admit and empiric antibiotics)	WBC >15,000 Band-neutrophil ratio >0.2 UA >10 WBC per hpf Urine gram stain positive CSF >8 WBC CSF Gram stain positive CXR with infiltrate Stool: blood, or moderate WBCs	WBC <5,000 or >15,000 Absolute bands >1500 UA >10 WBC per hpf Stool: >5 WBC	WBC >20,000 UA >10 WBC CSF >10 WBC CXR with infiltrate

Time for an update?

Let's put these guidelines into the perspective of time.

1984–1992	Data is collected for the Boston, Rochester, and Philadelphia criteria [9, 11, 12]
1987&1989	Release of Haemophilus influenzae type B (HIB) conjugate vaccines [13]
1993	CDC recommends HIB vaccine [13]
2000	7-valent pneumococcal conjugate vaccine (PCV7) is introduced [14]
2010	13-valent pneumococcal conjugate vaccine (PCV13) is introduced [15]

The epidemiology of serious bacterial infection (SBI) has changed since the HIB vaccine and pneumococcal vaccines. This is changing how physicians evaluate febrile infants, with the trend being a decline in frequency of ordering labs.[14] The overall rate of SBI has dramatically decreased since the widespread use of these vaccines in the United States.[13, 14, 16] In light of this, it seems to be time to reevaluate the data and develop new guidelines accounting for advances made in preventative medicine.

Greg Henry comments

"I have watched the pediatric fever evaluation change extensively during the course of my career."

It should be remembered that practice guidelines, written in broad and general terms, are a best guess of the science at any moment in time. We practice medicine on the specific patient in front of us. While it is important for physicians to be aware that guidelines exist, it is also reasonable to make deviations as necessary depending on the patient you are seeing; you are not a prisoner of guidelines. I have seen guidelines used many times in court, but if properly educated, a physician can duck the blows. It is important to document your management decisions which deviate from usual or customary care; your observations are excellent defensive postures should they be needed in court.

I have watched the pediatric fever evaluation change extensively during the course of my career. In the late 60's and early 70's, children three months and below were automatically septic work ups. Spinal taps, cath urines, cultures from every orifice were standard. IV, antibiotics and admission to the hospital were routine. Fortunately, someone actually looked at the statistics and found out that well-looking kids are well. The automatic work-up and admission has now gone from three months down to a month. A considerable number of children have been spared the tortures of a septic workup by applying some common sense and more data.

Pneumoniolitis?

What's the difference between bronchiolitis and pneumonia in infants? (Sounds like a bad joke!) There is a lot of overlap in how they have been defined.

Bronchiolitis—lower respiratory tract inflammation and bronchospasm commonly causing rhinitis, wheezing, cough, crackles, and signs of respiratory distress. Typically caused by viruses with the most common being RSV.[17]

Pneumonia—fever and/or acute respiratory symptoms with infiltrates on chest x-ray. Pathogens vary with age, most common in 3 weeks to 3 months being chlamydia trachomatis, RSV, parainfluenza 3, and strep pneumonia.[21]

This patient has significant risk factors, as her older sibling was recently RSV positive with pneumonia. Was it RSV pneumonia, or RSV with bacterial super-infection causing pneumonia? Either way, it would be difficult to justify an admission based on the initial ED visit. The bounceback visit is much easier because of the apparent life-threatening event (ALTE), fever, and infiltrate on chest x-ray. She's coming in!

Bronchiolitis and apparent life threatening events (ALTE)

ALTE is an episode that is frightening to the observer, characterized by apnea, color change (cyanotic or pale), change in muscle tone, choking, or gagging.[25] There is a known association between bronchiolitis and episodes of apnea.[23, 24] Risk factors for apneic episodes in infants include: prematurity, underlying chronic conditions, cardiac disease, pulmonary hypertension, and age <3 months with RSV, especially if the patient is hypoxic at presentation.[25] Apneic events are more common in infants <2–3 months with RSV, and within the first 5 days from onset of illness.[24]

In retrospect, there are several risk factors for this child: known exposure to RSV and age <2–3 months. Even if you had all of this information at your fingertips, what would you do differently? Routinely admitting her may be the most conservative action, but could lead to excessive and inappropriate admissions, though apnea is life threatening and observation in the hospital is very reasonable to do in high risk patients for apnea with bronchiolitis.

Prevention and treatment of bronchiolitis

The Cochrane Review from 2013 of vaccination to prevent bronchiolitis shows some data to support vaccination using Palivizumab in infants at increased risk for developing severe RSV infections. This would include infants born premature, or with chronic lung disease or congenital heart disease.[23] This is new and not yet the general practice. If this data translates to practice, this child would not have been a candidate for the Palivizumab vaccine.

Supplemental Oxygen

Treatment of bronchiolitis is based in supportive care—hydration and respiratory support. Supplemental oxygen should be started in hypoxic infants, with SpO2 <90–92%.[24] Heated humidified high-flow nasal cannula oxygen is a newer option for infants with worsening hypoxia or hypercapnia or increase in work of breathing, and may reduce the need for intubation.[25] No surprise, there is plenty of debate and no consensus about when to start supplemental oxygen, and what pulse oximeter number is the defined cut-off for hypoxia. If there is no consensus on fever, why would there be a consensus for hypoxia?!

Bronchodilators

Infants with respiratory distress may receive a trial of bronchodilators. This may help infants with underlying reactive airway disease that causes virally triggered wheezing or asthma.[26] However, there is little evidence showing benefit of bronchodilators in infants with bronchiolitis and no underlying reactive airway component.[27] A trial of nebulized bronchodilators may be appropriate if you suspect an underlying reactive airway disease, and if there is no improvement afterwards, further breathing treatments are likely futile. Racemic epinephrine nebulized treatment can be used in patients with bronchiolitis who meet admission criteria such as hypoxia, increased work of breathing, decrease oral intake due to respiratory distress (after nasal suction), and dehydration. The systematic review by Hartling, et al., concluded that epinephrine reduced hospitalizations compared with placebo on the day of the ED visit but not overall. Given that epinephrine has a transient effect and home administration is not routine practice, discharging an infant after observing a response in a monitored setting raises concerns for subsequent progression of illness. Studies have not found a difference in revisit rates, although the numbers of revisits are small and may not be adequately powered for this outcome. In summary, the current state of evidence does not support a routine role for epinephrine for bronchiolitis in outpatients, although further data may help to better define this question.[28, 29]

Discussion of this patient's bounceback

With an abundance of literature and guidelines applying somewhat arbitrary cut-offs, it can be easy to miss the big picture of what we are trying to do. The goal is to identify which patients may be at risk for serious bacterial illness, identify a source and treat them appropriately.

This is a case in which you want the child to bounce back. The ALTE, though frightening, was the clue that the baby was becoming more hypoxic. A bounce back means the parent listened to your return precautions. In this case, it led to the work-up that identified a source of infection, and an appropriate admission to the pediatric intensive care unit.

The details are important and useful, but with myopic focus on details it is easy to lose sight of the big picture. This is a well appearing child with a reliable caregiver and good follow-up, who was appropriately sent home with return precautions. Admission to the hospital is overkill and may even expose the child to worse pathogens. After reviewing the final outcome, it does not seem that anything could have been done differently on the initial visit to predict or to avoid the bounceback.

✔ Teaching points

- Obtain a detailed birth history regarding maternal perinatal infections, prematurity and immunization status, specifically against pneumococcal disease and pertussis.
- Accurate description and documentation of the general appearance, respiratory and hydration status in the febrile infant is important.
- Recognize the context of the Boston, Rochester, and Philadelphia criteria, and don't lose sight of your overall clinical impression.
- There is a known association between RSV and ALTE, especially if the patient is < 2–3 months, was born premature, and is hypoxic at the time of the visit.
- Hypoxic patients should get supplemental O2 and possibly a trial of bronchodilators if reactive airway disease is suspected. Deep nasal suction can markedly improve the respiratory status.
- Thorough instructions and indications for return should be discussed with a competent parent and might be the most life-saving intervention you provide. At-risk infants with borderline clinical findings or unreliable caregivers may benefit from observation.

References

1. Black S, France EK, Isaacman D, et al. Surveillance for invasive pneumococcal disease during 2000–2005 in a population of children who received 7-valent pneumococcal conjugate vaccine. Pediatr Infect Dis J. 2007;26(9):771–7.
2. Rudinsky SL, Carstairs KL, Reardon JM, et al. Serious bacterial infections in febrile infants in the post-pneumococcal conjugate vaccine era. Acad Emerg Med. 2009;16(7):585–90.
3. Mintegi S, Benito J, Sanchez J, et al. Predictors of occult bacteremia in young febrile children in the era of heptavalent pneumococcal conjugated vaccine. Eur J Emerg Med. 2009;16(4):199–205.
4. Kuppermann N, Bank DE, Walton EA, et al. Risks for bacteremia and urinary tract infections in young febrile children with bronchiolitis. Arch Pediatr Adolesc Med. 1997;151(12):1207–14.
5. Dagan R, Powell KR, Menegus MA. Identification of infants unlikely to have serious bacterial infection although hospitalized for suspected sepsis. J Pediatr. 1985; 107(6):855–60.
6. Baraff LJ. Management of the febrile child: a survey of pediatric and emergency residency directors. Pediatr Infect Dis J. 1991;10(11):795–800.
7. Harris M, Clark J, Coote N, et al. British Thoracic Society guidelines for the management of community acquired pneumonia in children: update 2011. Thorax. 2011;66 Suppl 2:ii1–23.
8. Mackowiak PA, Wasserman SS, Levine MM. A critical appraisal of 98.6 degrees F, the upper limit of the normal body temperature, and other legacies of Carl Reinhold August Wunderlich. JAMA. 1992;268(12):1578–80.
9. Baskin MN, O'Rourke EJ, Fleisher GR. Outpatient treatment of febrile infants 28 to 89 days of age with intramuscular administration of ceftriaxone. J Pediatr. 1992;120(1):22–7.
10. Jaskiewicz JA, McCarthy CA, Richardson AC, et al. Febrile infants at low risk for serious bacterial infection—an appraisal of the Rochester criteria and implications for management. Febrile Infant Collaborative Study Group. Pediatrics. 1994;94(3):390–6.
11. Hsiao AL, Chen L, Baker MD. Incidence and predictors of serious bacterial infections among 57- to 180-day-old infants. Pediatrics. 2006; 117(5):1695–701.
12. Baker DM, Bell LM, Avner JR. Outpatient management without antibiotics of fever in selected infants. N Engl J Med. 1993;329(20):1437–41.
13. Briere EC, Rubin L, Moro PL. Prevention and control of Haemophilus influenzae type b disease: Recommendations of the advisory committee on immunization practices (ACIP). MMWR Recomm Rep. 2014 Feb 28;63(RR-01):1–14.
14. Simon AE, Lukacs SL, Mendola P. National trends in emergency department use of urinalysis, complete blood count, and blood culture for fever without a source among children aged 2 to 24 months in the pneumococcal conjugate vaccine 7 era. Pediatr Emerg Care. 2013; 29(5):560–7.
15. Kaplan SL, Barson WJ, Lin PL. Early trends for invasive pneumococcal infections in children after the introduction of the 13-valent pneumococcal conjugate vaccine. Pediatr Infect Dis J. 2013;32(3):203–7.

16. Mistry RD, Wedin T, Balamuth F. Emergency department epidemiology of pneumococcal bacteremia in children since the institution of widespread PCV7 vaccination. J Emerg Med. 2013;45(6):813–20.
17. American Academy of Pediatrics Subcommittee on Diagnosis and Management of Bronchiolitis. Diagnosis and management of bronchiolitis. Pediatrics. 2006;118(4):1774–93.
18. McIntosh K. Community-acquired pneumonia in children. N Engl J Med. 2002; 346(6):429–37.
19. Little GA, Ballard RA, Brooks JG, et al. National Institute of Health Consensus Development. Course on infantile apnoea and home monitoring. Paediatrics. 1987;79:292–9.
20. Bruhn FW, Mokrohisky ST, McIntosh K. Apnea associated with respiratory syncytial virus infection in young infants. J Pediatr. 1977; 90(3):382–6.
21. Arms JL, Ortega H, Reid S. Chronological and clinical characteristics of apnea associated with respiratory syncytial virus infection: a retrospective case series. Clin Pediatr. 2008;47(9):953–8.
22. Bronchiolitis Guideline Team, Cincinnati Children's Hospital Medical Center. Bronchiolitis pediatric evidence-based care guidelines, 2010. http://www.cincinnatichildrens.org/service/j/anderson-center/evidence-based-care/bronchiolitis/ (Accessed on March 15, 2014).
23. Andabaka T, Nickerson JW, Rojas-Reyes MX, et al. Monoclonal antibody for reducing the risk of respiratory syncytial virus infection in children. Cochrane Database Syst Rev. 2013 Apr 30; 4:CD006602.
24. Panitch HB. Respiratory syncytial virus bronchiolitis: supportive care and therapies designed to overcome airway obstruction. Pediatr Infect Dis J. 2003; 22(2 Suppl):S83–7; discussion S87–8.
25. McKiernan C, Chua LC, Visintainer PF, et al. High flow nasal cannulae therapy in infants with bronchiolitis. J Pediatr. 2010;156(4):634–8.
26. Frey U, von Mutius E. The challenge of managing wheezing in infants. N Engl J Med. 2009;360(20):2130–3.
27. Gadomski AM, Bhasale AL. Bronchodilators for bronchiolitis. Cochrane Database Syst Rev 2006 Jul 19; (3):CD001266.
28. Hartling L, Fernandes RM, Bialy L, et al. Steroids and bronchodilators for acute bronchiolitis in the first two years of life: systematic review and meta-analysis. BMJ. 2011;342:d1714.
29. Wainwright C, Altamirano L, Cheney M, et al. A multicenter, randomized, double-blind, controlled trial of nebulized epinephrine in infants with acute bronchiolitis. N Engl J Med. 2003;349(1):27–35.

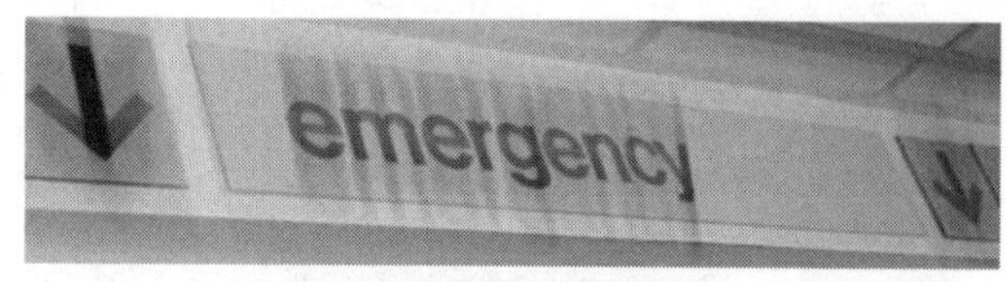

CASE 25

5-YEAR-OLD WITH FATIGUE AND SLEEPINESS

Stephen A. Coluccielo, MD, FACEP
Chief, Department of Emergency Medicine,
Carolinas Medical Center, Charlotte, NC
Professor, Department of Emergency Medicine,
University of North Carolina Charlotte Campus, Charlotte, NC

Jessica Baxley, MD
Department of Emergency Medicine, Resident
Carolinas Medical Center, Charlotte, NC
University of Maryland School of Medicine

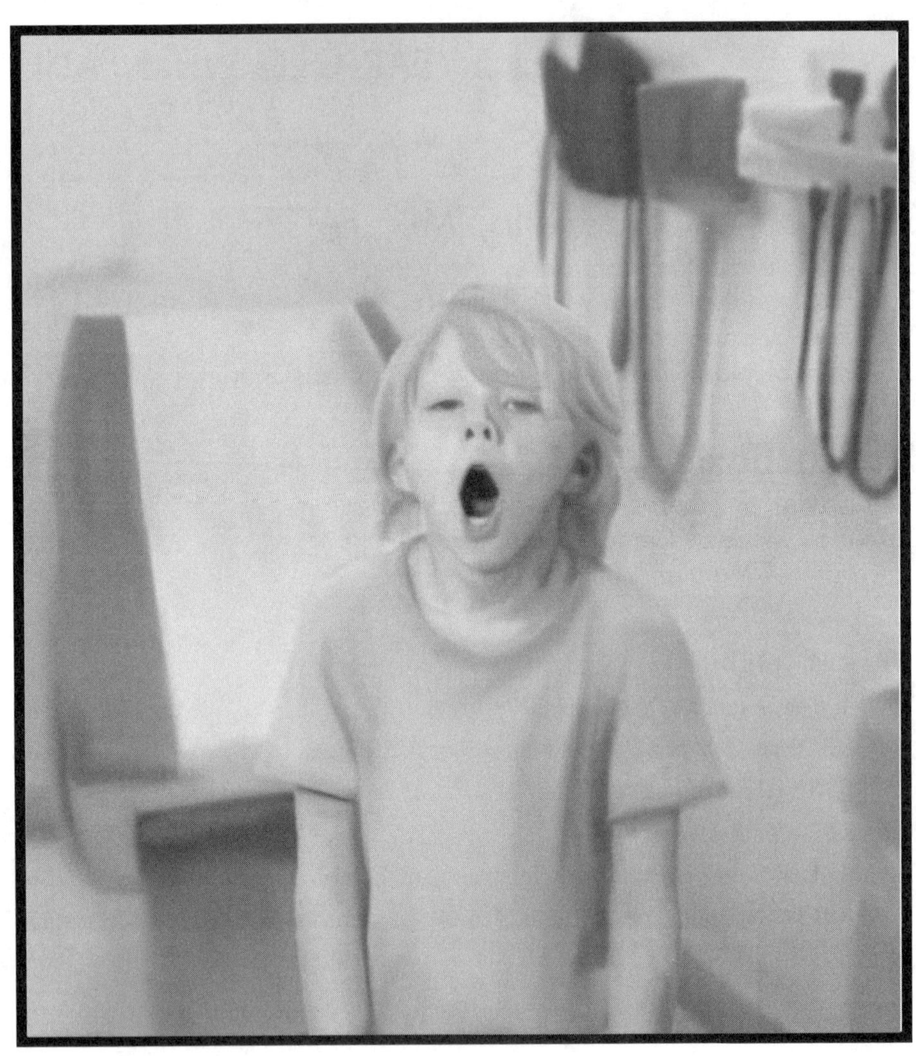

CASE 25

5-YEAR-OLD WITH FATIGUE AND SLEEPINESS

PART 1—MEDICAL

I. The Doctor's Version (the following is the actual documentation of the provider)

Date: January 21, 2014
Chief complaint: "Headache & fatigue"

PCP office:
HISTORY OF PRESENT ILLNESS "headache every day for the last several months, usually in the morning and decreased energy level for several weeks." (Patient was also documented to have short stature and questionable developmental delay.)

REVIEW OF SYSTEMS:
Constitutional: negative
Ears/Nose/Throat: negative
Respiratory: negative
Integumentary: needs eczema cream refilled
Neurologic: headache every day for the last several months, sometimes every other day, usually in the morning, never wakes him up in the middle of the night. Mother gives him Tylenol or Motrin 2-3 times a week

PAST MEDICAL HISTORY:
Allergies: Amoxicillin
Medications: Cetirizine, hydrocortisone topical
PMH: Eczema, short stature
Social History: vaccinations up to date
Family History: Asthma – brother; ADD – brother

EXAM:

VITAL SIGNS							
Tem(F)Rt	Pulse	Resp	Syst	Diast	SpO2	Height	Weight
NR*	NR*	NR*	88	42	NA	94.6cm	15.6kg

*NR=Not Recorded

General appearance – small but well developed
Eyes – Pupils are equal, round and reactive to light, Extraocular movements are intact, Normal conjunctiva.
HENT: Normocephalic, Tympanic membranes are clear, Oral mucosa is moist, No pharyngeal erythema, no pharyngeal exudate.
Neck: Supple, Non-tender, No lymphadenopathy.
Respiratory: Lungs are clear to auscultation, Respirations are non-labored, Breath sounds are equal, Symmetrical chest wall expansion.
Cardiovascular: Normal rate, Regular rhythm, No murmur, Good pulses equal in all extremities.
Gastrointestinal: Soft, Non-tender, Non-distended, Normal bowel sounds, No organomegaly, No masses.
Genitourinary: Bilateral Testes Descended; no inguinal hernia, Normal genitalia for age and sex.
Lymphatics: No lymphadenopathy.
Musculoskeletal: Normal Duck Walk; Normal Toe Walk; Normal Heel Walk; No scoliosis, Normal range of motion, Normal strength, Normal gait.
Integumentary: Pink, mild dry patches, old scratch marks on his abdomen, Warm, No rash.
Neurologic: Normal sensory, Normal motor function, No focal defects, Normal deep tendon reflexes.
Psychiatric: Cooperative.

OFFICE VISIT COURSE:
Patient received flu vaccination and was discharged home.

DIAGNOSIS: 1. Short stature for age 2. Headache

MDM: Small stature: likely familial (patient's parents with short stature). Headache is possibly attention seeking as the headache usually resolves with maternal attention

DISPOSITION: Patient was discharged home. Per the discharge note patient was to be evaluated in 2 weeks for bone age and blood work including CBC w/ diff, CMP, ESR, phosphate, TSH/T4/IGF-1, and IGFBP-3, anti tissue Transglutaminase, IgA and a possible endocrine referral

II.Discussion by Madeline Matar Joseph

Although the PCP was on the right track in test ordering, the MDM showed that the physician dismissed the importance of the combination of short stature and headache.

Causes of short stature fall into one of three major categories:

1. **Familial short stature:** Children with familial short stature have short parents. These normal children display normal growth velocity (speed of growth over time), and their bone development is normal (as indicated by the bone age corresponding to the calendar age). Children with familial short stature enter puberty at a normal time and typically complete growth with a height consistent with that of their parents.

2. **Constitutional delay of growth and development ("late bloomers"):** These are normal children who are small for their age but who have a normal growth rate. It is characterized by delayed bone age, normal growth velocity, and a predicted adult height appropriate to the family pattern. Children with constitutional growth delay typically have a close relative who displayed constitutional growth delay.
3. **Chronic disease:** Patients with chronic disease occur in a broad spectrum of disorders including endocrine disorders, such as hypothyroidism, growth hormone deficiency, and genetic diseases including Down syndrome and Turner syndrome.

"Attention seeking" should be diagnosed with caution and is less likely to occur spontaneously (i.e., not associated with a major life-event such as birth of a sibling, moving to a new home, or divorce).

III. The Bounceback

PHONE MESSAGE TO PCP:

2/26/14 15:46 – Nursing note "Mom says for the past few weeks patient has been unusually tired, sleeping an awful lot, not wanting to play. His schoolwork is suffering because he says he is too tired to do it. Mom says patient came in for blood work yesterday, "Any results from that yet?"

2/26/14 17:09 - PCP Addendum: Spoke with Mom and notified her of lab results. She said patient is sleeping "all day" and not eating much for past 2 weeks but seems worse past few days. Has had enuresis as well because he is too tired to get up. No sick contacts at home. Recommend go to ED now for evaluation. Mom states she will take him.

ED visit – February 26, 2014 – arrival in triage @ 20:00

- **HPI (20:45):** "5 yr old presents to emergency department with 2 weeks of increased fatigue and sleepiness. Mother states that two weeks ago the patient was out running around acting like a normal child and then became gradually more fatigue and sleepy. He states now that the child sleeps for most of the day. He is arousable. However, has begun peeing on himself because he is too tired to get out of bed to go to the bathroom. Mother also states that at times he will get up to walk and slump to the floor. Mother states that previously the patient would complain of frequent headache and was told by her pediatrician that it was most likely attention seeking. Mother denies any antecedent infection symptoms such as runny nose, cough, fevers or chills. Labs were drawn yesterday which showed a mild anemia and slightly decreased blood sugar and therefore the patient was sent to the emergency department for further evaluation."
- **ROS:** weakness, fatigue, decreased activity, no fever or chills, + headache, + altered level of consciousness
- **Vitals:** HR 74; RR 20; BP 94/65; O2 99% on RA
- **Physical Exam:**

  General: Asleep, arousable but then quickly falls back asleep.
  Developmental milestones: 4–5 years.
  Skin: Warm, intact, normal for ethnicity.
  Head: Normocephalic, atraumatic.
  Neck: Supple, trachea midline.

Eyes: Extra-ocular movements are intact, normal conjunctiva, No obvious papilledema
Ears, nose, mouth and throat: Tympanic membranes clear, oral mucosa moist, no pharyngeal erythema or exudate.
Cardiovascular: No murmur, Normal peripheral perfusion, No edema, Regular rhythm w/ rate.
Respiratory: Lungs are clear to auscultation, respirations are non-labored, breath sounds are equal, Symmetrical chest wall expansion.
Gastrointestinal: Soft, Nontender.
Genitourinary: Normal genitalia for age, no discharge, no lesions.
Musculoskeletal: Patient able to move bilateral upper and lower extremities. Not very cooperative with exam as patient falls asleep. Was able to lift arms and had good grip strength. Able to lift bilateral legs after much coaching. Diminished pulses in LE. 1+ biceps and brachialis reflex
Neurological: Sleepy but arousable. Falls back asleep quickly.

- **Labs (22:16):**
  - o CG4: pH 7.417; CO2 39.1, O2 48; Lactate 1.11
  - o WBC 4.8, Hgb 9.2/Hct 28%, PLT 351
  - o Metabolic: Na 136, K 4.0, Cl 102, CO2 26, BUN 20, Cr 0.4
- **Head CT (20:50):**

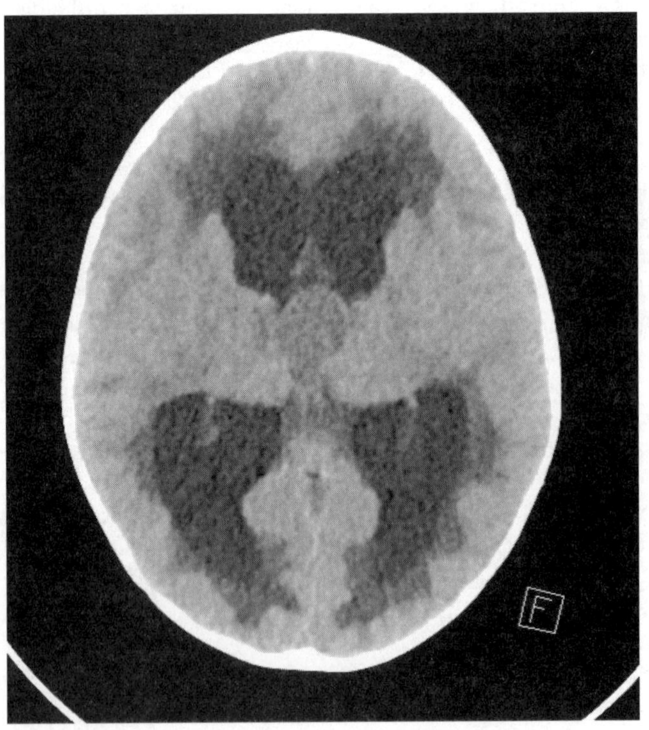

Rad reading: Large sellar/suprasellar mass causing severe obstructive hydrocephalus with transependymal CSF migration. Differential considerations include craniopharyngioma and, less likely, germinoma.

- Neurosurgery consulted
- PICU admission

Final ED diagnosis:

1. Altered Mental status
2. Sellar mass
3. Severe obstructive hydrocephalus

HOSPITAL COURSE

- Hospital Day (HD) #1: Admitted – underwent emergent bilateral ventricular catheter placement
- HD#6: Bifrontal craniotomy for resection of craniopharyngioma with placement of ventriculostomy
- HD#7: Developed post-operative diabetes insipidus
- HD#20: Bilateral burr hole craniotomy for evacuation of subdural hygromas
- HD #26: Discharged with shunt in place

PART 2—THE ANALYSIS

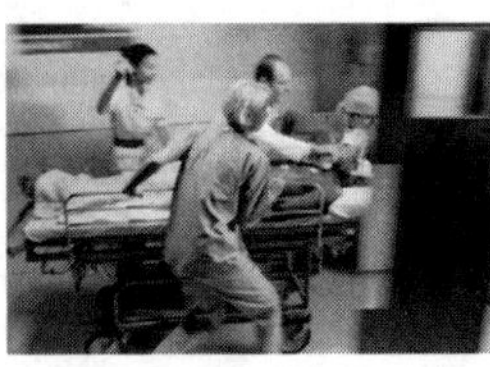

I. DIAGNOSIS AND MANAGEMENT OF PEDIATRIC FATIGUE/ALTERED MENTAL STATUS

Stephen A. Colucciello, MD, FACEP

Chief, Department of Emergency Medicine,
Carolinas Medical Center, Charlotte, NC
Professor, Department of Emergency Medicine,
University of North Carolina Charlotte Campus, Charlotte, NC

Jessica Baxley, MD

Department of Emergency Medicine, Resident
Carolinas Medical Center, Charlotte, NC
University of Maryland School of Medicine

Differential diagnosis of altered mental status (AMS)

Altered mental status (AMS) is one of the most common presenting symptoms seen in the adult emergency department.[1] However, it is less commonly encountered in the pediatric world. The diagnosis is complicated by the patient's inability to contribute to history taking and a wide range of potential etiologies. A brief reminder on pathophysiology: bilateral cerebral hemispheres and the ascending reticular activating system (ARAS) are needed in order to maintain consciousness and arousal. In order to impact cognition and arousal, both cerebral hemispheres or the ARAS need to be knocked out or impacted by global dysfunction.[2] The list of potential etiologies is overwhelming at best, and we've all learned a variety of mnemonics; the AEIOUTIPS is a favorite.[3]

A – Alcohol / Acidosis
E – Epilepsy/ Electrolytes
I – Infection
O – Overdose
U – Uremia
T – Trauma
I – Insulin (excess or deficiency), inborn errors of metabolism
P – Poisoning/ Psychosis
S – Stroke, shock, shunt, space occupying lesion

Infection, trauma, and toxins are the most common causes of altered level of consciousness in the pediatric population, with trauma increasing in incidence as children age.[4] In the pediatric population it may be easier to classify altered mental status etiologies based on age.

Infant

- Infection
- Congenital Malformation/ Hydrocephalus
- Metabolic Derangement
- Inborn error of metabolism
- Seizure
- Abuse

Childhood

- Infection
- Seizure
- Toxin
- Trauma
- Metabolic
- Abuse
- Space occupying lesion

Adolescence

- Toxin
- Trauma
- Infection
- Metabolic
- Space occupying lesions
- Psych

Approach to the Altered Pediatric Patient

ABCs first—always and forever

Evaluating mental status—alertness exists on a spectrum

- o Lethargy—arousable but decreased attention
- o Obtundation—decreased response to stimuli
- o Stupor—only arousable by repetitive and painful stimuli
- o Coma—nonresponsive

The progression from lethargy to coma can happen rather insidiously, as seen in our case presentation. The patient started out as "less energetic" than usual and became severely obtunded within weeks.

Clear as mud, right? Luckily we have a scale to allow us to adequately evaluate children's mental status: the Glasgow Coma Scale—the pediatric modified one to be exact. Though it was tough to memorize in medical school, it can be a useful tool in actual practice.[5]

Adult Glasgow	Pediatric Glasgow	Score
Eye Opening		
Spontaneously	Spontaneously	4
On command	To speech	3
To pain	To pain	2
None	None	1
Motor		
Follows commands	Spontaneously	6
Localizes	Withdraws to touch	5
Withdraws	Withdraws to pain	4
Decorticate	Abnormal flexion	3
Decerebrate	Abnormal extension	2
None	No response	1
Verbal		
Oriented	Coos, age appropriate verbalizations	5
Confused	Irritable cry	4
Inappropriate Words	Cries to pain	3
Incomprehensible	Moans/ grunts	2
No Response	No response	1

History: Though obtaining a history can be limited secondary to patient's mental status, there are some important clues that can lead to a diagnosis. The combination of altered mental status proceeded by or accompanying headache, blurred vision, nausea or vomiting should raise suspicion for an increase in intracranial pressure, and any focal neurologic findings on exam should prompt immediate neuro-imaging. This is complicated by the fact that some nonstructural etiologies of AMS, such as hypoglycemia, hypocalcemia or uremia can present with focal neuro deficits.[4] Hydrocephalus can be particularly difficult to pick up initially as it can present without focal neurologic findings or papilledema.

The rapidity of onset provides important clues to etiology. If there is a sudden onset change in mental status one should consider vascular catastrophes such as infarct or hemorrhage, cardiac etiologies such as arrhythmia or a toxic ingestion. A more insidious onset of symptoms, as was seen in this case, should raise concern for evolving structural mass or lesion.

Physical examination: Vital signs are important; hyperthermia, tachycardia and tachypnea can suggest toxic ingestion, metabolic abnormality or infectious process. The dreaded bradycardia and hypertension can represent impending herniation. Even normal vital signs can significantly narrow the differential.

- HEENT: evaluate for hematoma for possible evidence of trauma; in neonates feel for fullness or pulsations in the fontanel
- Eyes:
  - o Small & Fixed pupils—pontine lesion, opioid ingestions
  - o Small & Reactive pupils—medullary process, metabolic derangement

- o Dilated & Fixed
  - Bilateral—diffuse cerebral damage
  - Unilateral—space occupying lesion, herniation, third nerve palsy
- o Funduscopic
  - Evaluate for papilledema and retinal hemorrhages (indicative of abuse in young children) as well
  - Papilledema has a 98% specificity and 100% sensitivity for increased ICP in children over 8 yrs old[27]
- Ears/Nose—look for bleeding or CSF leak (trauma)
- Resp—Rate, odor—patients in DKA tend to have deep rapid breathing
- Skin
  - o Petechial rash and AMS should suggest meningococcemia, rocky mountain spotted fever (RMSF), sepsis, DIC, or TTP
  - o Bruising especially in infants and younger children may suggest non-accidental trauma (NAT)
- GI—splenomegaly, bruising, abrasions

Laboratory testing: Engrained in every provider caring for an altered patient should be an order for a stat bedside glucose. This is especially true in the pediatric population as it is a common cause of altered cognition, especially in neonates who have extremely low nutritional stores and cannot compensate to even the smallest of physical insults. A basic chemistry panel is useful to determine metabolic derangements including acidosis, DKA, and a CBC can help tease out infection or hematologic pathology. In the truly undifferentiated altered patient LFTs, ammonia, urine drug screen, and toxicological panels can be useful. Drug levels of any known anti-epileptic drug (AED) or antipsychotic should be drawn, and in the correct age group inborn errors of metabolism labs (plasma free fatty acids, serum carnitine, etc.) should be considered.

Imaging: Discussions about neuroimaging in the pediatric population are always surrounded by concern over radiation; which "altered" children require a CT scan, which need a MRI and who can get away without imaging? A complete discussion of preferred neuroimaging in children is beyond the scope of this chapter, but in general a CT scan is indicated if there is history or physical sequelae suggestive of trauma, focal findings on neurologic examination which could indicate mass or bleed, altered mental status (AMS) with unknown etiology, or unclear history/unsupervised child.

Back to our case

This was an admittedly difficult case initially—the moribund child is hard to miss, but a relatively well appearing 5-year-old with nonspecific complaints is much easier to overlook. However, there were several warning signs and management issues that could have been addressed. While the patient presented for a routine well child exam, the mom did raise concern over his nearly daily morning headaches as well as the associated fatigue. With this complaint, a more detailed history with consideration of carbon monoxide toxicity and a thorough neurological examination including assessment of gait (to rule ataxia since most of tumors in children are located in the posterior fossa) was mandated. Most damning in the original documentation is the suggestion that the patient's headaches are "attention seeking." Without an adequate history to justify the diagnosis, this is dangerous business!

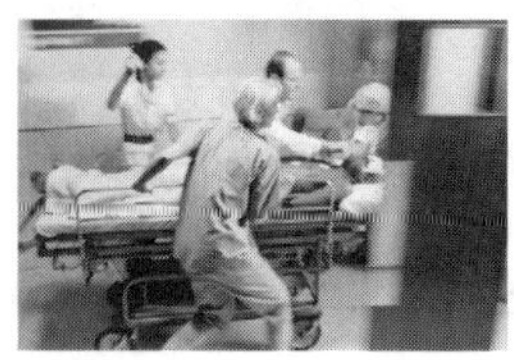

II. PEDIATRIC HYDROCEPHALUS

This is a relatively unusual etiology for altered mental status, however, it is associated with significant morbidity and mortality, and even brief delays in diagnosis can lead to worse outcomes.[6]

Definition—Hydrocephalus is caused by a mismatch between cerebrospinal fluid production and absorption and leads to enlargement of the ventricles, which compresses surrounding brain structures and cause increased intracranial pressure (ICP).[7] Hydrocephalus is divided into a variety of categories: communicating vs non-communicating, internal vs external, and congenital vs acquired.[8] While these classifications may impact long term treatment strategies and outcomes, they have little impact on our evaluation and emergent management of these patients.

Pathophysiology—The detrimental effects of hydrocephalus are not confined to the macroscopic changes seen on radiographic imaging. The increased pressure on the ventricles and brain tissue leads to perturbations in the basic physiology and ultrastructure of the brain. The associated morbidity created from these alterations depends on three major factors:

- The cause of hydrocephalus
- The age of onset
- The disease duration and rate of progression[9]

Etiology varies by age:

1. **Neonatal**—Congenital hydrocephalus has an estimated incidence of 3–4/1000 live births and has a variety of possible etiologies.[6] Most commonly it is caused by structural abnormalities such as Arnold Chiari malformations, Dandy Walker Malformations, and aqueductal stenosis. The TORCH intrauterine infections, especially CMV, syphilis, toxoplasmosis, and rubella, can lead to non-communicating hydrocephalus. Likewise, infectious disease contracted in the neonatal period can lead to inflammation in the subarachnoid space and lead to a non-communicating hydrocephalus. Trauma and prematurity can lead to intra-ventricular hemorrhage (IVH), which has seen an increasing incidence as neonatal care has improved over the past few decades.[10] Grade IV IVH involves ventricular dilation and bleeding into the surrounding brain parenchyma which can lead to immediate post hemorrhage hydrocephalus from blood clotting or a more insidious chronic obstructive secondary to fibrosis of the meninges.[11]
2. **School Aged/Adolescence**—Most commonly due to hemorrhage, post infectious, space occupying lesions, or shunt malfunction. The most common space occupying lesions include medulloblastoma, astrocytoma, and ependymoma.[12] Hydrocephalus can be either communicating or non-communicating from either pathology from debris blocking the flow of CSF acutely or long term scarring of the meninges. Our patient had severe obstructing hydrocephalus from a large supra-sellar mass.

***Presentations* vary by age:**

Symptoms are related to increased intracranial pressure, which leads to different clinical pictures in different age groups secondary to the plasticity and flexibility of the newborn's skull.

1. **Neonatal/infants**—Presentation in this group may be subtle, presenting with isolated increasing head size. As ICP increases, symptoms may progress to lethargy, fatigue, or poor sucking. Even in the ED, it's important to consider head circumference measurements in the undifferentiated "sleepy" baby; these measurements are not just for yearly checkups[13]! In addition: the "setting sun" eye phenomenon may also be seen. This is an ocular finding with a persistent downward gaze that is caused by aqueductal distention (secondary to ICP). It has been reported in up to 40% of children with hydrocephalus and can be seen earlier than increased head circumference or altered mental status.[14] Persistence of primitive reflexes may also be seen as well as spasticity and hyperreflexia secondary to increased pressure on motor pathways.[15] Even though neonates have open sutures and room to swell, if the onset of hydrocephalus is sudden and rapidly progressive, they can present with the classic ICP findings of vomiting, lethargy, and respiratory depression.
2. **School aged/adolescence**—Older children (with closed fontanels), present with symptoms of increased ICP impacted by the speed of onset and duration of hydrocephalus. There will be focal neurologic deficits when there is an obstructive mass or lesion. Papilledema and strabismus may result in the "bobble head sign" which is a rhythmic "bobbing" of the head (and occasionally the upper torso) that can be associated with ataxia possibly due to third ventricular obstruction.[16] Headaches (especially those worse in the morning), vomiting, visual disturbances (especially blurred or double vision), lethargy, and even emotional disturbances can be seen in school age and adolescent hydrocephalus. Growth abnormalities, stunted or accelerated sexual development, endocrine and thyroid derangements can result from disturbances in the hypothalamic pituitary access secondary to increased pressure.[8] In our case, the patient's "short stature" was pathologic and actually secondary to his intracranial mass.

Diagnosis

The most important part of making this diagnosis is having it on your differential! A good history and physical are imperative, but neuroimaging is the definitive study. In the neonatal population, ultrasonography has shown increasing sensitivity and specificity,[17] and in older children, noncontrasted head CTs are fast, readily available and do not require sedation. MRI is the preferred definitive imaging modality in the clearly stable patient as it allows for clearer imaging and identification of lesions.[18]

Management

- ABCs!!!!—If the patient is moribund, comatose, and/or showing signs of airway compromise or impending herniation, protect the airway first. Proceed with intubation and ventilator management as you would with any other massive head trauma; avoid hypoxia, hypovolemia, hyperthermia or medications that increase ICP. Consider mannitol, hypertonic saline or agents that decreased CSF production (acetazolamide, furosemide) as a temporizing measure while awaiting definitive intervention.[19]

- If there is no emergent indication for airway protection, consult neurosurgery. The majority will require a shunting procedure to decompress the ventricles.

Prognosis—Prognosis for pediatric hydrocephalus has improved dramatically in the past 50 years, with a 10-year survival rate that has nearly doubled. The age of presentation, duration of hydrocephalus and underlying etiology are important determinants of a patient's disease progression. Pediatric patients with hydrocephalus require lifelong follow up. The most common complications involve shunt malfunction and infection. Mortality is difficult to attribute solely to hydrocephalus but is estimated at 6–10% at 10 years.[20]

Recognition and evaluation of shunt malfunction

Over 15,000 pediatric patients undergo shunt placement for management of hydrocephalus each year.[21] Despite improvements over the past few decades, as many as one third fail within one year of placement and 60–80% of patients will experience shunt malfunction at some point in their lives.[22] Our patient has since been readmitted three times secondary to shunt malfunction and has required multiple shunt revisions.

Shunts can fail in a variety of ways, from infection to obstruction, excessive drainage, fracture, or migration.[23] Mortality associated with shunt malfunction is as high as 2%.[24] Unfortunately, many of the presenting symptoms of shunt malfunction are nonspecific and mimic common childhood illnesses and complaints. The complaints of headache, vomiting, lethargy, and shunt site swelling should mandate shunt evaluation. Shunt infection is seen more commonly within the first year of placement, however it accounts for upwards of 8% of all complications, and any fever of unknown source, particularly if associated with other unexplained symptoms such as lethargy, irritability to ambulate, vomiting or headache, should prompt shunt evaluation, especially within the first year of shunt placement.[22]

The correct imaging modality to evaluate for shunt malfunction has been debated. A shunt x-ray series is useful to evaluate for displacement or fracturing of the tubing. Head CT may show ventricular enlargement, however, it does not show an abnormality in nearly 50% of cases. Rapid sequence MRI is becoming more popular to quickly evaluate for shunt malfunction and has a high sensitivity.[25] Even in the absence of abnormal head CT or shunt series, a patient may still have shunt malfunction. If MRI is not readily available, it is incumbent on the emergency physician to maintain a high level of clinical suspicion for shunt malfunction and get the patient to a facility with MRI or neurosurgical intervention capabilities.

Chapter Summary

Altered mental status and fatigue are less commonly encountered in the pediatric emergency department than in the adult world. The exam, etiologies and outcomes vary in children based on age, and we need to keep the differential broad. This case demonstrates the insidious presentation of intracranial masses, increased ICP, and hydrocephalus and the importance of constant vigilance. Some pearls to keep in mind:

- Pediatric patients deserve neurologic examination too! Learn how to identify neuro deficits in even the youngest patients.
- Say it with me: "Altered mental status = BEDSIDE BLOOD GLUCOSE" = Forever and ever!

- Management of hydrocephalus should focus on emergent stabilization and quick consultation with neurosurgery for definitive intervention.
- Be cautious attributing neurologic symptoms to behavioral issues, especially emotional liability, decreased energy and emotional derangements as these can be the first evidence of an intracranial process.
- Shunt complications can present with nonspecific complaints that mimic benign childhood illnesses.

References

1. Kanich, et al. Altered mental status: evaluation and etiology in the ED. Am J Emerg Med. 2002; 20(7):613–7.
2. King D, Avner JR. Altered mental status. Clin Pediatr Emerg Med. 2003;4(3):171–8.
3. Koenig W. Altered level of consciousness. Prehospital care of pediatric emergencies (1997): 103.
4. Forti R, Avner J. Ch. 338. Altered Mental Status. American Academy of Pediatrics Textbook of Pediatric Care. Elk Grove Village IL: American Academy of Pediatrics, 2009.
5. Davis RJ, et al. Head and spinal cord injury. In Rogers MC, ed. Textbook of Pediatric Intensive Care. Baltimore: Williams & Wilkins, 1987; James H, Anas N, Perkin RM. Brain Insults in Infants and Children. New York: Grune & Stratton, 1985; and Morray JP, et al. Coma scale for use in brain-injured children. Critical Care Med. 1984;12:1018.
6. Pattisapu JV. Etiology and clinical course of hydrocephalus. Neurosurg Clin North Am. 2001;12(4):651–9.
7. Fishman MA. Ch. 396. Developmental defects. In: McMillan JA, et al, eds. Oski's Pediatrics: Principles and Practice, 3rd ed., 1999. Philadelphia: Lippincott Williams and Wilkins, 1906–9.
8. Ashwal S. Chapter 17: Congenital structural defects. In: Swaiman KF, Ashwal S (eds). Pediatric Neurology: Principles and Practice, 3rd ed. 1999, St. Louis: Mosby, 266–273.
9. Cinalli G, Maixner WJ, Sainte-Rose C, eds. Pediatric Hydrocephalus. Milano: 2004.
10. Wallace A, McConathy J, Menias C, et al. Imaging evaluation of CSF shunts. Am J Roentgenol. 2014; 202(1):38–53.
11. Hudgins RJ. Posthemorrhagic hydrocephalus of infancy. Neurosurg Clin North Am 2001;12(4):743–51.
12. Krause R. Hydrocephalus. In Schaider J, et al., eds. Rosen & Barkin's 5 Minute Emergency Medicine Consult. Philadelphia: Lippincott Williams & Wilkins, 2011.
13. Kestle J. Hydrocephalus. In Winn R, ed. Youmans neurological surgery. New York: Elsevier, 2011.
14. Boragina M, Cohen E. An infant with the "setting-sun" eye phenomenon. CMAJ. 2006;175(8):878.
15. Menkes JH, Sarnat HB. Ch. 4. Neuroembryology, Genetic Programming, and Malformations. In: Menkes JH, Sarnat HB, eds. Child Neurology. 6th ed. Philadelphia: Lippincott Williams and Wilkins. 2000;354–77.

16. Mussell H G, Dure L S, Percy A K, et al. Bobble-head doll syndrome: report of a case and review of the literature. Movement Disorders. 1997;12(5): 810–4.
17. Silverboard G, Horder MH, Ahmann P A, et al. Reliability of ultrasound in diagnosis of intracerebral hemorrhage and posthemorrhagic hydrocephalus: comparison with computed tomography. Pediatrics. 1980;66(4):507–14.
18. Bradley Jr WG. Diagnostic tools in hydrocephalus. Neurosurg Clin North Am 2001;12(4):661–84.
19. Kanev PM, Park TS. Treatment of hydrocephalus. Neurosurg Clin North Am 1993;4(4):611–9.
20. Vinchon M, Baroncini M, Delestret I. Adult outcome of pediatric hydrocephalus. Childs Nerv Syst. 2012;28(6):847–54. doi: 10.1007/s00381-012-1723-y. Epub 2012 Feb 19.
21. Bondurant CP, Jimenez DF. Epidemiology of cerebrospinal fluid shunting. Pediatr Neurosurg. 1995;23:254–8.
22. Kim T, et al. Signs and symptoms of cerebrospinal fluid shunt malfunction in the pediatric emergency department. Pediatr Emerg Care. 2006; 22(1): 28–34.
23. Piatt J, Garton, H. Clinical diagnosis of ventriculoperitoneal shunt failure among children with hydrocephalus. Pediatr Emerg Care. 2008; 24(4): 201–10.
24. Kang J, Lee I. Long term follow up of shunting therapy. Childs Nerv Syst. 1999;15:711–7.
25. Wallace A, McConathy J, Menias C, et al. Imaging evaluation of CSF shunts. Am J Roentgenol. 2014; 202(1):38–53.
26. Garton HJ, Kestle JR, Drake JM. Predicting shunt failure on the basis of clinical symptoms and signs in children. J Neurosurg. 2011; 94: 202–10.
27. Tuite GF, et al. The effectiveness of papilledema as an indicator of raised intracranial pressure in children with craniosynostosis. Neurosurgery. 1996; 38(2): 272–8.

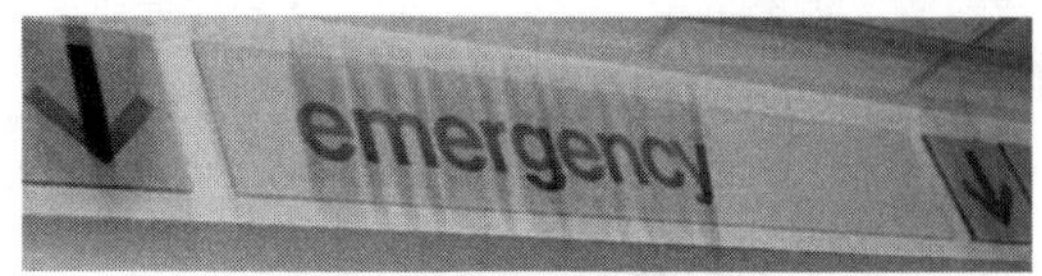

CASE 26

9-MONTH-OLD GIRL WITH FEVER AND RASH

Jennifer Maccagnano, DO
Emergency Medicine Resident
MSUCOM/Allegiance Health Emergency Medicine senior resident
Advanced Trauma Life Support (ATLS) Instructor, American College of Surgeons

PART 1—MEDICAL

PART 2—THE ANALYSIS

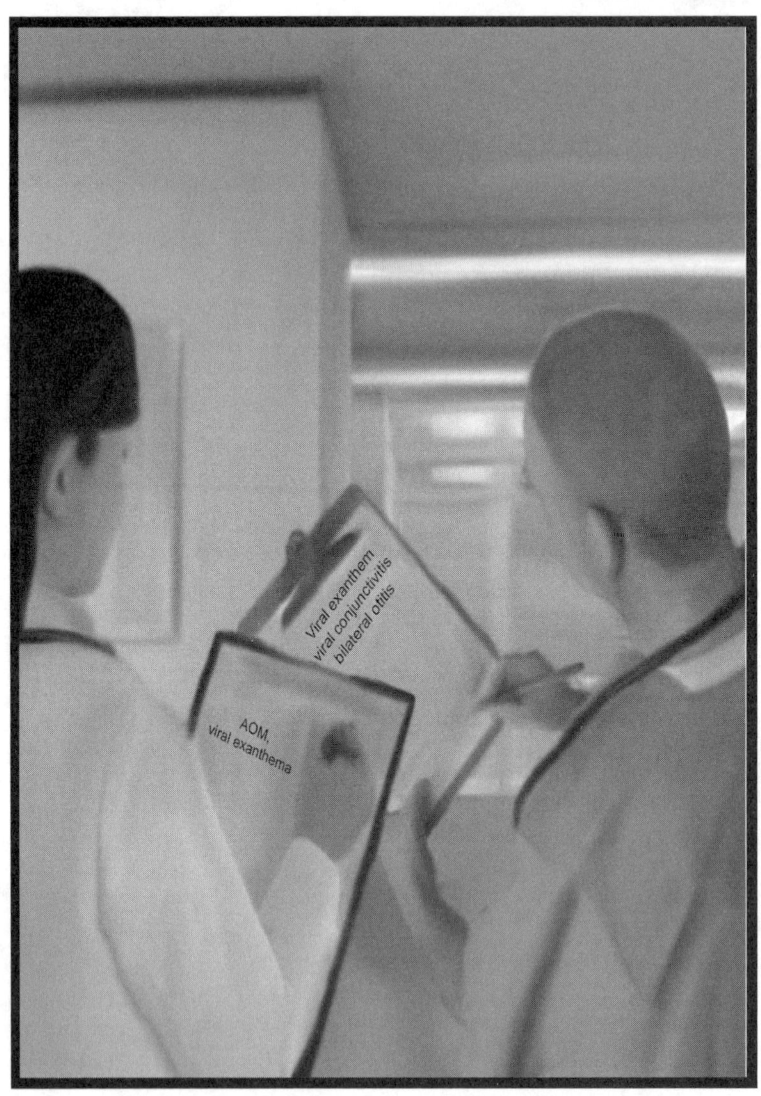
Viral exanthem
viral conjunctivitis
bilateral otitis
AOM,
viral exanthema

CASE 26

9-MONTH-OLD GIRL WITH FEVER AND RASH

PART 1—MEDICAL

I. The Doctor's Version (the following is the actual documentation of the provider)

Chief Complaint (triage): Fever

HPI (nurse practitioner): Pt. is a 9 months female who presents with a rash noted yesterday. Rash started around neck and has progressively worsened. Pt was started on Amoxicillin yesterday for bil AOM-rash started first though

Location: generalized
Severity: moderate
Course: acute
Associated local symptoms: swelling to hands and feet
Associated systemic symptoms: congestion
Previous treatment: none
New exposures: none although pt has never had Amoxicillin before
Sick contacts: none known
Immunization status: up to date per historian

PMH: Abnormal findings on newborn screening—Elevated 3-OH Isovalerylcarnitine
FH: Asthma in her brother and father.
Medications: None
Allergies: no known allergies.

PHYSICAL EXAM:

VITAL SIGNS				
Time	Temp(C)	Pulse	Resp	Weight
22:14	38.9	160	40	9kg

General: alert, well-appearing, no acute distress; pt sleeping but awakens with exam-age appropriate activity noted
Hydration: well-hydrated, mucous membranes moist, good skin turgor
Eyes: no eyelid swelling, both eyes: conjunctival exudate, conjunctival injection

Ears: no external swelling or tenderness, canals clear, Both TM's: abnormal light reflex, erythema, purulent fluid
Nose: nares patent, normal mucosa
Mouth/Throat: mucous membranes moist, no focal lesions, no tonsillar enlargement or exudate
Neck: nontender, full range of motion, no mass, no focal lymphadenopathy
Chest: Breath sounds clear and equal bilat, no distress, respir easy and regular
Cardiovascular: regular rate and rhythm, no murmur, brisk capillary refill
Abdomen: soft, nontender, nondistended, no HSM, no mass, normal bowel sounds
Skin: warm, dry, erythema, rash-maculopapular rash noted over entire body, bilateral hands and feet with swelling and redness to palms/soles

VITAL SIGNS

Time	Temp(C)	Pulse	Resp
23:40	37.7	139	30

ASSESSMENT/PLAN: 1) AOM 2) Viral exanthem
Plan: Follow up with PCP tomorrow afternoon, tylenol/motrin as needed, return if worse. Diagnosis and home care instructions explained to family/caregiver/patient; understanding is verbalized.

Attending Note: I have collaborated with the Nurse Practitioner. I have reviewed the nursing and nurse practitioner notes. My independent HPI is as follows: 9 mos female who presents with rash, fever, swelling of fingers and toes, red draining eyes and nasal discharge. On amoxicillin for one day for bilateral otitis media. Rash started before antibiotics and has spread and coalesced.

My independent physical exam included HEENT, Neck, Chest, Abdomen, Extremities, Neurologic and Skin exam and the only positives noted were as follows: alert, conjunctival erythema, conjunctival exudate, purulent rhinorrhea, diffuse exanthem: macular, coalescent on neck and lower abdomen, bilateral finger and foot edema with blanching erythema, no desquamation, moving those extremities well without appearance of pain or tenderness, hoarse voice noted.

My impression and plan is: Viral exanthem. viral conjunctivitis, bilateral otitis (per APN exam). Close followup with PCP. Watch for desquamation.

II. An Approach to Evaluating the Multiple Complaint Patient (Author note: Michael Weinstock)

Big surprise (spoiler alert...): The patient bounced back! In the context of this book, that is not surprising; but in the real world, we will see many patients with a viral exanthem before a serious cause is found. The evaluation noted above was well done in many ways, but the actual diagnosis was missed. Following is one approach to evaluating patients with multiple complaints.

First, let's localize the complaints:

1. Rash—noted first around the neck then generalized. This started prior to the amoxicillin
2. Fever—stated by triage and then as one word entry in the attending note
3. Conjunctival injection—documented in the physical exam but not in the history
4. Otitis media (initial dx the day previous at a community emergency department)

Next, let's look at each of these complaints to see how well each was evaluated and if there is a way to put them together into one diagnosis.

Rash

The primary complaint from the *triage* nurse was fever, but the complaint from the nurse practitioner (NP) was rash with no mention of fever. The first complaint mentioned by the attending ED physician was also rash though he did mention fever as the second item in his HPI. Does it matter which is the "chief complaint" and which was an "associated complaint?" Let's assume the patient actually gave a different chief complaint to the triage nurse and ED providers and first focus on the chief complaint of rash.

The nurse practitioner describes the location (generalized), severity (moderate) and course (acute), but it is not until the attending note that an actual *description* of the rash occurs. It is well done: "Diffuse exanthem: macular, coalescent on neck and lower abdomen, bilateral finger and foot edema with blanching erythema, no desquamation." The differential of this type of rash is broad:

1. Drug rash (though the rash preceded the use of amoxicillin)
2. Exposure/contact (not well explored)
3. Infectious: Scarlet fever, rheumatic fever, measles, rickettsial (Rocky Mountain Spotted Fever), Q fever (coxiella burnetii), Human Ehrlichiosis, mononucleosis and mycoplasma
4. Viral exanthem
5. Other: Kawasaki, Stevens Johnson syndrome (SJS), Henoch-Schönlein purpura (HSP)

Rash + fever

Bringing in the complaint of fever makes a drug rash less likely (compounded by the fact that the rash started after the amoxicillin). A consideration could still be a rash from a home remedy given for fever; this possibility was not explored in the history. The infectious causes listed above remain in play but some can be excluded based on timing or by obtaining a travel history. More serious causes of rash such as meningococcemia, thrombotic thrombocytopenic purpura (TTP), scalded skin syndrome, bullous pemphigoid are unlikely as the rash is not petechial or vesicular.

Viral exanthem remains in play; documentation of "congestion" by the NP and "nasal discharge" by the attending could support this diagnosis. Let's throw in another complaint and see if there is a way to narrow the differential:

Rash + fever + conjunctival injection

The third complaint listed by the attending, though not listed in the diagnosis of the nurse practitioner, is conjunctival injection. Now our ddx is narrowed: viral exanthema, SJS, Kawasaki, and measles remain in play (particularly if patient is unimmunized). Of note, there is no associated edema of hands and feet with measles.

Otitis media

OK. I'm racking my brain and just can't bring OM into the mix—maybe supporting a diagnosis of viral syndrome with exanthem... or just a red herring? Was it even present? Probably, but on the presentation listed above, for both the triage nurse, NP and attending EP, it was not a chief complaint.

Could this approach have changed the initial management by the NP and ED attending? Informing the family/caregivers that a definitive diagnosis has not been established can enable them to look for worsening or changed symptoms at home to prompt ED return.

III. Greg Henry Comments

"The concept of short-term interval follow up cannot be over emphasized. All of us have seen patients go from looking normal to near dead in 24 hours"

A 9-month-old should never be considered to have multiple complaints; there are large organisms who have been brought in by *somebody* who has multiple complaints. The history and physical exam as stated probably fits 90% of patients who present to the emergency department. Mild conjunctivitis. Viral exanthem. Fever.

It is interesting to note the diagnosis of otitis media is made on the basis of an abnormal light reflex; this is a finding that has never been confirmed to be of use and has gone the way of the buffalo. The correct way to look at tympanic membranes is movement with insufflations. One tympanic membrane always looks redder than the other, thus providing an excuse to give an antibiotic.

The follow up plan as described in the chart was excellent. Most children get better, and frequently the parents think they are so much improved they don't even take them back for re-examination. The concept of short-term interval follow up cannot be over emphasized. All of us have seen patients go from looking normal to near dead in 24 hours. The vast majority of children with fevers get better, but a sense of humility should guide our rapid return policies.

IV. PCP follow up: 11 AM the next day

HPI:

- The child has had a fever x 2 days and a rash x 3 days. Rash and fever are associated with swelling of the hands and feet. The rash started as tiny papules on the stomach and back and progressing to larger red raised areas. Associated with red eyes, decreased appetite, and fussiness. No amoxicillin since yesterday. Diagnosed with possible viral exanthem in our ED and advised to follow up today for re-check.
- Rash is worsening and progressing all over. No lesions in mouth or vaginal area. Swelling of hands and feet still present but maybe slightly improved - no skin peeling. No cough, difficulty breathing, vomiting, or diarrhea. Appetite is poor, but drinking well – took 2x6oz bottles and normal urine output. Very fussy and irritable. No sick contacts.

PE: Pulse = 136, Temp = 38.7 (101.6), Resp = 42.

- General – alert, ill appearing, irritable, consolable by mother
- Eyes = b/l conjunctival injection with periorbital redness
- Ears = b/l TMs erythematous, bulging, opaque with purulent effusion
- Mouth/Throat = no focal lesions, tacky mucous membranes, no erythema or cracking of lips
- Cardiovascular = no murmur, brisk capillary refill, tachycardic, regular rhythm
- Extremities = non-tender, +swelling of hands/feet
- Skin = diffuse erythematous raised wheals on trunk, extremities

IMPRESSION: Fever, rash, conjunctivitis, swelling – diff dx includes infectious etiology (viral syndrome-adeno, mycoplasma) but significant concern for Kawasaki disease or drug eruption. Spoke with ped ID attending on call. Return to ED ASAP

V. Bounceback Visit (24 Hours After Initial ED Visit)

CC: Rash, Swelling, Eye Problem, and Fever

HPI: Skin rash and fever, red eye

Today went to PCP who saw conjunctival injection, sent for possible Kawasaki.

- Fever first recorded yesterday with Tmax 102.4
- Decreased PO intake, 1 wet diaper today. No mucosal changes. No glandular swelling.

PE: BP 106/76 | Pulse 40 | Temp(Src) 100.2 °F (37.9 °C) | Resp 32

- Eyes: Bilateral injection, limbic sparring, no drainage or pus
- HEENT: No erythema of the lips or tongue. No strawberry tongue. No tonsillar exudates. L-TM: erythematous. Unable to fully visualize R – TM.
- Musculoskeletal: She exhibits edema (diffuse throughout arms, legs, digits, non-pitting.). She exhibits no tenderness. Swelling of hands/feet, no decreased ROM.
- Skin: Purpura and rash (maculopapular with coalescence, non-morbilliform, blanching on limbs, abd, groin, legs, face. no weeping) noted. No petechiae noted.

Results:

- Labs: WBC 8.4, Hb 10.5, plt 276, Sed rate 37 (0-13), LFT – WNL
- PCR negative for adenovirus, human metapneumovirus, rhinovirus, influenza A and B, RSV, and parainfluenza.
- Chest X-Ray – Normal

Impression/Plan

- Fever and maculopapular rash
- Viral Exanthem vs. drug reaction vs Kawasaki vs SJS spectrum

ED Fellow on day of admission: "Discussed with ID, does not yet meet Kawasaki criteria but due to age and probable need for echo will admit for close monitoring and treatment if needed."

Hospital course:

- The Infectious Diseases (ID) attending agrees the clinical picture suggests Kawasaki Syndrome and notes that adenovirus can cause similar symptoms but the very swollen hands/feet and conjunctival hyperemia are more suggestive of Kawasaki. It is common to have adenovirus co-infection with Kawasaki Syndrome. Due to high risk for aneurysms, pt was treated for Kawasaki.

- ECHO's were normal. EKG's were normal.
- Hospital Course: Patient given one dose of IVIG and aspirin in the hospital. Discharged home on low dose aspirin therapy

FINAL DIAGNOSIS: Kawasaki syndrome

PART 2—THE ANALYSIS

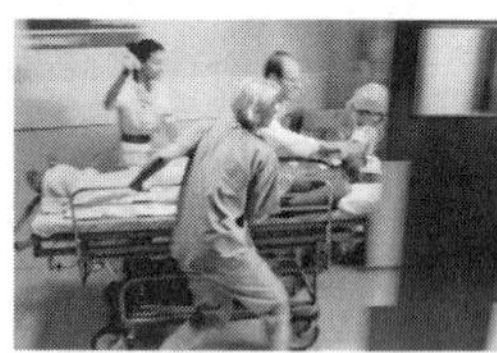

DISCUSSION OF FEVER, OTITIS MEDIA, RASH, AND INCOMPLETE KAWASAKI DISEASE

Jennifer Maccagnano, DO
MSUCOM/Allegiance Health Emergency Medicine senior resident
Advanced Trauma Life Support (ATLS) Instructor, American College of Surgeons

Pediatric Fever

On initial visit, our patient had documentation of a fever by the triage nurse, but this "chief complaint" was not explored further within the HPI of the NP. Further questions regarding fever could differentiate between tactile fever (feeling warm) and objective reading with a thermometer and use of antipyretics. It is unclear from the ED notes if the fever developed before the rash and otitis media, but becomes apparent at the PCP's visit on day two, where it is noted that the fever has been present for two days. The PCP gave Tylenol, so the patient did not manifest a fever on the second ED visit.

Pediatric Otitis Media

Patient was diagnosed at an outside hospital with otitis media, and on initial exam by the NP and PCP exam the next day, the patient has signs of otitis media. She has "b/l TMs erythematous, bulging, opaque with purulent effusion." Given that the PCP documented that her fever was for 2 days, we can conclude that she did not have a fever at the outside hospital. Although we do not have the exam from the outside hospital, given the PCP's ear exam and no complaints of otalgia in the HPIs, it seems as though the patient has non-severe bilateral otitis media and was an appropriate candidate for amoxicillin treatment. According to the American Academy of Pediatrics, antibiotic therapy is recommended for bilateral acute otitis media (AOM) in children 6 months through 23 months of age without severe signs or symptoms, i.e., mild otalgia for "less than 48 hours and temperature less than 39°C (102.2°F)."

Kawasaki Disease v. Incomplete Kawasaki disease

(Per CDC): KS is illness in a patient with fever of 5 or more days duration (or fever until the date of administration of intravenous immunoglobulin if it is given before the fifth day of fever), and the presence of at least 4 of the following 5 clinical signs:

1. Rash
2. Cervical lymphadenopathy (at least 1.5 cm in diameter)
3. Bilateral conjunctival injection
4. Oral mucosal changes
5. Peripheral extremity changes

Patients whose illness does not meet the above KS case definition but who have fever and coronary artery abnormalities are classified as having atypical or incomplete KS.[2]

On initial visit, our patient did have 2 of the symptoms of Kawasaki. She portrayed a rash as well as extremity changes with b/l finger and foot edema. Her conjunctivitis at the time was exudative, so her eye symptoms did not exactly fit with Kawasaki. Initially, this would have been a tough diagnosis.

Pediatric Ophthalmology

Acute conjunctivitis is very common and is usually due to bacterial, viral, or allergic etiology. More serious causes of conjunctival injection include acute iritis (an inflammatory condition), acute angle closure glaucoma and, oh yeah, Kawasaki ...

1. **Bacterial conjunctivitis**

   Bacterial conjunctivitis is usually caused by Haemophilis influenza, Streptococcus pneumonia, and Staphylococcus aureus.[3] Patients present with an abrupt, unilateral ocular onset, with spread to the opposite eye within 48 hours. Initially, the patient has tearing and irritation which progresses to mucopurulent discharge, and patients often describe tearing or gluing of the eyelashes. The conjunctivae are diffusely erythematous, but pre-auricular lymphadenopathy is not present.[3] In our patient, the NP does note: "both eyes: conjunctival exudate, conjunctival injection" but this finding is not correlated in the MDM or final diagnosis.

   Treatment for bacterial conjunctivitis is erythromycin, bacitracin-polymyxin B, or topical fluoroquinolone drops.[3] Children with purulent conjunctivitis may have otitis-conjunctivitis syndrome, and the bacterial cause is usually Haemophilis influenza.[4] Treatment for otitis-conjunctivits syndrome is with oral antibiotics; topical eye treatment is not necessary.[3] Since our patient was already taking amoxicillin, no additional treatment would have been necessary if this was the diagnosis.

2. **Viral conjunctivitis**

   Viral conjunctivitis is common and usually caused by adenovirus. Adenoviral conjunctivitis can be an isolated condition or part of a viral syndrome. Viral conjunctivitis includes red, profusely watery eyes, and when more severe, epidemic kerato-conjunctivitis. It starts unilateral and becomes bilateral within several days, with pre-auricular lymphadenopathy.[3]

   According to the attending physician on initial visit, the patient had viral conjunctivitis with "red draining eyes." However, in her physical exam, the attending noted conjunctival exudate without any comments on lymphadenopathy. A "can't miss" cause of viral conjunctivitis is herpetic conjunctivitis. Herpetic eye lesions are painful, usually unilateral and are associated with the classic dendritic pattern on fluorescein staining.

3. **Allergic conjunctivitis**
   Allergic conjunctivitis presents as pruritus of the eyes, injection of the conjunctival vessels, chemosis, and eyelid edema.[5] It is rare to have allergic conjunctivitis without pruritus of the eye.[5] Our patient did not have signs of allergic conjunctivitis.

4. **Acute iritis**
   Iritis is an inflammatory condition causing pain, redness, photophobia, excessive tearing, and sometimes decreased vision. Physical exam will show small pupils and a limbal flush—an injected circle around the iris but without generalized conjunctival injection. Slit lamp diagnosis is based on seeing cell and flare in the anterior chamber.[6] In the physical exam, the NP notes: "both eyes: conjunctival exudate, conjunctival injection." No comment was made about being irritated or crying with the lights in the exam room. Mother does not report any previous episodes of eye tearing or erythema which could be important as chronic uveitis is associated with juvenile idiopathic arthritis.[6]

5. **Acute angle closure glaucoma**
   Patients have an abrupt onset of eye pain that may be associated with headache, blurred vision, nausea and vomiting. On physical exam, patients have a fixed pupil with a cloudy/steamy cornea.[7] Patients also have conjunctival injection and elevated intraocular pressures. The patient did not have a fixed pupil or any cornea changes noted on her exam.

6. **Corneal Abrasion**
   In an irritated infant, it is important to consider corneal abrasion. Pain and foreign body sensation are the cardinal symptoms of corneal abrasion. Infants may present with excessive crying.[8] On initial exam, the patient did have exudate, not just crying, and was not irritable on initial exam.

Differential Diagnosis of Pediatric Rash

The differential diagnosis for rash in pediatric patients is very broad. Exanthems include Erythema Nodosum, Erythema Multiforme, Steven-Johnson Syndrome, Toxic Epidermal Necrolysis, Kawasaki Disease, Henoch-Schonlein Purpura, and Pityriasis Rosea.[9] In addition, viral exanthems are present in many pediatric patients with fevers and rash; drug rash can be a cause of skin changes in patients on medications. In children, it is very common to have viral exanthems with a viral illness.[10]

1. **Erythema Nodosum**
   In light of the patient's physical exam, she does not have palpable nodules, ruling out erythema nodosum.

2. **Allergy/Drug Rash**
   May manifest as morbilliform, urticarial, papulosquomous, pustular or bullous. Our patient's rash began before the antibiotic was started.

3. **Steven Johnson Syndrome**
   Steven Johnson Syndrome is severe and characterized by mucous membrane lesions, bullae, and toxic appearance.[11] The purulent conjunctivitis can be severe enough for the eyes to close shut.[11] Our patient did not have bullae on skin exam on either visit and although her illness progressed, she had a clear oropharynx on her second visit.

4. **Toxic Epidermal Necrolysis**
Characterized by mucous membrane involvement, macular rash, and Nikolsky's sign (slight rubbing of the skin causing a blister within a few minutes).[11] Although the patient had a maculopapular rash, she did not portray mucous membrane involvement or a Nikolsky's sign.

5. **Henoch-Schonlein Purpura (HSP)**
HSP is a vasculitis that presents with palpable purpura, renal disease, abdominal pain, and poly-arthralgias.[9] HSP can be associated with upper respiratory infections, streptococcal infections, or medications .

6. **Pityriasis rosea**
Often seen in older children and adults, ages 10–35 years, and characterized by a herald patch.[9]

7. **Erythema multiforme**
Characterized by acute onset of violaceous macules, papules, vesicles, or bullae with a symmetrical distribution most commonly found on the soles and palms, backs of the hand and feet, and extensor surfaces of the extremities. The hallmark is a "target" lesion comprised of three zones of color: a central, dark papule or vesicle surrounded by a pale zone, and a halo of erythema.[11] The patient had erythema on the palms and soles, but did not have a target lesion. Of note, erythema multiforme can be an initial sign with incomplete Kawasaki Disease.

8. **Viral exanthems**
Skin eruptions that occur as a symptom of a general disease usually are maculopapular, although they have varying characteristics.[11] Since otitis media and conjunctivitis are typically of viral etiology, patients with ear and eye infections can have a viral exanthem. Initially, the patient was described as having a maculopapular rash, and she was diagnosed with viral exanthem; however she also had edema, which is not a characteristic of viral exanthems, eye infections, or ear infections.

Diagnosis of Kawasaki Disease

Kawasaki Disease is a clinical diagnosis, and if patients do not meet the full clinical criteria, it can be easily missed. Kawasaki Disease is associated with bilateral non-exudative conjunctivitis.[13] Initially, it was reported that the patient had exudative conjunctivitis. As her disease progressed and she was seen by additional healthcare providers, her PCP noted "b/l conjunctival injection with periorbital redness," and on the same day, the attending pediatric emergency physician notes, "+conjunctival injection with limbic sparing bilaterally, no drainage," which correlates with the ocular findings of Kawasaki.

Dermatological Changes in Kawasaki

The rash in Kawasaki Disease can vary in its presentation. It usually appears within five days of the fever.[13] The most common rash seen in Kawasaki is a nonspecific, diffuse, maculopapular eruption.[13] On initial ED presentation, our patient portrayed the most common rash of Kawasaki; an erythematous, maculopapular rash. The rash was spreading from initial presentation to second presentation.

It has been noted that children with Kawasaki Disease are often more irritable than children suffering from other febrile diseases.[13] Although this is not part of the diagnostic criteria, it can help physicians when trying to decide between viral exanthem and Kawasaki. She was not noted to be irritable on the initial ED visit, but at her PCP's office the next day, she was.

Extremity Changes in Kawasaki Disease

Changes in the extremities in Kawasaki Disease can be very distinctive ranging from erythema and induration to desquamation of the fingers and toes.[13] The patient did not exhibit erythema or desquamation at the initial visit; however, the patient had bilateral hand and feet edema, not typically seen with viral syndromes.

Diagnosis of Incomplete Kawasaki

The American Heart Association has determined clinical criteria for incomplete Kawasaki as patients having fever for 5 or more days and 2–3 of the principal criteria of Kawasaki Disease.[13] On initial visit, the patient had 2 of the criteria of Kawasaki (diffuse rash and extremity changes since she had b/l finger and foot edema) and on her second visit, she had 3 criteria (rash, extremity edema, and conjunctival injection without purulence) and in addition, fever continued the next day. Incomplete Kawasaki is more common in younger infants and older children.[13] The diagnosis of incomplete Kawasaki leads clinicians to look for evidence of systemic inflammation and coronary artery aneurysms.

Echocardiography and IVIG are considered when the CRP is 3 mg/dL or higher or if the Erythrocyte Sedimentation Rate is 40 mm/hr or more.[14] Laboratory studies were not done on the patient's initial visit; on her return ED visit, her CRP was 5.0 and her ESR was 37.

Cardiac Disease with Kawasaki and Kawasaki Treatment

Evaluation by echocardiography is performed for patients diagnosed with either Kawasaki or incomplete Kawasaki as both diseases place patients at risk for coronary artery aneurysms.[14]

Infants are more likely to be diagnosed without meeting criteria, to receive IVIG later, and to have coronary artery abnormalities than older children.[15] Since the risk of developing coronary artery abnormalities increases between onset of symptoms and administration of treatment,[15] it is critical to start treatment as early as possible. However, unnecessary treatment is not ideal due to expense, side effects from the medication, and perception of vulnerability when parents are told the child's illness might affect his or her heart.[15] As with all medications/medical treatment, it is important to assess the risk/benefit ratio in conjunction with the parents.

✔ Teaching Points

- All red eyes are not infectious conjunctivitis.
- Coronary artery aneurysms can occur with incomplete Kawasaki disease.
- Early follow up is essential as the disease progresses over time.

References

1. Lieberthal AS, Carroll AE, Chonmaitree T, et al. The diagnosis and management of acute otitis media. Pediatrics. 2013;13 (3):e964–e99.
2. http://www.cdc.gov/kawasaki/
3. Prentiss KA, Dorfman DH. Pediatric ophthalmology in the emergency department. Emerg Med Clin N Am. 2008; 26: 181–98.
4. Pfaff, James A., Moore, Gregory P. Otolaryngology. In: Marx JA, et al., eds. Rosen's Emergency Medicine: Concepts and Clinical Practice. Philadelphia: Mosby; 2010: 877–87.
5. Ahrens WR. Chapter 69. Common Allergic Presentations: Allergic Conjunctivitis/Rhinitis. In: Strange GR, Ahrens WR, Schafermeyer RW, et al., eds. Pediatric Emergency Medicine, 3e. New York: McGraw-Hill; 2009. http://accessemergencymedicine.mhmedical.com
6. Gerstenblith AT, Rabinowitz MP, et al., eds. The Wills Eye Manuel: Office and Emergency Room Diagnosis and Treatment of Eye Disease. 6th ed. Philadelphia: Lippincott Williams & Wilkins; 2012.
7. Walker RA, Adhikari S. Eye Emergencies. In: Tintinalli JE, et al., eds. Tintinalli's Emergency Medicine: A Comprehensive Study Guide. New York: McGraw-Hill; 2011. http://accessemergencymedicine.mhmedical.com
8. Lazzaro DR. Chapter 8. Ophthalmology. In: Shah BR, et al., eds. Atlas of Pediatric Emergency Medicine, 2nd ed. New York: McGraw-Hill; 2013. http://accessemergencymedicine.mhmedical.com
9. Bonfante, Gary, Rosenau, Alexander M. Rashes in Infants and Children. In: Tintinalli JE, et al., eds. Tintinalli's Emergency Medicine: A Comprehensive Study Guide. 7th ed. New York: McGraw-Hill; 2011: 910–29.
10. Lam, Joseph M. Characterizing viral exanthems. Pediatric Health. 2010;4(6):623–35.
11. Cydulka, Rita K., Garber, Boris. Dermatologic Presentations. In: Marx JA, et al., eds. Rosen's Emergency Medicine: Concepts and Clinical Practice. Philadelphia: Mosby; 2010: 1529–56.
12. Shah BR. Chapter 12. Rheumatology. In: Shah BR, et al., eds. Atlas of Pediatric Emergency Medicine, 2nd ed. New York: McGraw-Hill; 2013. http://accessemergencymedicine.mhmedical.com
13. Newburger JW, Takahashi M, Gerber MA, et al. Diagnosis, treatment, and long-term management of Kawasaki disease: a statement for health professionals from the Committee on Rheumatic Fever, Endocarditis, and Kawasaki Disease, Council on Cardiovascular Disease in the Young, American Heart Association. Pediatrics. 2004; 114(6):1708–33.
14. Yeom JS, Woo H, Park JS, et. al. Kawasaki disease in infants. Korean J Pediatr. 2013;56(9): 377–82.
15. Witt MT, Minich L, Bohnsack JF, Young PC. Kawasaki disease: more patients are being diagnosed who do not meet American Heart Association criteria. Pediatrics. 1999; 104(1):1–5.

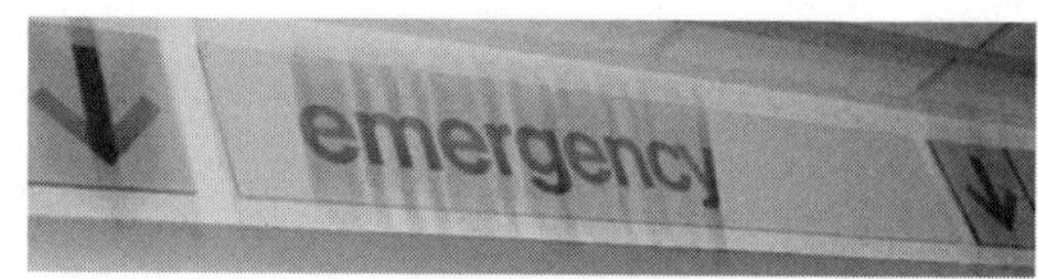

CASE 27

5-YEAR-OLD BOY WITH HEADACHE AND SORE THROAT

Annalise Sorrentino, MD, FACEP, FAAP
Professor of pediatric emergency medicine
Division of Emergency Medicine, University of Alabama, Birmingham
Assistant Dean of students, University of Alabama School of Medicine

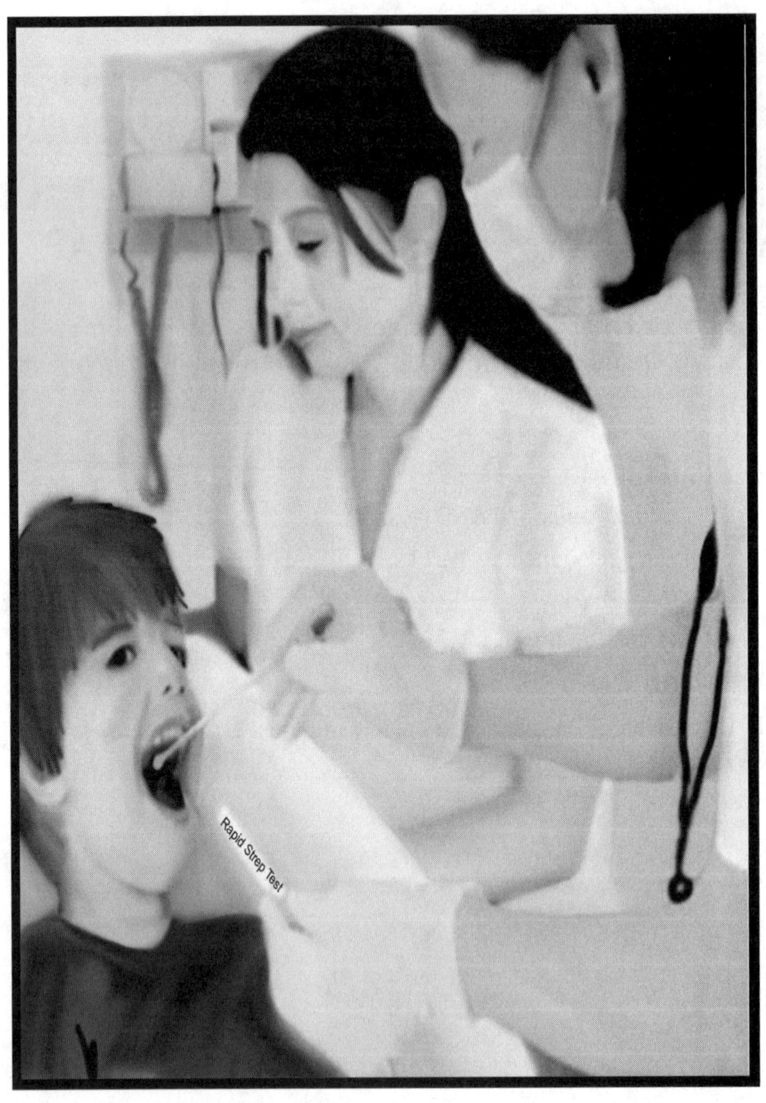
Rapid Strep Test

CASE 27

5-YEAR-OLD BOY WITH HEADACHE AND SORE THROAT

PART 1—MEDICAL

I. The Doctor's Version (the following is the actual documentation of the provider)

Date: Tuesday, 01/02/2001
Time: 09:10
Chief Complaint: Headache and sore throat
Nurse note: Triage category Green (non-urgent). Airway-Breathing-Circulation Assessment: Clear breath sounds, no increased WOB; skin pink and warm, CR < 3 seconds; Alert and interactive, normal for age. Ibuprofen 200 mg po given under patient care guidelines (weight 21.5 kg)

HPI (09:15): 5 yo with headache "off and on" x 7 days. No fever. Also with sore throat, cough, and congestion x 3 days. Emesis x 3 today, felt to be post-tussive. Describes headache as frontal and responds to ibuprofen at home. Came to the ED because he was "crying in pain" this morning. He does have associated sore throat, congestion, is sleeping more and is less active. He denies wheezing, decreased intake, neck stiffness. Ill contacts include his grandmother with URI and headache

PAST MEDICAL HISTORY:
NKDA
PMH: Asthma
Meds: Ibuprofen, albuterol
Immunizations: UTD according to AAP guidelines
Social History: Lives with mother, aunt, grandmother

VITAL SIGNS

Time	Temp(F)	Pulse	Resp	Syst	Syst	Sat
09:14	97.8	112	20	121	66	99%

General: Alert, playful, non ill-appearing; well-hydrated, smiling
HEENT: Sclera clear, PERRL, lids normal; + clear rhinorrhea, tonsils 2+ and erythematous without pus; TMs clear, membranes moist
Neck: Supple, no meningismus
Pulmonary: End-expiratory wheezes bilaterally; no increased WOB
Cardiac: Regular without murmur
Abdomen: Soft, NT, no masses

Neurological: CNs intact, DTRs 2+ symmetrically, normal strength, normal cerebellar exam
Lymph: Shotty lymphadenopathy anterior cervical chain
Skin: Clear, no petechiae

ED COURSE:

- Rapid strep obtained: results negative (Culture sent)
- Albuterol 5mg nebulized treatment given
- Patient given oral fluids

MDM: After aerosol, patient with clear breath sounds, tolerating oral fluids

DISPOSITION (10:50) - Discharge to home, continue home meds, including albuterol and ibuprofen, Follow-up with PMD

DISCHARGE DIAGNOSES: headache, URI, bronchospasm, cough

II. Greg Henry Comments—Part 1

"An ED complaint of HA should be approached from a red flag's basis"

Though the vast majority of ED headaches are benign, most in children are not; a 5-year-old rarely complains of a headache. An ED complaint of HA should be approached from a red flag's basis. First, history should explore for increased intracranial pressure with questioning for vomiting and any neurological findings. Second, an excellent neurological examination is needed, which was not well documented in this case. Bacterial meningitis and encephalitis are disasters but usually have accompanying findings; an increased temperature, altered mental status, or stiff neck to let us know that there is evil lurking in the land.

Note: Greg Henry comments continue after bounceback visit

III. The Bounceback

Date: Wednesday 1/3/01 (one day later)
Chief Complaint: Headache and vomiting

VITAL SIGNS					
Time	Temp(F)	Pulse	Resp	Syst	Syst
11:25	98.7(oral)	129	24	132	69

HISTORY OF PRESENT ILLNESS (13:00): Headache since 12/25 with development of NBNB emesis; slight fever, some loose stools, normal UOP; + ST and abdominal pain, rash that has developed since ED visit yesterday; Grandmother and Aunt with similar symptoms of headache, vomiting and decreased energy; Mom confirms the use of space heaters in the home.

PHYSICAL EXAM

- Alert, not ill-appearing; well-hydrated
- Oropharynx erythematous
- Neurological: CNs intact, DTRs 2+ symmetrically, normal strength, normal cerebellar exam
- Skin: generalized papular rash, no petechiae

ED COURSE

- 13:00 - VBG with co-oximetry - Result: Carbon Monoxide (MO) level 16.3 (H)
- 14:00 - Patient placed on 100% FIO2 via NRB
- 17:00 - Repeat VBG with co-oximetry drawn
  1. Result: CO level 0.0
  2. Patient asymptomatic
- Family members were tested at another facility with similar results and outcome

DISPOSITION

- Discharge home with Dad until patient's home cleared
- Follow-up PMD
- Diagnosis: Headache, emesis, carbon monoxide toxicity

FINAL DIAGNOSIS: Acute Carbon Monoxide Toxicity

IV. Greg Henry Comments—Part 2

"No one can disagree with the work up which was done."

How do we diagnose carbon monoxide poisoning? Usually people come in as family clusters or groups. In fact, a given during heating season is that a collection of family members is carbon monoxide poisoning until proven otherwise. Unfortunately, in this case we only had the single child. No one can disagree with the work up which was done.

The other real difficulty is bringing the child to the emergency department means he is removed from the carbon monoxide source; of course he feels better when he gets to the emergency department ... his carbon monoxide level has fallen!

I will freely admit to having been deceived by a teenager with multiple visits for headache, which seem to occur during the school week. His headaches resolved on weekends when he was away at wrestling tournaments. I came to find out he lived in converted attic space, away from the rest of the family, where an old chimney with poor mortar joints exposed him to carbon monoxide.

The emergency personnel in this case did an excellent job given the history and physical findings, and I applaud them for coming up with the correct diagnosis.

PART 2—THE ANALYSIS

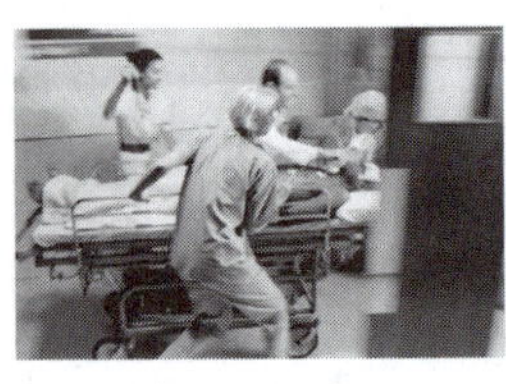

EVALUATION OF CARBON MONOXIDE TOXICITY

Annalise Sorrentino, MD, FACEP, FAAP
Professor of Pediatric Emergency Medicine
Division of Emergency Medicine, University of Alabama, Birmingham
Assistant Dean of students, University of Alabama School of Medicine

Living in Alabama, you wouldn't expect that I would encounter too many cases of carbon monoxide toxicity, and I don't. Whether it stems from a space heater, a generator or barbecuing in the living room (true story), it won't be diagnosed if you don't think to ask the right questions.

Etiology and Pathogenesis

Carbon monoxide (CO) is a colorless, tasteless, odorless, non-irritating gas that is most commonly created from incomplete combustion of hydrocarbons.[1] Although it has been present since the formation of the planet, it was first truly identified in 1800 by William Cruikshank. Later in the 19th century, John Scott Haldane demonstrated that the resultant hypoxia was due to displacement of oxygen from hemoglobin molecules.[2]

CO is the most common cause of poisoning deaths among children, and a large majority of them are unintentional and preventable.[3] When associated with a house fire or other inhalation injury, it is easier to suspect CO toxicity, but often times symptoms are vague, and the diagnosis can be difficult to make without a high index of suspicion.

CO toxicity is most commonly encountered in the winter and after natural disasters, due to the increased use of space heaters and generators from power outages. In the warmer months, it can be seen after riding in the back of a truck or behind a boat. Intentional exposures have been described, primarily in adolescent males.[1]

When inhaled, CO has a 210-times greater affinity for hemoglobin than oxygen. Therefore, with exposure, hemoglobin delivers a highly reduced amount of oxygen to tissues (remember the oxygen dissociation curve shift-to-the-left?), resulting in tissue hypoxia. This, coupled with the direct cellular damage caused by the oxidative stress on mitochondrial cytochrome oxidase, results in toxicity. End organs with the highest sensitivity to CO toxicity are those with the highest metabolic demands including the central nervous system, myocardium and fetal tissue.[2]

Clinical Presentation

Known as "the great imitator," the clinical presentation of CO toxicity can be subtle and resemble several other common illnesses commonly seen in the ED. Especially in the absence of external signs of burns, the physical exam is most often normal. It has been thought that symptomatology depends on the duration of exposure and the level of toxicity, although adult studies have shown that despite considerable differences in CO levels, there was minimal difference in clinical symptoms.[4] A pediatric study showed that levels > 25% strongly correlated with more severe symptoms, and that the severity of symptoms increased with patient age.[5]

Headache is the most common presenting symptoms in patients with CO toxicity, as seen in our patient. In retrospect, it was evident that her symptoms improved when she was removed from the environment; she was essentially asymptomatic on presentation to the ED. Other symptoms with CO toxicity include nausea and vomiting, dizziness, and malaise ... the "flu-like illness" we often attribute to viral etiology instead of CO toxicity.

It is important to note if there have been others ill in the household, including pets. Interestingly, in one study, the presence of fever and/or diarrhea did not exclude the presence of high levels of CO in pediatric patients.[1] More concerning signs and symptoms may include syncope, chest pain, dyspnea, hypotension, pulmonary edema, seizures and coma.[6]

The physical exam in the majority of patients with known CO toxicity is completely normal, or consisting of findings unrelated to the exposure, also seen in our patient. Specific findings attributable to CO poisoning would be seen in end-organ damage. Vital signs may demonstrate tachycardia, tachypnea or hypotension. Pulse oximetry remains normal despite tissue hypoxia, as the wavelength read by the oximeter is very similar between oxy- and carboxyhemoglobin. Traditionally, the diagnosis could be considered in the presence of "cherry red lips," although this is typically a post-mortem finding.[1]

Diagnostic Evaluation

The cornerstone of diagnosis is a carboxyhemoglobin (COHb) level by CO-oximetry. This can be done on an arterial or venous sample, or by a noninvasive CO-oximetry monitor. A COHb level of > 3% in nonsmokers and > 10% in smokers confirms the diagnosis, and treatment should be initiated.[6]

Other testing should be done on a patient-by-patient basis. If the exposure was a result of a fire, the patient may need a full trauma evaluation or emergent airway attention. All females of child-bearing age should have a pregnancy test performed, as CO crosses the placenta and fetal tissues are much more highly affected. More aggressive treatment may be indicated on a pregnant patient at lower measured levels.[7]

Cardiac tissue is highly sensitive; electrocardiography, echocardiography and cardiac markers may be obtained in certain patients.[6] One pediatric study showed that myocardial injury was seen more consistently in children who presented with hypotension and a Glasgow Coma Scale score of 14 or less, even with a normal ECG.[8] In the setting of the patient with neurological symptoms, brain imaging may be warranted.[1]

Treatment and Prognosis

Once the diagnosis of CO toxicity is suspected, the patient should be removed from the source and placed on 100% FIO_2 via a well-fitting non-rebreather mask, even before the diagnosis is confirmed.[1] This is a case where there is no harm in starting the proposed therapy prior to confirming the diagnosis. The half-life of CO is 4–5 hours on room air, but with the addition of normobaric 100% oxygen, the half-life is decreased to approximately 1 hour. It has been generally accepted that treatment should continue until the CO levels are $< 10\%$, but it is more important to continue the treatment until the patient is asymptomatic, especially since levels poorly correlate with symptoms.[2] Our patient was asymptomatic and had negligible levels at 3 hours.

The use of hyperbaric oxygen (HBO) has been around for years, although there is still some controversy that surrounds it. The half-life of CO on HBO is about 30 minutes, and is felt to be attributable to increasing the amount of oxygen dissolved in plasma (shifting the curve back to the right), improving mitochondrial oxidative processes, and causing vasoconstriction, leading to decreased cerebral edema.[6] The disadvantages include availability of a HBO chamber, barotrauma, decompression sickness and claustrophobia/anxiety. Limited patient access could also make it undesirable for more unstable patients.

The American College of Emergency Physicians maintains that HBO is a therapeutic option for CO toxicity, although its use cannot be mandated, and after extensive literature review, was unable to identify a specific group of patients that it would receive the greatest benefit. None of the studies reviewed included any patients under the age of 15,[9] and there continues to be insufficient information regarding its use in children.[1]

Overall prognosis is often dependent on the initial clinical picture. The more severe the presentation, the more likely there will be longstanding effects, especially myocardial and neuropsychiatric.

A well described long term sequelae of CO toxicity is a delayed neuropsychiatric syndrome (DNS). Although there is no reliable way to predict who will develop this syndrome, some feel that if there are seizures, hypotension, and significant metabolic acidosis on presentation, one is more likely to develop these sequelae.[1] It can occur days to months after the exposure, and symptoms can range from mild cognitive issues to severe signs of dementia and Parkinson's-like effects.[6] One study demonstrated complete resolution in 100% of pediatric patients with DNS, although further investigations needs to be performed to truly understand this condition in the pediatric population.[1]

Conclusions

Often referred to as the "silent killer," CO toxicity can be difficult to identify, and impossible if it is not suspected. One hundred percent of deaths by CO poisoning are preventable and, as with many things pediatric, education is the key to prevention. Make sure families know the dangers of space heaters and generators (or of barbecuing in the living room), and remind them of the importance of CO detectors...even in Alabama.

Acknowledgments: Special thanks to Dr. Kathy Monroe for letting me use her case ... again!

References

1. Williams A. An evidence-based approach to pediatric carbon monoxide poisoning. Pediatr Emerg Med Pract. 2011;8(9):1–16.
2. Huzar TF, George T, Cross JM. Carbon monoxide and cyanide toxicity: etiology, pathophysiology, and treatment in inhalation injury. Expert Rev Respir Med. 2013;7(2):159–70 (doi:10.1586/ers.13.9).
3. Riordan M, Rylance G, Berry K. Poisoning in Children 5: Rare and Dangerous Poisons. Arch Dis Child. 2002;87:407–10.
4. Hampson NB, Hauff NM. Carboxyhemoglobin levels in carbon monoxide poisoning: do they correlate with the clinical picture? Am J Emerg Med 2008;26:665–9.
5. Kurt F, Bektas O, Kalkan G, et al. Does age affect symptoms in children with carbon monoxide poisoning? Pediatr Emer Care. 2013;29:916–21.
6. Guzman JA. Carbon monoxide poisoning. Crit Care Clin. 2012;28:537–48.
7. Kind T. Carbon monoxide. Pediatr Rev. 2005;26:150–1.
8. Teksam O, Gumus P, Bayrakci B et al. Acute cardiac effects of carbon monoxide poisoning in children. European J Emerg Med. 2010;17:192–6.
9. Wolk SJ, Lavonas EJ, Sloan EP, Jagoda AS. Clinical policy: critical issues in the management of adult patients presenting to the emergency department with acute carbon monoxide poisoning. Ann Emerg Med. 2008;51:138–52.

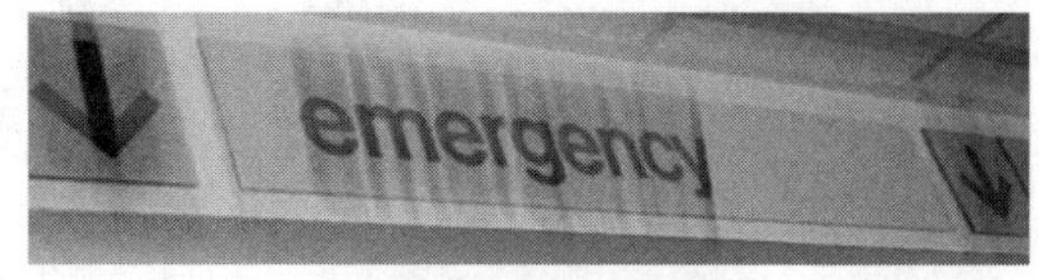

CASE 28

16-YEAR-OLD GIRL WITH FLANK PAIN

Leah S Honigman, MD, MPH
Assistant Professor, Department of Emergency Medicine
George Washington University School of Medicine and Health Sciences

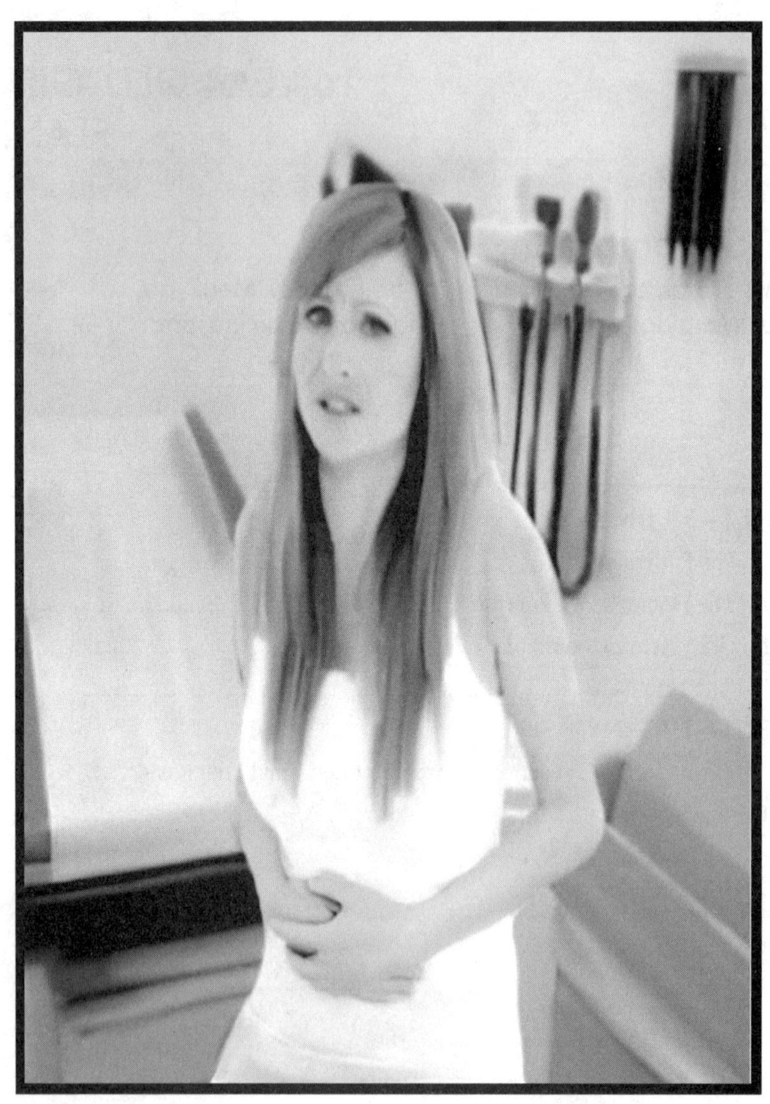

CASE 28

16-YEAR-OLD GIRL WITH FLANK PAIN

PART 1—MEDICAL

I. The Patient's Story

Madison comes from an athletic family. Her father played hockey, mother ran track, and she has an older sister at a local university who plays varsity college soccer. Since her early childhood, Madison has followed in the family footsteps and been very healthy and participated in many athletic activities.

II.The Doctor's Version (the following is the actual documentation of the provider)

CHIEF COMPLAINT: Right Flank Pain
Date: January 20, 2014 22:39

HISTORY OF PRESENT ILLNESS

16-year-old female, nonsmoker, comes into the emergency department with report of right flank pain. Patient reports that she noted that the pain started this morning around 7 AM. It has waxed and waned throughout the day. At one point it went away completely. It then returned this evening around 6 PM. The pain was severe earlier, but now has decreased in intensity. She did take some Tylenol prior to arrival. She reports the pain currently is 4/10. It is persistent in her right flank. She denies any abdominal pain. No dysuria or hematuria. No fevers or chills. She did vomit once earlier today. Denies any trauma to her back. Denies any history of kidney stones. No numbness or weakness of her extremities and no radiation of pain into her legs.

PAST MEDICAL HISTORY

Allergies: NKA
Medications: None
PMH/PSH: none
Social history: No Data Available

PHYSICAL EXAMINATION

VITAL SIGNS

Time	Temp (F)	HR	BP	Resp	Pulse Oximetry	Pain
22:39	97.8 (Oral)	68	122/88	16	100% RA	8/10

Constitutional: Alert F in no acute respiratory distress, appropriate with exam
Eyes: PERRL, no scleral icterus.
Oropharyngeal: MMM
Nose: The nose is normal in appearance without rhinorrhea
Resp: Normal chest excursion with respiration; breath sounds clear and equal bilaterally; no wheezes, rhonchi, or rales
Card: Regular rhythm, without murmur, rub or gallop
Abd: Non-distended; non-tender, soft, without rigidity, rebound or guarding
Back: no CVAT bilaterally, no evidence of trauma/rash
Ext: 2+ radial/PT pulses bilaterally; no edema; no calf tenderness

Vital Signs

Time	HR	BP	Respir	Pulse Oximetry	Pain
23:32	74	122/73	20	98% RA	3/10
01:00	57	105/61	18	99% RA	1/10
02:42	62	100/64	18	99% RA	

RESULTS:
Urine dip: Blood 3+, Leukocytes 1+, Nitrite-neg, Glucose-neg, Protein-trace, pregnancy-neg
Urine micro (23:31): Blood 300/UL, Protein 30mg/dl, WBC 11/HPF, RBC 144/HPF, Squamous epi-many, bacteria-occasional
Renal u/s: No hydronephrosis and normal appearing kidneys

MEDICAL DECISION MAKING:
Patient has no flank pain and feels well. I discussed with the patient and her father the urine results and the ultrasound results. I asked her to f/u with her PCP for any continued pain and to return for worsening pain. They are aware of the reasoning behind not performing a CT scan on this patient at this time particularly, as she had a head CT 10/13 for a concussion.

DIAGNOSIS: Flank pain, Hematuria

DISPOSITION: Discharged home. Follow up with PCP within 1 to 2 days; Return to Emergency Department Within Follow-up as needed. Instructions for: Flank Pain, Kidney Stones, School Release1 day

PRESCRIPTIONS: Ibuprofen 600 mg oral tablet (Prescribe): 1 Tab, PO, Q6h, 20 Tab, PRN, for pain

III. Greg Henry Comments

"It is rare that you see a case in the Bouncebacks! series where the initial evaluation has been so intelligently done"

A 16-year-old who still has their appendix has appendicitis till proven otherwise. A 16-year-old girl could be pregnant despite their negative answers to your questions; I don't really care if they are having sex, I just want to know if they are pregnant. Flank pain with blood in the urine in a woman not currently menstruating is pyelonephritis or stone.

The one test with no downside and a tremendous upside is the ultrasound. Without the risk of radiation exposure sustained from a CT scan, the US can evaluate the ovaries for cyst, torsion, ectopic, or free fluid, the aorta for aneurysm, the gall bladder for stones, and the kidneys for hydronephrosis. Whether an actual stone is found or not is beside the point, we are really looking for obstruction of the ureter.

With adequate pain control and no symptoms or signs of a urinary infection, these patients can be sent home. The physician who ordered the US made a good move. Instructing the family that the pain of ureterolithiasis can wax and wane and that some people will need to return, was a prudent decision. It is rare that you see a case in the Bouncebacks! series where the initial evaluation has been so intelligently done.

IV. Bounceback Visit—1 Day Later

CHIEF COMPLAINT: R Flank Pain

- **HPI:** I reviewed the record from yesterday. Pain began suddenly yesterday and is sharp and intermittent. Blood in the urine. LMP 2 weeks ago. No dysuria or urinary frequency, vaginal bleeding, fevers. Vomited once yesterday
- **Vital signs:** Temp 98.8, Pulse 91, Respiratory Rate 20, BP 123/82
- **PE:** A&O, NAD, abdomen soft and NT, Back with right CVAT, no left CVAT
- **MDM**
  - o **10:42 -** Ultrasound result was reviewed. At this point as there is continued pain and blood in the urine a CT will be done to look for stone or other etiology to establish a definitive diagnosis.
  - o **12:36 -** I did review the CT scan which shows a 3 mm right UPJ stone. She does appear comfortable. I'll have her follow up with urology later this week
- **DIAGNOSIS**: Ureteral colic
- **DISPOSITION:** Discharged home. Stable condition. Follow up with PCP as needed, follow up with urologist within 3 to 4 days, call for an appointment. Instructions for ureteral Colic, Rx Percocet

PART 2—THE ANALYSIS

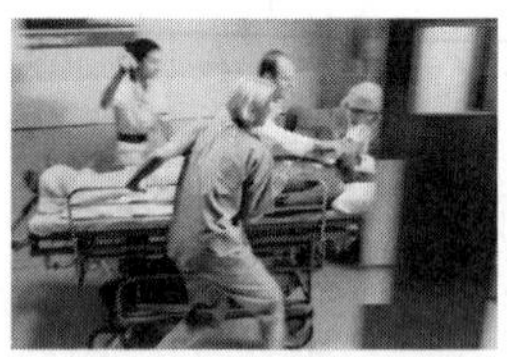

EVAULATION OF FLANK PAIN, MANAGING URETEROLITHIASIS, BALANCING RISKS AND BENEFITS OF RADIATION EXPOSURE IN CHILDREN

Leah S Honigman, MD, MPH

Assistant Professor, Department of Emergency Medicine
George Washington University School of Medicine and Health Sciences

Flank pain

This adolescent female presented with sudden onset of intermittent flank pain over a 12–14 hour period. Although there were many elements of the history that would suggest nephrolithiasis (sudden onset of colicky flank pain in a patient without trauma) there were other aspects that were not classic (no radiation, no urinary symptoms including hematuria or urinary urgency, not doing the "kidney stone dance").

Classically, the pain from nephrolithiasis tends to be sudden and severe and it often radiates from the flank to the groin (in boys/men often radiating to the testicle). Patients cannot get comfortable and are often pacing around the room. Patients will also frequently report nausea and vomiting. They can be tachycardic and hypertensive with an exam positive for costo-vertebral angle tenderness (CVAT) with a benign abdominal exam.

Differential diagnosis

Other conditions that are important to consider in patients with right-sided flank pain include:

- Pyelonephritis
- Renal abscess
- Renal tumor
- Appendicitis
- Biliary colic
- Constipation
- Musculoskeletal problems

For adolescent female patients other serious genitourinary conditions should be considered including:

- Ectopic pregnancy
- Ovarian torsion
- Tubo-ovarian abscess
- Pelvic inflammatory disease

Evaluation

It is important to obtain a thorough sexual history in an adolescent female as well as a pregnancy test. In our patient, a pregnancy test was done, but the sexual history was not obtained in either the initial or the follow-up visits. A pelvic exam was not done. Of note, The American Academy of Pediatrics does not recommend a pelvic exam in an adolescent patient who is not sexually active and does not report concerning symptoms such as persistent vaginal discharge, lower abdominal pain, abnormal vaginal bleeding or reported sexual assault or abuse. Note that some adolescents may be afraid to come forth on their own.[38]

Epidemiology of nephrolithiasis

Calcium stones are the most common but stones can also be formed from uric acid, struvite or cysteine. While nephrolithiasis is relatively common among adults and is estimated to affect approximately 5% of the population, it is significantly less common in children; approximately one-tenth of the rate in adults, or 0.5%.[1] Stone disease accounts for 1 in 685 pediatric hospitalizations in the US; there has been a significant increase in the number of children diagnosed with and treated for nephrolithiasis over the last decade [2,3] In the adult population, stones occur more frequently in males, however in the pediatric population the prevalence is more equally divided.[2]

Approximately 40% of pediatric patients with nephrolithiasis have a positive family history.[4] Hypercalciuria, or excessive urinary calcium excretion, is the most common identifiable cause of calcium kidney stone disease. Idiopathic hypercalciuria is diagnosed when clinical, laboratory, and radiographic investigations fail to delineate an underlying cause of the condition. Secondary hypercalciuria occurs when a known process produces excessive urinary calcium including absorptive hypercalciuria, renal phosphate leak hypercalciuria, and resorptive hypercalciuria—this is almost always caused by hyperparathyroidism.

Diseases associated with stone formation include:

- Hyperparathyroidism
- Gastrointestinal disorders (i.e., jejuno-ileal bypass, intestinal resection, Crohn's disease, malabsorptive conditions)
- Sarcoidosis
- Cystinuria
- Primary hyperoxaluira
- Renal tubular acidosis
- Lesh-Nyhan Syndrome
- Cystic fibrosis
- Anatomic abnormalities of the urinary system system[5]

This patient did not have any clear risk factors for development of a kidney stone, although many of these risk factors were not ascertained by the providers.

Diagnosis of nephrolithiasis

The initial evaluation of this patient involved a urine analysis (UA) and renal ultrasound. Presence of hematuria on a microscopic UA has a high sensitivity (81%) for kidney stones, but only a moderate specificity (49%).[6] Additionally, hematuria is more common earlier in presentation of nephrolithiasis.[7] Other labs to consider on initial evaluation can include a basic metabolic panel to check renal function, however this test does not need to be done with uncomplicated ureteral stone. Depending on the level of suspicion of type of stone, further electrolytes including calcium, phosphorous, magnesium and uric acid can also be obtained.

For patients with a first presentation for suspected nephrolithiasis, it is often recommended to establish the diagnosis with imaging. New patients most often undergo non-contrast abdominal CT scans. However, there is debate about the best form of imaging for the pediatric population.

Radiographic imaging for suspected nephrolithiasis

Radiography can establish the diagnosis of nephrolithiasis as well as providing information about the size, orientation, radiolucency, location of the stone, and evidence of hydronephrosis. Options include:

- Abdominal x-rays
- Intravenous urography (IVU)
- Renal ultrasound
- Non-contrast abdominal CT scan

In the past, plain radiographs in combination with IVU were performed, however due to the high radiation dose, frequent rate of allergic reactions to the dye, and increased availability of other modalities, IVU has fallen out of favor.[8] Plain abdominal radiography can be useful to assess total stone burden and is sometimes used to track stone movement. Plain films are 59% sensitive for visibility of stones, which are more radiolucent if they are composed of calcium oxalate.[9]

Renal ultrasound can be obtained by experienced providers at the bedside or for others in the radiology department. However, it can be difficult to directly visualize a stone. Instead it relies on indirect markers of ureteral obstruction including renal or ureteral dilation and absence of ureteral ejaculation into the bladder.[8]

In recent years, abdominal CT scans have become the most common initial radiographic study for patients with suspected uretero/nephrolithiasis and are considered by many to be the first line imaging study.[9] The use of CT scans in evaluating patients with acute flank pain increased ten-fold from1996–2006 in the adult ED population, while the use of ultrasound has remained stable and the use of x-rays has declined.[10, 11] CT scans have likely increased in utilization given the high sensitivity and specificity for detecting ureteral stones.[8, 12-17] Particularly relevant to the pediatric population, CT scans can be obtained quickly which reduces the need for procedural sedation.[18, 19] While CT has the advantage of diagnosing other potential sources of flank pain, there is also a high rate of incidental findings, which can lead to inappropriate downstream diagnostic testing and treatment.[20, 21]

CT vs. Ultrasound for nephrolithiasis

Despite the increasing use of CT, the proportion of patients who present with flank pain diagnosed with a kidney stone has remained unchanged over time.[10] Furthermore despite increased use of radiographic studies there is no associated improvement in patient outcomes as the vast majority of patients are discharged home. [10, 11, 22] While there is a difference in detection of stones between CT and renal ultrasound, a trial found no significant difference in patient outcome including the diagnosis of high-risk conditions and complications.[23]

In a recent study by Smith-Bindman, et al.,[39] a total of 2759 patients underwent randomization: 908 to point-of-care ultrasonography, 893 to radiology ultrasonography, and 958 to CT. The incidence of high-risk diagnoses with complications in the first 30 days was low (0.4%) and did not vary according to imaging method. The mean 6-month cumulative radiation exposure was significantly lower in the ultrasonography groups than in the CT group. The study concluded that initial ultrasonography was associated with lower cumulative radiation exposure than initial CT, without significant differences in high-risk diagnoses with complications, serious adverse events, pain scores, return emergency department visits, or hospitalizations. This study was conducted in the adult population (>18 years of age), but results might be applicable to adolescents.

Imaging considerations in the pediatric population

Consideration of the best imaging modality in the pediatric population is particularly important due to the long-term risks of radiation exposure. Children have more years of life ahead of them and are more sensitive to radiation due to a higher proportion of actively dividing cells.[24] There is a small but significant increase in the development of neoplasm associated with radiation exposure.[25-30]

It is common for patients with kidney stone disease to have future radiographic studies given the recurrent nature of the disease, resulting in excessive radiation exposure from overuse of CT scans.[31-33] It is estimated that a fifth of patients with kidney stones exceed the recommended annual safety limits for radiation exposure.[34] In order to balance the concerns of radiation exposure with the necessity to accurately diagnose nephrolithiasis, investigation into accuracy of CT scans with reduced radiation dose has found similar detection rates in the pediatric population.[35]

While there is no clear guideline for evaluation of suspected nephrolithiasis in the pediatric population, it seems reasonable to use ultrasound as a first line imaging study to evaluate for stone visualization or secondary signs such as hydronephrosis. If either is found and there is a high suspicion for kidney stone, the patient should be managed as an outpatient in conjunction with urology. If the diagnosis is less certain or there is evidence of infection/acute illness, then CT may be necessary. Ideally, a low dose protocol should be employed. Once a stone is diagnosed, CT scans are rarely needed for recurrent stones or to follow the course of the disease.

Management of nephrolithiasis

Initial management should include adequate hydration and pain control including NSAIDs and opioid analgesics. A meta-analysis has demonstrated better pain control with NSAIDs than opioids.[36]

In adults, the American Urologic Association estimates that the majority of stones will pass within 4–6 weeks. Smaller stones will pass more easily and an estimated 68–80% of stones that are less than 5mm will pass spontaneously. That rate of spontaneous passage diminishes with increasing size but nearly half (47%) of stones between 5–10mm will pass without intervention. In the pediatric population, the smaller size of the urinary tract may make the rate of spontaneous passage lower.[37]

Indications for intervention include:

- Presence of any infection with obstruction
- Intractable pain or vomiting
- Potential for renal deterioration

For patients with a new diagnosis of kidney stone that is less than 10mm, initial expectant management with observation and pain control is recommended.[37] Patients should be given a strainer to facilitate stone analysis. Pediatric patients with a new diagnosis of nephrolithiasis should be referred to urology for further evaluation.

✔ Teaching Points

- Nephrolithiasis is less common in the pediatric population than among adults but should be considered for patients with concerning symptoms or a positive family history.
- Diagnosis of nephrolithiasis can be confirmed with a UA and selective imaging.
- While CT scans have a high sensitivity in the diagnosis of nephrolithiasis, there is significant potential for adverse downstream effects of radiation in the pediatric population.
- Renal ultrasound should be considered as initial imaging study for pediatric patients with suspected nephrolithiasis.
- Expectant management of nephrolithiasis includes fluid hydration and pain control.

References

1. Hoppe B, Kemper MJ. Diagnostic examination of the child with urolithiasis or nephrocalcinosis. Pediatr Nephrol. 2010;25(3):403–13.
2. Bush NC, Xu L, Brown BJ, et al. Hospitalizations for pediatric stone disease in United States, 2002–2007. J Urol. 2010;183(3):1151–6.
3. Routh JC, Graham DA, Nelson CP. Epidemiological trends in pediatric urolithiasis at United States freestanding pediatric hospitals. J Urol. 2010;184(3):1100–4.
4. Diamond DA, Menon M, Lee PH, Rickwood AMK, Johnston JH. Etiological factors in pediatric stone recurrence. J Urol. 1989;142(2):606–8.
5. Guidelines on urolithiaisis. European Association of Urology. March 2011. http://www.uroweb.org/gls/pdf/18_Urolithiasis.pdf
6. Bove P, Kaplan D, Dalrymple N, et al. Reexamining the value of hematuria testing in patients with acute flank pain. J Urol. 1999;162(3):685–7.
7. Kobayashi T, Nishizawa K, Mitsumori K, et al. Impact of date of onset on the absence of hematuria in patients with acute renal colic. J Urol. 2003;170(4):1093–6.
8. Heidenreich A, Desgrandschamps F, Terrier F. Modern approach of diagnosis and management of acute flank pain: Review of all imaging modalities. Eur Urol. 2002; 41(4):351–62.
9. Coursey CA, Casalino DD, Remer EM, et al. ACR Appropriateness Criteria ® acute onset flank pain-suspicion of stone disease. Ultrasound Q. 2012;28(3):227–33.
10. Hyams ES, Korley FK, Pham JC, et al. Trends in imaging use during the emergency department evaluation of flank pain. J Urol. 2011;186(6):2270–4.
11. Westphalen AC, Hsia RY, Maselli JH, et al. Radiological imaging of patients with suspected urinary tract stones: national trends, diagnoses, and predictors. Acad Emerg Med. 2011;18(7):700–7.

12. Cullen IM, Cafferty F, Oon SF, et al. Evaluation of suspected renal colic with noncontrast CT in the emergency department: a single institution study. J Endourol. 2008;22(11): 2441–5.
13. Eshed I, Kornecki A, Rabin A, et al. Unenhanced spiral CT for the assessment of renal colic. How does limiting the referral base affect the discovery of additional findings not related to urinary tract calculi? Eur J Radiol. 2002;41(1):60–4.
14. Boulay I, Holtz P, Foley WD, et al. Ureteral calculi: Diagnostic efficacy of helical CT and implications for treatment of patients. Am J Roentgenol. 1999;172(6):1485–90.
15. Yilmaz S, Sindel T, Arslan G, et al. Renal colic: comparison of spiral CT, US and IVU in the detection of ureteral calculi. Eur Radiol. 1998;8(2):212–7.
16. Worster A, Preyra I, Weaver B, et al. The accuracy of noncontrast helical computed tomography versus intravenous pyelography in the diagnosis of suspected acute urolithiasis: a meta-analysis. Ann Emerg Med. 2002;40(3):280–6.
17. Edmonds ML, Yan JW, Sedran RJ, et al. The utility of renal ultrasonography in the diagnosis of renal colic in emergency department patients. Can J Emerg Med. 2010;12(3):201–6.
18. Larson DB, Johnson LW, Schnell BM, et al. National trends in CT use in the emergency department: 1995–2007. Radiol. 2011;258(1):164–73.
19. Linton OW, Mettler FA Jr. National conference on dose reduction in CT, with an emphasis on pediatric patients. Am J Roentgenol. 2003;181:321–9.
20. Lumbreras B, Donat L, Hernandez-Aguado I. Incidental findings in imaging diagnostic tests: a systematic review. British J Radiol. 2010;83(988):276–89.
21. Thompson RJ, Wojcik SM, Grant WD, et al. Incidental findings on CT scans in the emergency department. Emerg Med Inter. 2011:Article ID 624847. doi:10.1155/2011/624847
22. Dalziel PJ, Noble VE. Bedside ultrasound and the assessment of renal colic: a review. Emerg Med J. 2013;30(1):3–8.
23. Smith-Bindman R, Miglioretti DL, Johnson E, et al. Use of diagnostic imaging studies and associated radiation exposure for patients enrolled in large integrated health care systems, 1996–2010. JAMA. Jun 2012;307(22):2400–9.
24. Health risks from exposure to low levels of ionizing radiation—BEIR VII. Washington, DC: National Academies Press, 2005.
25. Brenner DJ, Doll R, Goodhead DT, et al. Cancer risks attributable to low doses of ionizing radiation: assessing what we really know. Proceedings of the National Academy of Sciences of the United States of America. 2003;100(24):13761–6.
26. Brenner DJ, Elliston CD, Hall EJ, et al. Estimated risks of radiation-induced fatal cancer from pediatric CT. Am J Roentgenol. 2001;176(2):289–96.
27. Preston DL, Ron E, Tokuoka S, et al. Solid cancer incidence in atomic bomb survivors: 1958–1998. Radiation Res. 2007;168(1):1–64.
28. Pearce MS, Salotti JA, Little MP, et al. Radiation exposure from CT scans in childhood and subsequent risk of leukaemia and brain tumours: a retrospective cohort study. Lancet. 2012;380(9840):499–505.
29. Mathews JD, Forsythe AV, Brady Z, et al. Cancer risk in 680 000 people exposed to computed tomography scans in childhood or adolescence: data linkage study of 11 million Australians. BMJ. May 21, 2013;346:f2360. http://www.bmj.com/content/346/bmj.f2360

30. Fazel R, Krumholz HM, Wang Y, et al. Exposure to low-dose ionizing radiation from medical imaging procedures. New Eng J Med. 2009;361(9):849–57.
31. Mettler FA, Jr., Wiest PW, Locken JA, et al. CT scanning: patterns of use and dose. J Radiolog Protect. 2000;20(4):353–9.
32. Katz SI, Saluja S, Brink JA, et al. Radiation dose associated with unenhanced CT for suspected renal colic: impact of repetitive studies. Am J Roentgenol. 2006;186(4):1120–4.
33. Sodickson A, Baeyens PF, Andriole KP, et al. Recurrent CT, cumulative radiation exposure, and associated radiation-induced cancer risks from CT of adults. Radiol. 2009;251(1):175–84.
34. Ferrandino MN, Bagrodia A, Pierre SA, et al. Radiation exposure in the acute and short-term management of urolithiasis at 2 academic centers. J Urol. 2009;181(2):668–72.
35. Karmazyn B, Frush DP, Applegate KE, et al. CT with a computer-simulated dose reduction technique for detection of pediatric nephroureterolithiasis: comparison of standard and reduced radiation doses. Am J Roentgenol. 2009;192(1):143–9.
36. Holdgate A, Pollock T. Systematic review of the relative efficacy of non-steroidal anti-inflammatory drugs and opioids in the treatment of acute renal colic. BMJ. 2004;328:1401–9.
37. Guidelines for the Management of Ureteral Calculi. European Association of Urology and American Urological Association. 2007.
38. Braverman PK, Breech L. The Committee on Adolescence. Gyneocologic examination for adolescents in the pediatric office setting. Pediatrics. 2010;126,31:583–90.
39. Smith-Bindman R, Aubin C, Bailitz J, et al. Ultrasonography versus computed tomography for suspected nephrolithiasis. N Engl J Med. 2014;371:1100–10.

Afterword located on last page of book

Notes

Notes

Notes

Notes

Notes

Notes

Notes

NOTES

Notes

Notes

Notes

Notes

Notes

- spelling errors
- title errors
- "I'm glad I was not the third physician"

AFTERWORD

Whew! Glad I didn't pick up that patient!

After reading about 28 children whose initial diagnosis was missed, the tendency may be to work-up every URI, back pain, headache and fever with blood tests, X-rays, and a total body CT… but that is not the message we are trying to convey. Many of these patients could have been best managed with a more complete history and physical, expanded differential, or longer period of observation; not high-tech stuff.

As Mel Herbert said, "If you have a high index of suspicion with everyone, pretty soon, all you have is an index of suspicion." We hope these true stories will focus attention on the recognition of abnormal vital signs, red flags of serious disease, and an expanded pediatric-centric differential. We advocate against defensive medicine, but for an evaluation and documentation which is logical and complete and therefore defensible.

We thank the chapter authors who have shared their patient's stories as well as their own. The courage to share an adverse outcome is inspiring; you have made us better clinicians.

Michael Weinstock
Kevin Klauer
Madeline Matar Joseph
Greg Henry
March, 2015

www.embouncebacks.com